# Health and Medicine

# 1994

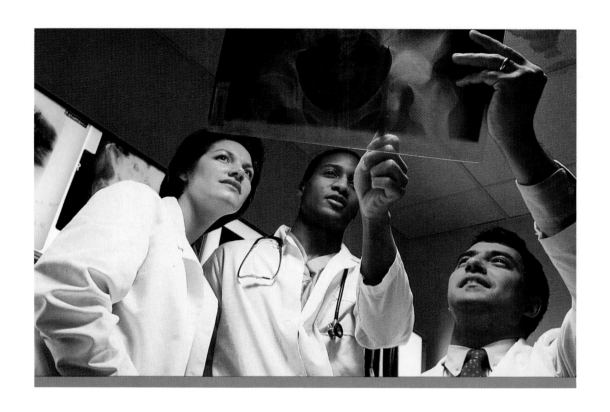

# Health and Medicine

# 1994

The *Health and Medicine Annual* should not be used in lieu of professional
medical advice. The editors urge all readers to consult a physician
on a regular basis as part of their normal health-care routine and
to seek medical attention should symptoms arise that require
professional diagnosis or treatment.

PUBLISHED BY THE SOUTHWESTERN COMPANY 1994

# Board of Advisors

**JOSEPH DeVITO,** Freelance writer
VIDEO GAMES: VICTIM OR VILLAIN?

**HERBERT S. DIAMOND, M.D.,** Chairman, Department of Medicine, Western Pennsylvania Hospital, Pittsburgh, PA
ARTHRITIS AND RHEUMATISM

**MICHELLE M. EMERY, R.Ph.,** Drug Information Specialist, University of Rhode Island Drug Information Center, Roger Williams Medical Center, Providence, RI
coauthor, MEDICATIONS AND DRUGS

**BRENDAN M. FOX, M.D.,** Clinical Associate Professor, Department of Urology, University of Connecticut, Farmington, CT
UROLOGY

**LAURA FRASER,** Contributor, *Health* magazine
GETTING THROUGH GRIEF

**SUE GEBO, M.P.H., R.D.,** Consulting nutritionist in private practice; author, *What's Left to Eat?* (McGraw-Hill, 1992)
GOING WILD! GAME IN THE KITCHEN

**MARIA GUGLIELMINO, M.S., R.D.,** Registered dietitian and exercise physiologist
ACCENT ON ANTIOXIDANTS
NUTRITION AND DIET

**MARY HAGER,** Correspondent, *Newsweek* magazine
HEALTH-CARE COSTS

**LINDA HUGHEY HOLT, M.D.,** Department Chairman, Obstetrics and Gynecology, Rush North Shore Hospital, Skokie, IL
OBSTETRICS AND GYNECOLOGY

**IRA M. JACOBSON, M.D.,** Associate Clinical Professor of Medicine, Cornell University Medical College, New York, NY
LIVER

**JAMES F. JEKEL, M.D., M.P.H.,** Professor of Epidemiology and Public Health, Yale University School of Medicine, New Haven, CT
AIDS
PUBLIC HEALTH

**KENNETH L. KALKWARF, D.D.S., M.S.,** Dean, University of Texas Health Science Center at San Antonio Dental School, San Antonio, TX
TEETH AND GUMS

**LARRY KATZENSTEIN,** Senior Editor, *American Health* magazine
ALLERGIES: NOTHING TO SNEEZE AT

**JENNIFER KENNEDY, M.S.,** Johns Hopkins Hospital "Live for Life" health promotion program, Baltimore, MD
HOUSECALLS: FITNESS AND HEALTH

**CHRISTOPHER KING,** Managing Editor, *Science Watch,* Institute for Scientific Information, Philadelphia, PA
AIL TO THE CHIEF?
NOBEL PRIZE: PHYSIOLOGY OR MEDICINE

**ROBERT L. KNOBLER, M.D., Ph.D.,** Professor of Neurology; Associate Director, Division of Neuroimmunology, Jefferson Medical College, Philadelphia, PA
BRAIN AND NERVOUS SYSTEM

**PREETHI KRISHNAMURTHY,** Freelance writer based in New Haven, CT
THE GROWING CONTROVERSY OVER GENDER PSYCHOLOGY

**RALPH LaFORGE,** Exercise Physiologist, University of California, San Diego; Contributing Editor, *Executive Health's Good Health Report*
EXERCISE MYTHS

**ARNON LAMBROZA, M.D.,** Assistant Professor of Medicine, Division of Digestive Diseases, The New York Hospital-Cornell Medical Center, New York, NY
DIGESTIVE SYSTEM

**ROBERT LAUFER,** Freelance medical writer based in South Nyack, NY
ANESTHESIOLOGY
BLOOD AND LYMPHATIC SYSTEM

**THOMAS H. MAUGH II,** Science writer, *The Los Angeles Times*
GENETICS AND GENETIC ENGINEERING

**ELIZABETH McGOWAN,** Freelance writer based in New York, NY
ERGONOMICS

**ALISON A. MOY, M.D.,** Postdoctoral Fellow, Department of Endocrinology and Metabolism, Yale University School of Medicine, New Haven, CT
ENDOCRINOLOGY

**RICHARD L. MUELLER, M.D.,** Cardiovascular Center, The New York Hospital-Cornell Medical Center, New York, NY
HEART AND CIRCULATORY SYSTEM

**WILLIBALD NAGLER, M.D.,** Chairman, Rehabilitation Medicine, The New York Hospital-Cornell Medical Center, New York, NY
REHABILITATION MEDICINE

**ALICE NAUDE,** Freelance writer based in New York, NY
CAFFEINE: THE HIDDEN INGREDIENT

**SUSAN NIELSEN,** Freelance writer specializing in consumer advocacy and health issues
HOT TUBS AND SPAS: HEALTHY OR HAZARDOUS?

**MARCY O'KOON,** Freelance writer and editor based in Atlanta, GA
CULTS: THE ULTIMATE MIND TRAP
THE HEALTHY TRAVELER
SEXUAL HARASSMENT: WHAT IS THE LAW?

**MARIA LUISA PADILLA, M.D.,** Associate Professor of Medicine, Pulmonary Division, Mount Sinai School of Medicine, New York, NY
RESPIRATORY SYSTEM

**DEVERA PINE,** Freelance writer based in New York, NY
AGING
BONES, MUSCLES, AND JOINTS
THE MYSTERY OF MENOPAUSE

**ABIGAIL W. POLEK,** Freelance writer and editor
KIDNEY DIALYSIS
MEDICAL TECHNOLOGY

**EDMUND A. PRIBITKIN, M.D.,** Assistant Professor, Department of Otolaryngology — Head and Neck Surgery, Thomas Jefferson University, Philadelphia, PA
EAR, NOSE, AND THROAT

**MICHAEL X. REPKA, M.D.,** Associate Professor of Ophthalmology and Pediatrics, Johns Hopkins University School of Medicine, Baltimore, MD
EYES AND VISION

**CYNTHIA PORTER RICKERT, Ph.D.,** Assistant Professor of Pediatrics, University of Arkansas for Medical Sciences, Little Rock, AR
CHILD DEVELOPMENT AND PSYCHOLOGY

**MACE L. ROTHENBERG, M.D.,** Assistant Professor of Medicine, University of Texas Health Science Center at San Antonio, TX
CANCER

**JAMES A. ROTHERHAM, Ph.D.,** Senior Associate, Chambers Associates, Inc., Washington, D.C.
GOVERNMENT POLICIES AND PROGRAMS

**C. ANDREW SALZBERG, M.D.,** Assistant Professor of Plastic and Reconstructive Surgery, New York Medical College, Valhalla, NY
PLASTIC SURGERY

**KAREN M. SANDRICK,** Freelance medical writer
HEALTH PERSONNEL AND FACILITIES

**COLLEEN SAUBER,** Contributor, *Harvard Health Letter*
UNKIND MILK

**MARIAN SEGAL,** Food and Drug Administration
WOMEN AND AIDS

**NEIL SPRINGER,** Freelance writer covering health and science matters
OCCUPATIONAL HEALTH

**CHERYL A. STOUKIDES, Pharm.D.,** Director, University of Rhode Island College of Pharmacy Drug Information Center, Providence, RI
coauthor, MEDICATIONS AND DRUGS

**MONA SUTNICK, Ed.D., R.D.,** Spokesperson, American Dietetic Association; Consultant in nutrition communication and education
HOUSECALLS: NUTRITION

**ROBERT M. SWIFT, M.D., Ph.D.,** Associate Professor, Department of Psychiatry, Brown University Medical School, Providence, RI
SUBSTANCE ABUSE

**FRANK M. SZIVOS,** Freelance medical writer based in Fairfield, CT
PROBLEMS "DOWN THERE"

**JANET C. TATE,** Senior Editor, Special Reports Network, Whittle Communications, Knoxville, TN
TOURETTE SYNDROME
WHAT'S COOKING IN COOKWARE?

**STEPHEN G. UNDERWOOD, M.D.,** Associate Faculty Member in Psychiatry, University of Pennsylvania School of Medicine, Philadelphia, PA; Consulting Psychiatrist, Bryn Mawr College Child Study Institute, Bryn Mawr, PA
HOUSECALLS: PSYCHOLOGY

**GEORGE VALKO, M.D.,** Instructor, Department of Family Medicine, Jefferson Medical College, Thomas Jefferson University, Philadelphia, PA
HOUSECALLS: MEDICINE AND THE HUMAN BODY

**LESLIE VREELAND,** Freelance writer specializing in health care and finance
DO YOU NEED A NUTRITIONIST?

**BARBARA ALDEN WILSON,** Freelance writer specializing in health and medicine in Seattle, WA
MARTIAL ARTS

**CONNIE ZUCKERMAN, J.D.,** Assistant Professor of Humanities in Medicine and of Family Medicine, State University of New York Health Science Center, Brooklyn, NY
MEDICAL ETHICS

# Contents

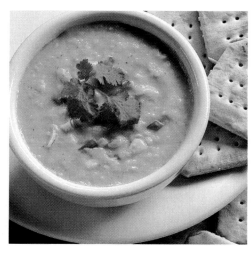

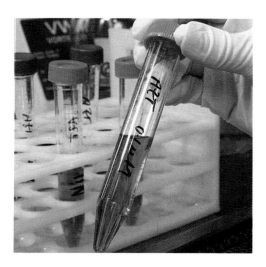

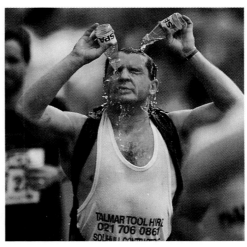

# Reports '94 ...................................229

# Review '94

People are enjoying longer, healthier lives as researchers unravel ever more secrets of the human body and as health-care professionals put this new knowledge to work. Life expectancy at birth in the United States has reached a record 75.5 years. The death rate for cardiovascular disease has declined dramatically over the past 15 years. And more people are surviving cancer now than several decades ago. While much of the credit for such improvements belongs to medical science, a significant share belongs to ordinary individuals, who are exercising more, eating better, getting regular checkups, and practicing other wholesome habits.

Even in developing nations, life expectancy has increased, jumping to 63 years from only 46 years as recently as 1960. World Health Organization (WHO) officials credit basic public-health measures, such as improved water supply sanitation, standard immunizations, and distribution of inexpensive drugs that combat nutritional deficiencies and intestinal infections, for the improvement. UNICEF (the United Nations Children's Fund) notes that there have been major reductions in infant deaths from pneumonia, diarrhea, tetanus, and whooping cough. Worldwide deaths from measles among children under 5 have fallen to just over 1 million a year.

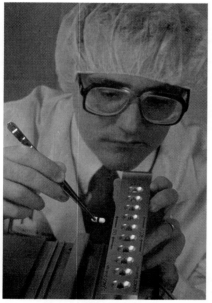

*Researchers continue to work feverishly to find a cure or a vaccine for AIDS and to discover the genetic basis of many untreatable disorders.*

Further advancements are anticipated during the coming years as new medical procedures become available. Particular attention is being paid to gene therapy, which, although still in its infancy, is beginning to revolutionize medicine. The idea is simple: a patient is given the normal genes that he or she lacks. In 1993 gene therapy was used for the first time on a patient with cystic fibrosis, the most common genetic killer in the United States. In the procedure the patient inhaled harmless viruses that had been altered to contain copies of the cystic-fibrosis gene. Other medical pioneers were three children, including two young infants, with severe combined immunodeficiency, a rare hereditary disease that leaves people defenseless against infections. Cells containing normal genes were injected into the children's bloodstreams in hopes of curing the disease and enabling the children's immune systems to function properly.

Before gene therapy is possible, the genetic defects that underlie a disease must be identified. Important discoveries during 1993 included finding the genes that cause two fatal neurodegenerative disorders: Huntington's disease and amyotrophic lateral sclerosis (more commonly known as "Lou Gehrig's disease"). Scientists also found a genetic defect that may predispose some men toward aggressive, violent behavior. It is the aim of the Human Genome Project, an international effort involving dozens of laboratories, to isolate all 100,000 human genes by 2005—a goal some researchers believe is optimistic, although by late 1993 it was reported that researchers had produced preliminary maps of all 23 pairs of human chromosomes.

The cost of medical care continued to grow, rising approximately 5.5 percent in 1993—about double the general inflation rate. The number of people without health insurance also continued to grow, reaching 38.9 million in 1992, according to a recent report from the Employee Benefit Research Institute.

Such statistics increased pressure on public officials to overhaul the U.S. health-care system. Several plans for health-care reform were presented during 1993. The most ambitious of these was President Clinton's plan, which called for comprehensive health benefits for all Americans "that can never be taken away." But as 1994 began, it was unclear whether Congress would soon pass a major health-care bill, especially one that guarantees coverage for all Americans.

A major area of concern among public-health officials is the mounting menace of infectious diseases, both old and new. Tuberculosis, which doctors had hoped to eradicate in the United States by 2010, has instead spread, with the number of cases jumping 20 percent from 1985 to 1993; among children under 15, cases increased 35 percent during that time. Worldwide, tuberculosis kills 3 million people annually. WHO's Arata Kotchi, M.D., calls it "the world's most neglected health crisis," pointing out that the tuberculosis bacterium "already infects one in every three people on the planet."

The AIDS pandemic, caused by HIV (human immunodeficiency virus), continued to spread. Some 14 million people worldwide were believed to have been infected with HIV by 1993, and experts fear that unless stronger preventive measures are taken, this number will soar to 30 million to 40 million by the year 2000. An estimated 1 million HIV-infected people live in the United States, where more than 200,000 people have died from AIDS since it was first recognized in 1981. Although several medications extend survival, no treatment is yet available to vaccinate against infection or to cure the disease.

A new or previously unrecognized strain of hantaviruses was found to be the cause of a deadly disease that surfaced in 1993, primarily among people in the American Southwest. The virus, which causes severe respiratory illness, appears to spread through airborne particles from the urine, droppings, and saliva of deer mice and other rodents.

Another public-health concern in the United States that received growing recognition from both health officials and the general public was violence, particularly the growing number of deaths from guns and the rampant spread of teenage homicide. "Violence is the leading cause of lost life in this country today. If it's not a public-health problem, why are all those people dying from it?" asked David Satcher, M.D., the new director of the Centers for Disease Control and Prevention (CDC). The possible contributions to real-life violence by violence in video games and on television were vociferously debated, as were the effects of poverty, drugs, lack of family structure, and weak gun-control laws.

Many billions of dollars are being spent as researchers seek solutions to the growth of violence, the spread of AIDS, and other medical crises. Additional sums are being spent to disseminate and put into practice already-proven solutions to health problems. Many of these efforts will bear fruit during the coming years. Thanks to the 1993 discovery of a gene that predisposes people to colon cancer, it will soon be possible to screen people with a family history of the disease, and to provide treatment during curable stages. Because of a new multidrug treatment program, WHO believes that it may be possible to wipe out leprosy by the year 2000. And because preventive therapies are proving effective in treating everything from heart disease to premature aging, many experts foresee people enjoying even longer, healthier lives than they do today.

*The Editors*

# Health and Medicine: Features '94

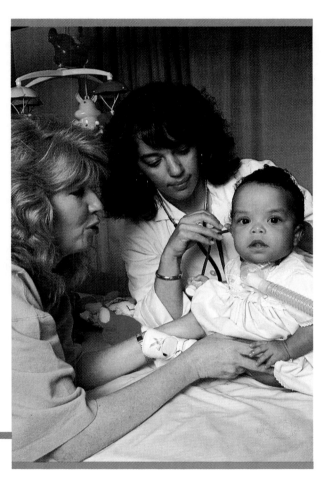

# Medicine and the Human Body

**See also:**
Individual articles in the second half of this book, arranged in alphabetical order, for additional information.

The human body is equipped with marvelous defense mechanisms. But sometimes these mechanisms are unable to cope with invading microbes, environmental pollutants, injuries, and other stresses. To regain good health, people call on the tools and techniques of medicine. The range of these therapies continuously broadens, as scientists increase their understanding of the human body. For instance, in 1993 researchers reported that they had developed a new magnetic resonance imaging (MRI) technique that provides clear images of nerves. They are hopeful that the technique will lead to improved diagnosis of chronic back pain and other nerve conditions, and will reduce the need for exploratory surgery to locate compressed and injured nerves.

Sometimes research leads to important modifications in medical practices. The Diabetes Control and Complications Trial, scheduled to be a 10-year study comparing two treatments for Type I (juvenile-onset) diabetes, was stopped earlier than planned so that its dramatic findings could be shared with all diabetics. The study compared conventional treatment, in which diabetics received one or two shots of insulin daily, with a more rigorous therapy, in which diabetics were put on a special diet and either received three or more injections daily or relied on an insulin pump to continuously deliver insulin to their bloodstream. The latter procedure reduces fluctuations in blood-sugar levels and, in the study, significantly prevented or delayed blindness, kidney failure, and other complications.

In other cases, scientists have presented new evidence of the efficacy of current practices. A 13-year study involving 46,551 Minnesota residents shows that people who are annually tested for blood in the feces experience 33 percent fewer deaths from colorectal cancer than people who are not tested. The test helps physicians detect cancer at an early, curable stage; it also helps detect adenomatous polyps. The decade-long National Polyp Study, conducted on 1,418 adults who had had at least one adenomatous polyp removed from their colons, demonstrates that finding and removing these polyps cut the risk of colon cancer by 90 percent.

Two vaccines show early promise of providing immunity against disease, though researchers caution that it may take years to perfect the compounds. Initial safety tests of a vaccine for Lyme disease were successful, and clinical trials are scheduled to begin in 1994. A vaccine against multiple sclerosis also appeared to be safe, and it cut attacks by 50 percent among a small group of patients who have the relapsing form of the disease. In mid-1993 the U.S. Food and Drug Administration (FDA) approved Betaseron, the first drug ever approved for the treatment of multiple sclerosis. The FDA also approved Pulmozyme, a genetically engineered drug to treat cystic fibrosis—the first new treatment in 30 years for the life-threatening genetic disease.

People who live in areas that lack medical specialists can anticipate improved care thanks to the new field of telemedicine—the use of video and telephone technology to deliver health-care services. New products introduced during 1993 included Medtel, an interactive video system marketed by Raytheon that can be used for medical examinations, diagnosis, and treatment. Physicians or nurses use electronic stethoscopes and other electronic instruments to gather

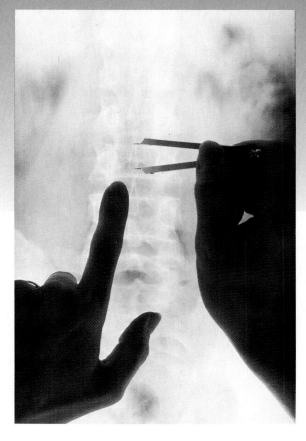

data from a patient. The data are sent via telephone to one or more specialists, who help interpret the data and suggest treatment.

In medicine, as in any field, the path to progress is often steeped with frustrations. Nowhere is this more evident— and worrisome— than in the fight against HIV, the virus that causes AIDS. "Our progress seems desperately slow," says Michael H. Merson, M.D., director of the World Health Organization's (WHO's) AIDS program. "Our scientific advances today are coming in small steps, not in leaps and bounds."

But even though progress against AIDS has slowed, breakthroughs continue to be made. In late 1993 a team headed by Ara Hovanessian, M.D., at the Pasteur Institute in Paris, France, announced that it had identified a protein on the surface of immune cells that enables the HIV to enter and infect the cells. Researchers now hope to find a way to inhibit the action of the surface protein, which could be a step toward developing a vaccine against AIDS.

*As researchers gain a better understanding of the human body, therapies for treating illness will also improve.*

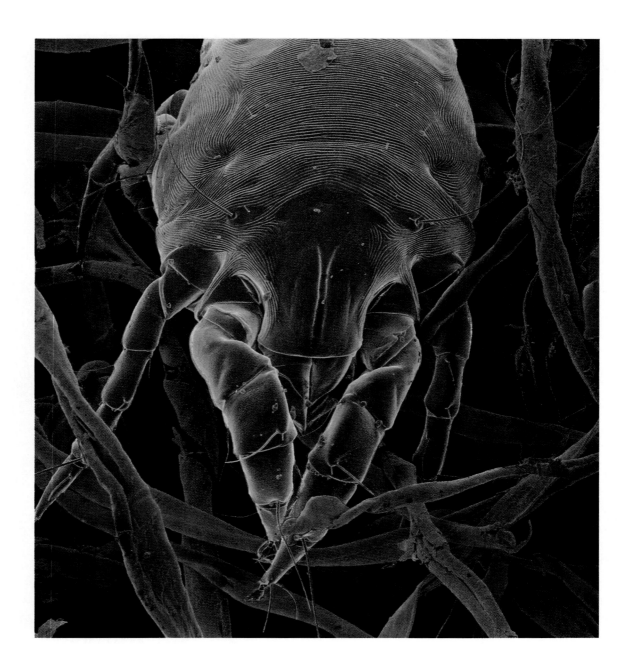

# Allergies: nothing to *sneeze* at

*by Larry Katzenstein*

Bill Clinton's 1992 fall campaign was rigorous, but the following spring and summer proved even tougher. That's when some of the president's most formidable adversaries breezed into the nation's capital: weed pollen, grass pollen, and mold spores. (President Clinton is moderately allergic to cat dander as well, but Socks, the First Feline, seems in no danger of a presidential veto.)

Allergies afflict not only presidents—former President Reagan has them, too—but also more than 50 million of their constituents, who are tormented by the same garden-variety allergens that affect President Clinton, plus numerous others, including copper coins, nickel-coated earrings, mangoes, insect stings, heat, cold, and even sperm. Reactions range from the merely annoying to the life-threatening.

The tendency to develop allergies is clearly inherited: If one of your parents has allergies, you have a one-in-three chance of developing them, too (although not necessarily the same ones); with two allergic parents, it's almost a guarantee. Allergies usually show up by the time you're 30, although even people well into their 80s can become first-time sufferers. On the other hand, people tend to outgrow allergies as they age.

### Confused Immune System

All allergies result from the same basic cause: an immune system unable to distinguish between the benign and the harmful. The immune system's crucial task is to produce antibodies that protect the body from disease-causing bacteria and viruses. But in allergic people the system also makes antibodies against seemingly innocuous substances, such as pollen grains.

The antibodies responsible for allergies belong to a class known as immunoglobulin E (IgE). Everyone makes some IgE, but allergic people make about 10 times as much as people unaffected by allergies.

The first encounter with an allergen —the name for a substance that triggers an allergic response—may prompt the body to begin churning out IgE against it. These antibodies attach to special cells known as mast cells, millions of which line the respiratory and digestive tract; millions more are found in the skin. The mast cells with their antibody coatings resemble mines bristling with detonators,

ready to ambush the allergen if it reappears. And they can wait a long time.

Most antibodies last in the body only about three weeks, but IgE's can persist for months or years—and so can the mast cells they sit upon. "That's why someone who had an allergic reaction to penicillin as a child could still be allergic to the drug as an adult," explains Michael Kaliner, M.D., from the National Institute of Allergy and Infectious Diseases in Bethesda, Maryland. "The IgE antibody he made as a six-year-old could still be present at age 40, sitting on mast cells and conveying incredibly long-lived sensitivity to the allergen."

*A growing arsenal of sprays and tablets can make allergies bearable for most people.*

Generally, however, it takes several exposures to an allergen—two to five seasons in the case of tree or ragweed pollen, for example—before a person makes enough IgE to produce allergic symptoms. Then, when the allergen comes along, its encounter with IgE will trigger mast cells to release powerful chemicals—such as histamine—that engage the "enemy" allergen, but also inflame and damage surrounding tissue.

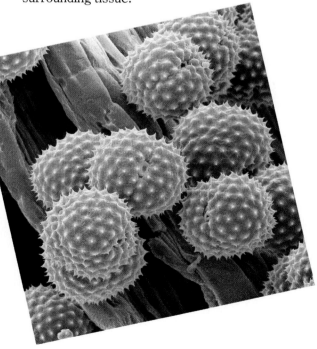

**Diminutive but dastardly, the dust mite (left) and the ragweed pollen (right) are just two of the many allergens that cause 22 million Americans to sneeze and wheeze.**

### Types of Tissue

A person's symptoms depend on where in the body these chemicals are released. Allergies to foods or drugs can manifest themselves in hives (itchy skin welts) or intestinal upsets, including vomiting and diarrhea. Inflammation of tissue lining the air passages results in the wheezing, coughing, and labored breathing of asthma.

And then there's the champion allergic malady, hay fever, which inflames the lining of the nose, sinuses, and eyelids, producing watery, puffy, or itchy eyes; sneezing fits; and a runny, stopped-up, or itchy nose. The culprits in hay fever are microscopic airborne allergens. They affect 35 million Americans, making hay fever the most common of all chronic diseases.

Hay fever is singularly misnamed, since it isn't caused by hay and doesn't involve fever. The more accurate term is allergic rhinitis, meaning nasal inflammation due to allergy. For most sufferers, hay fever is a seasonal

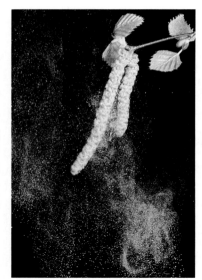

*Mild winters, increased rainfall, and cool springs produce concentrated pollen production that wreaks havoc in May and June.*

torment caused by pollen. But thanks largely to indoor contaminants, hay fever can affect people year-round as well.

Seasonal hay-fever victims are usually afflicted in the fall or spring, or both, when the air is awash in pollen: grass and tree pollens in the spring, and ragweed in late summer or early fall. Summer allergies can be caused by mold spores spawned by humidity, and winter allergies from dust in tightly shut houses.

In some people, dust and mold can also cause year-round hay fever, a problem that can be brought on by household pets as well—particularly cats, whose skin and saliva are notorious for provoking misery. (President Clinton's puffy eyes, for example, probably are as much due to his cat Socks as to his propensity for burning the midnight oil.)

The best way to treat any allergy is to avoid the allergens that cause it. Seasonal hay-fever sufferers know that avoiding pollen is easier said than done, but staying inside for

# LEADING CAUSES OF ALLERGIC REACTION

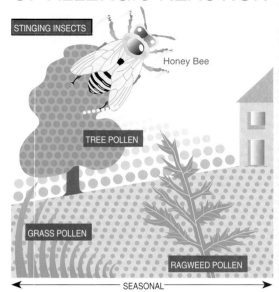

STINGING INSECTS

Honey Bee

TREE POLLEN

GRASS POLLEN

RAGWEED POLLEN

←——— SEASONAL ———→

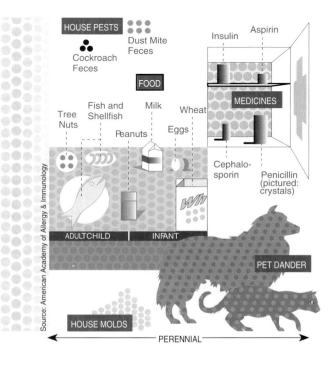

HOUSE PESTS

Dust Mite Feces

Cockroach Feces

FOOD

Tree Nuts

Fish and Shellfish

Milk

Peanuts

Eggs

Wheat

Insulin

Aspirin

MEDICINES

Cephalosporin

Penicillin (pictured: crystals)

ADULT CHILD

INFANT

PET DANDER

HOUSE MOLDS

←——— PERENNIAL ———→

Source: American Academy of Allergy & Immunology

## Of Mites and Men

Do motes dance in the shaft of sunlight streaming through your bedroom window? If so, they could be causing your year-round hay fever or your child's asthma.

House dust is now recognized as a major cause of allergic disease. Inhaling it can cause symptoms ranging from mild irritation to incapacitating airway constriction. Forty to 80 percent of all asthmatics react to one or more of dust's unsavory ingredients.

House-dust components include human and animal dander, mold, lint, and—most important of all—dead dust mites: their powdery remains, and especially their airborne feces, are the main provokers of dust-mite allergy. The microscopic mites thrive in the summer, feasting primarily on human dander, and die in the winter.

"Dust mites are probably the most important allergen in the world," says Michael Kaliner, M.D., head of the allergic-diseases section of the National Institute of Allergy and Infectious Diseases. "All temperate regions are afflicted with the pests, which live in carpeting, mattresses, pillows, and upholstery." (Arid areas are spared, since mites can't survive when the relative humidity is below 50 percent.)

"Most people can't control the dust conditions under which they work," says Kaliner, "but they can do something about the bedroom, where they spend six to eight hours a night, and where dust mites most often reside." To this end, he offers the following suggestions for maintaining a dust-free bedroom:

• Keep carpets out of the bedroom. They trap dust—particularly shag rugs, the worst type for a dust-sensitive person.
• Buy products that kill dust mites, known as acaricides, which are now available in drugstores and can help control mites in carpets as well as in mattresses and sofas.
• Encase the bed's box springs, mattress, and pillows in dustproof zippered covers.

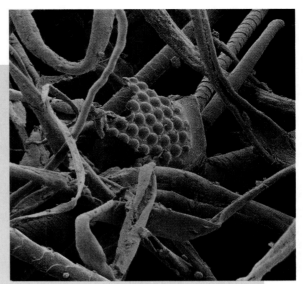

*Household dust and the mites and animal dander that inhabit it (above) can make the atmosphere a veritable land mine, triggering explosive reactions in sensitive people.*

(You can buy dustproof fabric covers, which are more comfortable than the plastic variety.)
• Use window shades instead of venetian blinds, which are dust traps. Other dust magnets include down-filled or fuzzy wool blankets or comforters, feather pillows, closets full of clothing, and dogs and cats. Keep all animals with fur or feathers out of the bedroom.
• Use only washable materials on the bed, and wash bedding weekly in hot water (above 130° F). Warm or cold water won't kill mites.
• Keep toys that gather dust—particularly stuffed ones—out of any bedroom that belongs to a dust-sensitive child.
• Clean the room daily, wiping down surfaces with a damp cloth or oil mop. Do a thorough cleaning once a week. Dust-sensitive people should avoid vacuuming, which may churn up more dust than it removes.
• Try to eradicate cockroaches, prime felons in causing allergies and asthma, particularly among urban children, who are more often exposed to them.
• Consider purchasing a high-efficiency particulate arresting (HEPA) filtering unit, a device that can help reduce airborne allergens.

part of the day and turning on the air conditioner can help. Pollen counts are highest in the early morning, and air-conditioning filters out more than 99 percent of pollen in the air.

For some allergic people—particularly those with year-round hay fever and asthma —staying inside just makes things worse. Microscopic menaces in household air play key roles in perpetuating symptoms, and eliminating them can markedly improve health. (For advice on vanquishing some common offenders, see "Of Mites and Men" on page 21.)

If avoidance isn't feasible or doesn't work, the next choice should be medication to relieve symptoms. Recently introduced drugs have revolutionized hay-fever treatment, but many people don't know about them.

### Allergy Medications

*Antihistamines* are the most frequently used drugs in hay-fever treatment. As their name implies, antihistamines counteract histamines, the chemicals responsible for several hay-fever symptoms, including runny nose, sneezing, and itching eyes and throat.

First-generation antihistamines include several types of nonprescription tablets such as brompheniramine (available in Dimetane and Nasahist B), chlorpheniramine (Chlor-Trimeton), and diphenhydramine (Benadryl and Benylin). Many of these products are also sold in generic form. All begin providing relief within 15 to 30 minutes, but they have a serious drawback: drowsiness. Several antihistamine ingredients, in fact, are also sold as sedatives.

Two newer, prescription-only antihistamines—terfenadine (Seldane) and astemizole (Hismanal)—don't cause that problem. These nonsedating antihistamines are as effective as their older brethren, but are also much more expensive. They're not identical: Although Seldane starts working faster than Hismanal (within one or two hours versus up to four hours), a dose of Seldane doesn't last as long (about 12 hours versus 24 hours or longer). The recently introduced Seldane-D adds a dollop of decongestant. You can economize on antihistamine by taking a nonsedating antihistamine during the day, and one of the less expensive sedating varieties before bed. A word of caution: Last year the Food and Drug Administration (FDA) warned that Seldane, Seldane-D, and Hismanal can cause abnormal heart rhythms when taken in excessive doses or when used in combination with either ketoconazole (an antifungal drug) or the much-prescribed antibiotic erythromycin.

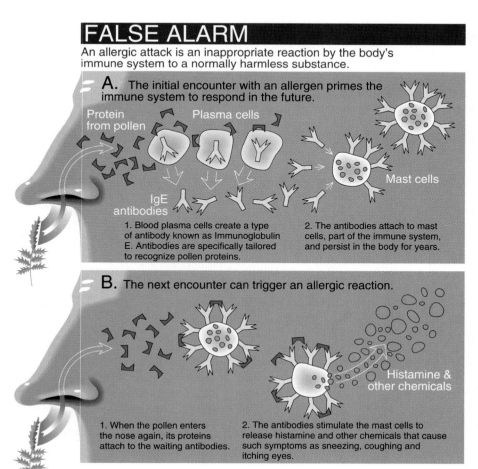

## FALSE ALARM

An allergic attack is an inappropriate reaction by the body's immune system to a normally harmless substance.

**A.** The initial encounter with an allergen primes the immune system to respond in the future.

Protein from pollen

Plasma cells

IgE antibodies

Mast cells

1. Blood plasma cells create a type of antibody known as Immunoglobulin E. Antibodies are specifically tailored to recognize pollen proteins.

2. The antibodies attach to mast cells, part of the immune system, and persist in the body for years.

**B.** The next encounter can trigger an allergic reaction.

Histamine & other chemicals

1. When the pollen enters the nose again, its proteins attach to the waiting antibodies.

2. The antibodies stimulate the mast cells to release histamine and other chemicals that cause such symptoms as sneezing, coughing and itching eyes.

*Decongestants* relieve another symptom: nasal congestion, so common in hay fever and often not helped by antihistamines. Decongestants come in tablets, sprays, and drops.

The decongestant sprays and drops typically contain either xylometazoline (Neo-Synephrine II long-acting nasal spray) or oxymetazoline (Afrin, Allerest 12-Hour, Dristan long-lasting nasal sprays, and many others). They start acting immediately, but must be used sparingly; if taken for more than three or four days in a row, the nasal decongestants often cause rebound congestion worse than the original problem.

Decongestant tablets don't work as rapidly as sprays, but can be used for a longer time,

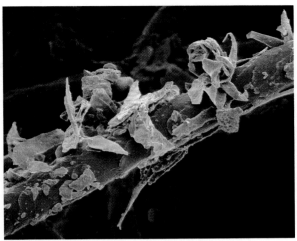

*Dander (above) from pets can produce a host of allergy symptoms. Sensitive people should keep their bedrooms off limits to cats and dogs.*

## Asthma and the Allergy Connection

Asthma, a disease marked by shortness of breath and wheezing, is affecting more Americans, especially younger ones. Some 3.7 million children and adolescents now have asthma, up sharply from 2.4 million in 1980. Possible reasons for the increase include tighter, better-insulated homes (which trap allergens and other pollutants), and respiratory infections linked to day care. About 15 million Americans have asthma, and more than 4,000 die from it each year.

Asthma affects the tubes that bring air to the lungs, known as bronchi, which become narrowed in several ways: The muscles surrounding them constrict; their lining becomes inflamed and swollen; and excess mucus threatens to clog whatever space is left.

While asthma and allergy are distinct conditions, they do overlap, especially among asthmatics 15 years old and younger. Ninety percent of asthmatic children have allergies, and evidence suggests that their allergies are often the cause of their asthma. A recent study, for example, found that children exposed to high levels of airborne dust mites as infants were at increased risk of developing asthma; another study found that childhood exposure to cat dander had the same effect.

But while allergies seem responsible for many cases of asthma, not all asthmatics have them. Other causes include respiratory infections, chemicals in the workplace, and childhood exposure to cigarette smoke.

The big news in asthma is the change in the way it's treated—or should be treated. Until recently, treatment emphasized bronchodilators—drugs that widen the airways by relaxing their surrounding muscles. But researchers have discovered that asthma is primarily a disease of airway *inflammation,* which persists even when the asthmatic person seems fine. Inflamed bronchial tissue is hyperactive to things that can trigger asthma attacks, including pollen and other airborne allergens, exercise, aspirin, sulfites, and pollutants such as cigarette smoke.

In 1991 recognition of asthma as an inflammatory disease led experts at the National Institutes of Health (NIH) to call for greater use of anti-inflammatory drugs to treat the disease. For most asthmatics, that means regular use of inhaled steroids or inhaled cromolyn sodium to control airway inflammation.

# Cat Advice

A few simple measures can permit many cat-sensitive people to co-exist relatively comfortably with Miss Puss or Mister Boots. Thomas Platts-Mills, M.D., head of the allergy and clinical immunology division at the University of Virginia Medical School in Charlottesville, has recommended a two-pronged strategy. "For many people, taking these measures means they can live with their cat," Platts-Mills says.

**Attack the Places Where Cat Allergen Lurks.** Cat allergen is a protein known as Felid I, made primarily by sebaceous glands in the cat's skin; the protein coats the fur, is transferred to the animal's saliva through grooming, and then becomes airborne. (Short-haired cats shed just as much allergen as longhairs, and possibly even more, Platts-Mills says.) He urges allergic cat owners to get rid of carpets and upholstered furniture, wipe down walls, and filter the air.

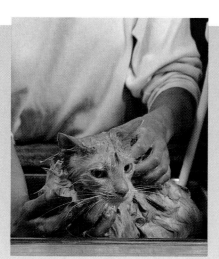

**Wash Your Cat.** Studies by Platts-Mills have shown that washing a cat once a week reduces the level of allergen coming off the cat by 90 percent. A formal bath isn't necessary: Just pouring some water over the cat and then wiping it off can suffice. (For the free brochure "Protocol for Cat Washing," send an SASE to *Dr. H. James Wedner, Washington University School of Medicine, 660 South Euclid Ave., Box 8122, St. Louis, MO 63110.)*

Martin Valentine, M.D., a professor of medicine at Johns Hopkins Asthma and Allergy Center in Baltimore, Maryland, recommends that people allergic to *anything*—pollen, for example—should avoid getting a cat, since prolonged exposure will probably bring out cat allergy as well. "It will take six months to determine if they're sensitive, and by then they'll be attached to the animal," he says. "Get a snake instead, or a lizard, fish, or turtle." Even dogs, he says, are less likely to cause problems than cats.

although some people find their effectiveness diminishes after a couple of weeks. The tablets typically contain either pseudoephedrine (Sudafed and generic versions) or phenylpropanolamine (Propagest), which are equally potent. Oral decongestants can cause side effects including nervousness, restlessness, and insomnia.

Drugstore shelves are swamped with cold and allergy tablets that combine a decongestant and an antihistamine: Chlor-Trimeton Decongestant, Contac 12-Hour, Dimetapp, Drixoral, Sudafed Plus, Tavist-D, Triaminic-12, and many others. If you really need both an antihistamine and a decongestant, these two-in-one products make sense. The decongestant's "hyper" side effect may counteract the antihistamine's drowsiness effect.

*Steroid nasal sprays*, introduced several years ago and available only by prescription, are the most effective of all hay-fever drugs. Indeed, a recent article in the *New England Journal of Medicine* concluded that the drugs offer "excellent symptomatic relief" to "more than 90 percent" of hay-fever patients. Steroid sprays work by reducing inflammation in the nasal passages. They complement antihistamines by relieving the nasal congestion that so often occurs in hay fever. Steroid sprays include preparations containing the steroids beclomethasone (Beclovent, Beconase, Vancenase AO, and Vanceril), flunisolide (AeroBid and Nasalide), and triamcinolone (Nasacort).

These steroids are completely different than the hazardous anabolic steroids used by some athletes to gain strength. In addition, very little of the steroid in these sprays is absorbed into the body, making them much safer for regular use than oral steroid preparations, which can delay growth in children and cause bone thinning and other serious side effects when used for long periods.

The major drawback to steroid sprays is the long wait—about a week or more before they become fully effective. (So it's best to start using them a few days before symptoms are expected—before the fall ragweed season, for example.) They're also expensive, and they cause sneezing, nasal irritation, or burning in about 10 percent of users.

*Cromolyn sodium* is another type of antiinflammatory drug used in treating respiratory problems. It comes in several forms, including an inhaler (Intal) and a nasal solution (Nasalcrom). Cromolyn sodium is somewhat less potent than steroid sprays, but its lack of side effects makes it appropriate for children.

*Nobody is exempt from allergies, not even Bill Clinton. His puffy eyes are more likely caused by allergens than by burning the midnight oil.*

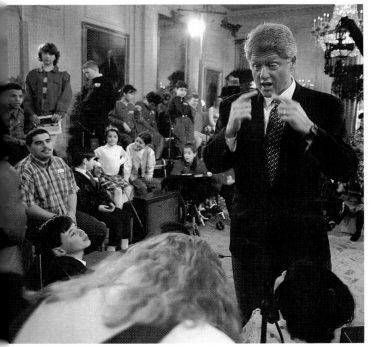

## A Shot of Relief

Most hay-fever sufferers should obtain considerable relief from the drugs now available, either over-the-counter or by prescription. Unlike allergy shots, these drugs work against the symptoms caused by a wide variety of allergens, from pollen to dust mites. In some cases a combination may be needed: an antihistamine for a runny nose, and a steroid spray to relieve congestion, for example.

Although today's drugs excel at handling symptoms, allergy shots are the only known "cure" for allergies. Patients receive regular injections of extracts of the allergens that irk them. "The shots desensitize a person to these allergens by reducing the production of IgE antibodies and increasing levels of another class of antibodies, the IgG's, which actually protect people from allergic disease," Dr. Kaliner says.

Shots are especially useful for people strongly allergic to stings from bees and other insects. They're also suited for people who, like President Clinton, have year-round allergy symptoms. "We generally use shots when people have problems for two seasons of the year or longer," Kaliner says. "Those with single-season allergies are usually treated with medication, but if they're really bothered in a major way, we'll use shots to lower their need for drugs."

Shots reduce symptoms in about 85 percent of people who receive them for hay fever caused by grass, ragweed, trees, and dust mites. And people whose asthma is provoked by such allergies can also benefit from shots. On the negative side, shots are expensive, occasionally cause allergic reactions themselves, and require frequent office visits. What's more, it usually takes a year or more after the allergy shots have been initiated before a patient experiences maximum symptom relief. ◇

**For More Information:**

**The National Jewish Center for Immunology and Respiratory Medicine,**
800-222-LUNG.

**The Allergy and Asthma Network,**
800-878-4403.

**American Academy of Allergy and Immunology,**
800-822-ASMA.

**University of California at Davis's Pet Loss Support Hotline,**
916-752-4200.

**Allergy-Control Products,**
800-422-DUST.

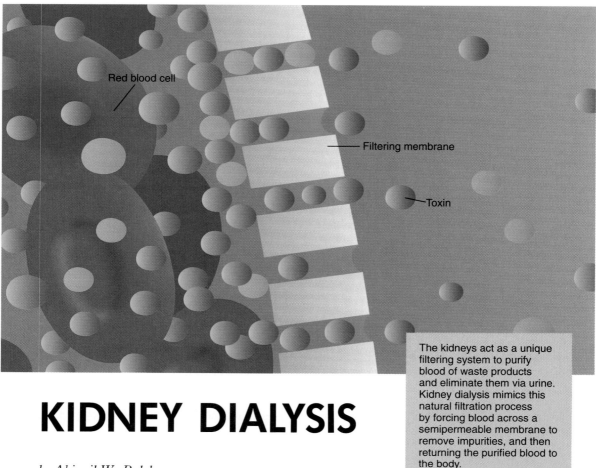

Red blood cell

Filtering membrane

Toxin

The kidneys act as a unique filtering system to purify blood of waste products and eliminate them via urine. Kidney dialysis mimics this natural filtration process by forcing blood across a semipermeable membrane to remove impurities, and then returning the purified blood to the body.

# KIDNEY DIALYSIS

*by Abigail W. Polek*

Each year, some 45,000 Americans suffer kidney failure. In the not-too-distant past, these people would have died, but not after first experiencing a sometimes-prolonged period of misery as the toxins usually filtered out by the kidneys instead accumulated in their bodies. Medical science today offers a new lease on life for victims of kidney disease through a process called dialysis, a procedure that artificially filters impurities from the blood. For some people, dialysis becomes a lifelong routine. For others, it represents a temporary measure until an appropriate kidney becomes available for transplant. For all of the more than 130,000 patients currently on one form or another of this therapy, dialysis has become—at least for a brief time—a way of life.

### Kidney Function and Disease
The kidneys are twin, fist-sized, bean-shaped organs located in the middle back area

of the body. In a healthy person, these organs perform three important functions: They excrete urine, which contains waste products and excess water; they produce hormones; and they break down protein and amino acids. The kidneys also maintain the balance of *electrolytes*—substances such as sodium, potassium, and calcium that take on an electric charge when mixed in liquid. Electrolytes affect how muscles and nerves function—an imbalance of any one of these substances can cause symptoms as mild as muscle fatigue or as serious as an irregular heartbeat. Together, these three functions allow the kidneys to maintain fluid balance in the body.

When a kidney is damaged by disease or injury, it may stop functioning altogether or function at a decreased capacity. *Acute renal failure* is the sudden and complete shutdown of both kidneys. It may occur after surgery or be caused by shock, toxic drugs or chemicals, a blood transfusion, or a severe injury.

If treated immediately with medication or dialysis, it can usually be reversed, and full or partial kidney function restored.

*Chronic renal failure* is a long-term decrease in kidney function. It takes place over a period of months or years, and results from repeated kidney infections, damage caused by kidney stones, injuries, and various diseases. It is permanent and irreversible. Chronic renal failure eventually leads to *uremia,* or *end-stage renal failure* (ESRF). The kidneys stop functioning, and toxins begin to accumulate at dangerously high levels in the blood. A person with ESRF cannot live without dialysis.

## Types of Dialysis

Dialysis is based on the natural process of *osmosis,* the tendency of substances to move from an area of greater concentration to an area of lesser concentration, until the two areas are balanced. During dialysis the blood is moved across a *semipermeable membrane* —one with many microscopic holes—that separates it from a sterile fluid. Small particles of impurities pass easily through the membrane, while larger molecules, such as red blood cells and undigested proteins, do not. In this way the blood is purified only of toxins.

Dialysis takes two forms: *Hemodialysis* filters the blood outside of the body, while *peritoneal dialysis* cleans the blood inside the body, in the peritoneal cavity, or abdomen.

Hemodialysis. The more common procedure, hemodialysis requires the use of a dialysis machine and is usually performed at a hospital or dialysis center. A dialysis machine consists of two compartments separated by a semipermeable membrane made of cellulose. One compartment holds the blood, while the other contains a sterile solution called the *dialysate,* which is enriched with electrolytes.

In hemodialysis a patient is hooked up to a dialysis machine using two needles. One is placed in an artery to direct the blood into the machine; the other is attached to a vein to return the refreshed blood to the body. These needles are usually attached to the patient's arm at a *fistula,* an area where an artery and a vein have been surgically joined together, or at a *shunt,* a section of silicone-rubber tubing permanently implanted in the skin. The blood is pumped out of the body; before entering the dialysis machine, the blood is treated with an anticoagulant to prevent it from clotting when it mixes with other substances. The blood is then moved across the cellulose membrane in the dialysis machine, and the impurities it contains pass through this membrane into the dialysate. The purified blood is then returned to the body, and the cycle is repeated.

Each time the blood flows through the body, it picks up more waste products. Filtering the blood several times over the course of one dialysis treatment ensures that the majority of toxins are removed. The whole process lasts from three to five hours, and it is usually repeated three times a week, or every other day.

Peritoneal dialysis. In peritoneal dialysis, a dialysate is put into the kidney patient's abdomen. As the blood circulates through the body, it passes over the *peritoneal membrane,* the sac that covers the stomach, the intestines, and other organs in the abdomen. The impurities the blood contains pass through this membrane and into the dialysate in the abdomen. The dialysate is then drained from the patient's abdomen and discarded. Three types of peritoneal dialysis are in use today: *continuous ambulatory peritoneal dialysis, continuous cyclic peritoneal dialysis,* and *intermittent peritoneal dialysis.*

Continuous ambulatory peritoneal dialysis (CAPD) is the most common of the three. It occurs continuously, and the individual can move around freely while it is happening. Patients on this form of dialysis have a tube, or catheter, implanted in their abdomen, near the navel. A plastic bag containing the dialysis solution is then hooked up to the catheter, and the solution is drained into the abdomen. When the bag is empty, it is simply folded up under the clothes, though left attached. Four to six hours later, the individual unfolds the empty bag and drains the fluid from the abdomen back into it. The bag is then removed, and a new one containing fresh dialysate is attached to the catheter. The entire process is then repeated.

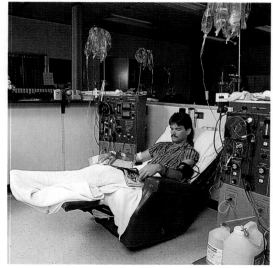

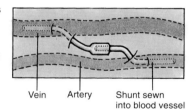

## Hemodialysis

1. A doctor makes a shunt connecting an artery to a vein. This permits access to the bloodstream for rapid removal and return of blood.

Vein    Artery    Shunt sewn into blood vessel

2. Blood is passed to the artificial kidney and back to the patient via a needle connected to plastic tubing. The artificial kidney contains many membrane layers that separate the blood from a special fluid called dialysate. Toxins pass from the blood into the dialysate.

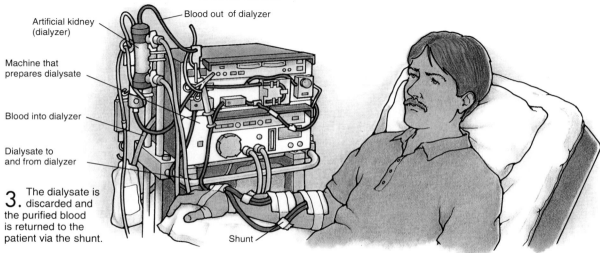

Artificial kidney (dialyzer)

Blood out of dialyzer

Machine that prepares dialysate

Blood into dialyzer

Dialysate to and from dialyzer

3. The dialysate is discarded and the purified blood is returned to the patient via the shunt.

Shunt

In continuous cyclic peritoneal dialysis (CCPD), the patient also has a catheter implanted in the abdomen. However, the catheter is hooked up to a cycling machine rather than a portable bag, and the dialysis is performed overnight. The cycling machine pumps the dialysate into the abdomen, and then pumps it back out after several hours. New fluid is then pumped into the abdomen and emptied out two more times over the course of the night; a third batch is pumped in at the end of the treatment and allowed to remain in the patient's abdomen during the day. The process is repeated each night.

The third type of peritoneal dialysis, *intermittent peritoneal dialysis* (IPD), also requires an individual to be hooked up to a cycling machine. This type of dialysis takes 8 to 12 hours and is performed three times a week. The cycling machine pumps a small amount of dialysate into the abdomen, allows it to remain for 10 minutes, and then pumps it back out over a 15-minute period. The process is then repeated as many times as possible over the next 8 to 12 hours.

### Deciding Which Type of Dialysis to Use

Choosing a dialysis method is based on a variety of factors, including proximity to a hospital or dialysis center and lifestyle. CAPD, while the most convenient form of dialysis, carries a high risk of infection—every time a bag is changed, the catheter is exposed to bacteria. Most CAPD patients get *peritonitis*, an infection of the peritoneal membrane, at least once a year.

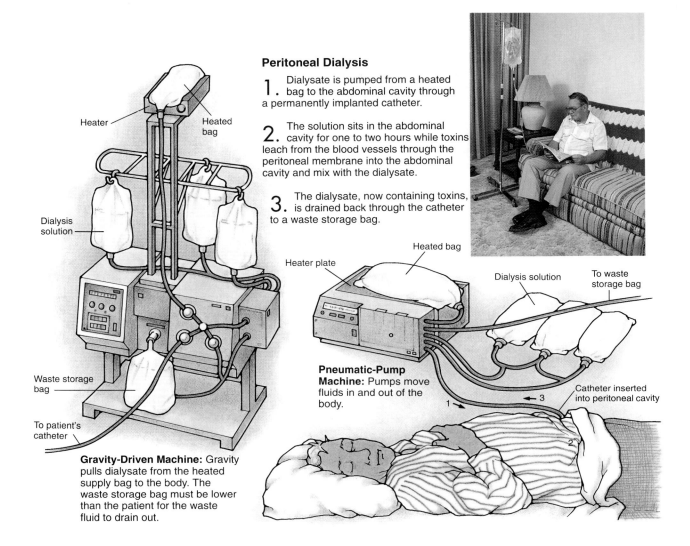

**Peritoneal Dialysis**

1. Dialysate is pumped from a heated bag to the abdominal cavity through a permanently implanted catheter.

2. The solution sits in the abdominal cavity for one to two hours while toxins leach from the blood vessels through the peritoneal membrane into the abdominal cavity and mix with the dialysate.

3. The dialysate, now containing toxins, is drained back through the catheter to a waste storage bag.

Heater

Heated bag

Dialysis solution

Waste storage bag

To patient's catheter

**Gravity-Driven Machine:** Gravity pulls dialysate from the heated supply bag to the body. The waste storage bag must be lower than the patient for the waste fluid to drain out.

Heater plate

Heated bag

Dialysis solution

To waste storage bag

**Pneumatic-Pump Machine:** Pumps move fluids in and out of the body.

Catheter inserted into peritoneal cavity

Doctors tend to recommend hemodialysis for pregnant women and patients with bowel disease or nutritional deficiencies. Peritoneal dialysis is better for children waiting for a transplant, people who travel frequently, and those with an aversion to needles. Individuals with acquired immune deficiency syndrome (AIDS) and hepatitis are also better suited for peritoneal dialysis.

Cost is *not* a factor in determining dialysis use in the United States. Since 1972 Medicare, the federal health-insurance program for the elderly and severely disabled, has covered dialysis (and kidney transplants) as part of the End-State Renal Disease Program. This program pays up to $32,000 a year for every kidney patient who requires maintenance dialysis to survive.

**New Options**

Recently a *Y-set catheter* was introduced in Europe for use with CAPD. This device allows a new bag of dialysate to be attached to the catheter before the fluid in the abdomen is returned to the old bag. Once the new bag is firmly in place, the old fluid is drained; any bacteria that might have entered the catheter when the new bag was attached are flushed into the old bag with the fluid, which is then discarded. The Y-catheter reduces the potential for infection in CAPD patients.

The introduction of Epogen, a genetically engineered form of the hormone *erythropoietin,* marked another significant advance in dialysis treatment. Erythropoietin, responsible for the production of red blood cells, is normally produced by the kidneys.

Kidneys that have stopped functioning, however, no longer secrete it. As a result, patients with ESRF frequently develop anemia. Until Epogen was created, the supply of natural erythropoietin was limited, and dialysis patients had to cope with the side effects of anemia as well as the effects of dialysis.

### Living with Dialysis

Once an individual is diagnosed with ESRF and begins receiving dialysis, the treatment may continue indefinitely or until a donor kidney becomes available for transplant (see sidebar). However, the average patient lives for only three years after beginning dialysis, according to the Health Care Financing Administration. The average life span is longer for patients who start dialysis at a young age

(the average age is 56); the life span is also greater for dialysis patients in Germany, France, and Japan, for reasons that are not understood. However, several explanatory theories have been proposed recently. For example, in the United States, the length of each dialysis treatment is shorter than in Europe and Japan. New research indicates that such short treatment times may increase the mortality rate of dialysis patients. A 1991 study by Philip Held of the Renal Research Program of the Urban Institute, Washington, D.C., analyzed data for 600 patients who underwent hemodialysis in the United States from 1984 to 1988. The study concluded that patients who received treatments lasting less than 3.5 hours were twice as likely to die as were patients who underwent longer dialysis

## Kidney Transplants

For many patients, dialysis is a temporary treatment while they wait to receive a new kidney. "There is no question that dialysis, as good as it is, is not nearly as good as a human kidney," says Aaron Spital, M.D., a kidney specialist at the University of Rochester in New York. But not everyone who relies on dialysis is a good candidate for this relatively simple operation. Elderly patients and individuals at high risk for surgery, for example, are considered unsuitable for transplant operations.

Once a doctor clears a dialysis patient for a transplant, there is still no guarantee that a new kidney will be available—at least not right away. The candidate's blood and tissue types must first be determined. The patient's name and blood and tissue types are then added to a national computer registry of waiting patients and available organs. This list is maintained by the United Network for Organ Sharing (UNOS) in Richmond, Virginia. As organs become available, UNOS matches them with candidates, based on blood and tissue types, the length of time patients have been waiting for a transplant, and medical urgency.

The number of kidneys needed far exceeds the number available. For example, in 1991 more than 20,000 Americans waited for a kidney transplant, but only 10,000 received a new organ that year. Organs donated by relatives are best (blood and tissue types are more likely to match), but they represent a very limited source. In 1991 only 2,300 people received kidneys from relatives. The greatest single supply of donor kidneys comes from victims of untimely death. Over 7,500 "cadaver" kidneys, as they are called, were transplanted in 1991.

Fortunately for kidney recipients, the chance for survival is high. Of the nearly 10,000 kidneys transplanted in the United States each year, 80 percent are still functioning a year later. One reason for this high success rate is the use of drugs such as cyclosporine that suppress the body's antitransplant immune response. If a patient's body rejects the transplanted kidney, however, he or she can return to dialysis—and begin waiting for a new kidney. In general, there is no reason why a kidney patient cannot receive another transplant if the first one fails.

## A Brief History of Dialysis

Hemodialysis was developed in the mid-1880s by Scottish chemist Thomas Graham. Using the basic principle of osmosis, he used a semipermeable membrane and a neutral fluid to filter the blood of a sick patient.

Hemodialysis was first performed in the U.S. in 1913 on animals. Although the process worked in principle, the blood tended to clot, or coagulate, as it passed to and from the body. This remained a problem until heparin, the first anticoagulant, was introduced in 1926.

The first hemodialysis machine was developed in the 1940s by Willem Kolff, a Dutch physician. Designed for use in patients with acute renal failure, Kolff's machine filtered impurities from the blood using a coiled semipermeable membrane. Hemodialysis machines as they exist today were developed in the 1960s, when pumps were added to help move the blood in and out of the machine. At the same time, rubber tubing was replaced by the more sanitary plastic tubing.

As early as the 1920s, physicians were aware that the body's own peritoneal membrane could be used for dialysis. The high rate of infection that accompanied peritoneal dialysis was too great, however, for it to be considered a viable treatment. The introduction of disposable polyvinyl chloride (PVC) tubing, prepackaged dialysis solutions, and an automatic peritoneal-dialysis cycling machine in the 1950s and 1960s finally reduced the risk of contamination by bacteria, and the use of peritoneal dialysis became more widespread. In 1968 catheters that could be permanently implanted in the abdomen were developed. The mid-1970s heralded the introduction of CAPD.

---

treatments. According to Held, treatment times have steadily declined from an average of six hours to three hours. Experts attribute the decrease, in part, to cost cutting by Medicare, which reimburses dialysis providers for the treatments they administer. Between 1983 and 1990, the average Medicare payment was reduced by 44 percent; treatment times at reimbursed centers declined proportionately.

The reuse of hemodialysis machine parts also appears to negatively affect mortality rates of dialysis patients. This practice is much more common in the United States than in other industrialized countries. Two 1992 studies, one by the Urban Institute and the other by the National Institutes of Health (NIH), revealed a higher death rate among patients whose dialysis machines were disinfected with germicides between treatments. The studies did not, however, identify whether the problem was with the germicides or with the way the germicides were used. Nor did the studies determine if the reuse of dialysis machines was unsafe.

Diets low in phosphorus, potassium, and sodium are very important. Fluids are allowed only in decreased quantities to reduce swelling and high blood pressure.

### Psychology of Dialysis

Moral support from family and friends appears to be critical in helping dialysis patients adjust to dietary and lifestyle restrictions. It also helps these individuals move through the three phases of adjustment associated with dialysis. During the *honeymoon* phase, the patient experiences a measurable physical and emotional improvement as the dialysis begins to remove the accumulated toxins from the blood. When the second phase of adjustment begins—*disenchantment and discouragement*—the initial euphoria of feeling better has faded, and the frustration of the inescapable routine of dialysis has set in. This phase may last from a few months to a year. Eventually the patient moves into the third and final phase, called *long-term adaptation*, in which the dependence on dialysis is accepted and coped with as well as possible. ◇

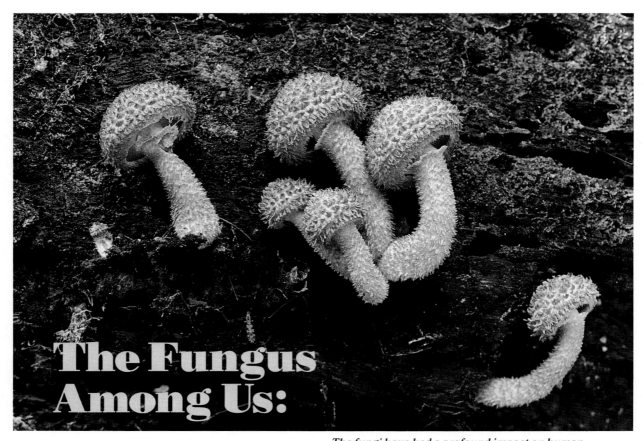

# The Fungus Among Us:

## friend or foe?

The fungi have had a profound impact on humanity, from the great potato famine in Ireland to the lifesaving penicillin antibiotics to the edible mushrooms, such as those from the species Pholiota *above, that have graced many menus.*

*by James A. Blackman, M.D.*

W hat grows on the bottom of feet, is added to spaghetti sauce, and can cure pneumonia? The answer: fungus (the plural is *fungi*), one of the simplest and yet most interesting forms of life. Some fungi cause disease (athlete's foot); one type produces penicillin, a lifesaving antibiotic; and other varieties are considered delicacies (shiitake mushrooms).

The majority of fungi are molds composed of a network of threadlike branches (hyphae) that form a fluffy, colorful growth visible to the naked eye. Yeasts (which make bread dough rise and promote fermentation of grape juice) are microscopic, single-celled fungi. Some fungi, such as mushrooms, produce large, aggregated structures that sprout from moist soil or decaying tree

stumps. Most animals instinctively know which fungi are edible and which are deadly, but humans have to learn from experts which are safe to eat.

### What Are Fungi?
Fungi, of which there are more than 300,000 species, are simple, nongreen organisms. Unlike plants, fungi have no leaves, roots, or stems. Instead, they are composed of masses of filaments. A fungal filament is called a *hypha,* and all the hyphae of a single organism are called collectively a *mycelium.* Since they contain no chlorophyll (the green pigment that plants use to convert light energy into chemical energy and store it until needed), fungi depend on other organisms for sustenance, feeding on dead plant or animal

material. In this way, they play a key role in the natural process of decay. A few types of fungi function as parasites on a variety of living organisms.

In the evolutionary scheme, fungi have done well. While humans are at the top of the evolutionary ladder, and fungi near the bottom, they definitely have what it takes to survive. Retired University of Minnesota fungus expert Clyde Christensen, Ph.D., put this into a poignant and slightly unnerving perspective: "Molds were on the scene and doing well long before man appeared, and many of them are pretty certain to be around in the remote future, long after man has played his part and groped his way into the dark wings or fallen through the trapdoor on the stage."

### The Good Fungi

For most people, the word "fungus" evokes ugly, smelly, or deadly images: black mold along the tiles of the shower, mildew in a pile of damp clothes, or the highly poisonous amanita toadstools in the backyard. Some fungi are good, some bad, others ugly. Yet fungi are essential to the survival of our ecosystem, and they produce lifesaving drugs.

Fungi, along with bacteria, are nature's recyclers. Without them, life on Earth would be impossible. Because fungi cannot produce their own food, they must extract proteins, carbohydrates, and other nutrients from the animals, plants, or decaying matter on which they live. Fungi discharge chemicals called enzymes into the material on which they feed. The enzymes break down complex carbohydrates and proteins into simple compounds that the fungal hyphae can absorb. As a result of this process, decaying matter is converted into rich soil. Without fungi, most green plants could not survive, since they depend upon the products of fungus decay in the soil. Without green plants, there would be no life on Earth, since green plants are the only living things able to use the energy from the Sun to manufacture products on which all other life depends.

### Fungi as Factories

Quite by accident, scientists found that fungi manufacture chemicals that are of consider-able importance to human health (see the sidebar about Scottish bacteriologist Alexander Fleming and the discovery of penicillin on page 34).

The success of penicillin touched off one of the biggest searches in the history of medicine. Scientists continue to examine fungi and bacteria in the hope of discovering other important medicinal chemicals. Today penicillin and its improved relatives remain a mainstay in antibiotic therapy. Furthermore, other antibiotics such as cephalosporin and griseofulvin (an antifungal medication) are harvested from fungi.

*Fungi are survivors— they will still be around long after humanity is gone.*

In 1970 Jean Borel, a scientist in Basel, Switzerland, isolated a new fungus from soil samples obtained in Wisconsin and Norway. He found that the fungus synthesizes cyclosporine, a potent suppressor of the body's immune system. Cyclosporine revolutionized human organ transplantation by preventing a recipient's body from rejecting transplanted tissue (such as kidney or heart) from donors.

*Penicillin was initially obtained from a strain of* Penicillium notatum, *but most commercial penicillins today are produced from high-yielding strains of* P. chrysogenum *in aerated tanks.*

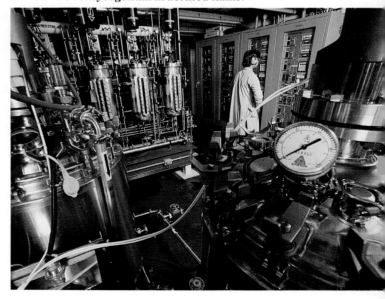

## The Bad Fungi

Despite improved methods of food production, transportation, and storage, molds still infect our grain crops, grow in our refrigerators, turn our bread green, and make tomatoes fuzzy. There are dozens, perhaps hundreds, of species of mold that can affect our food. Most of them are not harmful. As a matter of fact, some are used to enhance the flavor of such foods as Roquefort cheese or Auslese wine.

The riskiest molds are those that produce toxic substances called *mycotoxins*. They do not grow in our refrigerators, but in the fields and storage bins—on peanuts, corn, and other grains, particularly in times of excessive dampness.

Aflatoxins are a group of carcinogenic mycotoxins produced by the mold *Aspergillus flavus*. These mycotoxins have been found to cause liver damage and cancer in laboratory animals. They are believed to be responsible for a high incidence of liver cancer among people in tropic regions of Africa and Asia who may consume moldy grains, peanuts, or other *Aspergillus*-contaminated foods.

In 1987 thousands of people in India's Kashmir Valley suffered abdominal pain and other symptoms after eating bread made from moldy wheat. The outbreak was apparently caused by mycotoxins called trichothecenes.

A kidney disease known as Balkan endemic nephropathy, which primarily affects people

## The Discovery of Penicillin

In the early 1920s, two young scientists in the laboratories of the Pasteur Institute in Paris were studying *Staphylococcus aureus*, a germ responsible for boils and impetigo. One of the cultures became covered with a mold, and the surprised research workers discovered that the mold had killed the bacteria. They identified the mold as a member of the *Penicillium* genus, and wrote two short reports on their finding. Unfortunately, their discovery was overlooked, and both Andre Gratia and Sara Dath missed immortality by a hair.

The same fate nearly befell Sir Alexander Fleming, the second discoverer of penicillin, but the individual who is credited in history. In 1928 Fleming found that a *Penicillium* mold had accidentally con-

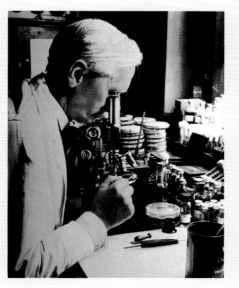

taminated a staphyloccocus culture and stopped the bacteria's growth. No one paid attention to Fleming's subsequent 1929 report either. Ten years later, however, Drs. Howard Florey and Ernst Chain at Oxford University ran across Fleming's old paper. They revived the research on penicillin, and had the chance to experiment on a 48-year-old London policeman who had nicked himself while shaving. After a few days, the policeman's face became swollen and red, and his temperature rose to 105° F. The first injections of penicillin into a human proved to be a

*Alexander Fleming accidentally discovered penicillin while examining a bacteria culture contaminated with mold.*

partial success. Within five days the man's temperature dropped, and he seemed to be recovering. Unfortunately, the doctors ran out of penicillin, and the patient died.

living in rural areas of Bulgaria, Romania, and Yugoslavia, has been linked with ochratoxin A, a mycotoxin that is known to contaminate beans, grains, and pork from pigs that eat tainted grain. People in these regions are 88 times more likely to develop kidney cancer than people living in areas where ochratoxin A is not common.

Fortunately, there have been no documented outbreaks of human poisoning or death from mycotoxins in the United States.

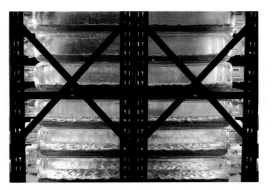

*In 1943 only 29 pounds of penicillin were produced. Improved methods for mass production made penicillin widely available virtually everywhere by 1945.*

However, the effects of low-level exposure to these chemicals over time are not known. A 1990 *Consumer Reports* analysis found higher levels of aflatoxin in fresh-ground peanut butters from supermarkets or health-food stores than in the prepackaged major brands. The analysis estimated that if,

The lack of availability of sufficient quantities of this new wonder drug dogged scientists for years. "You can get more gold out of ordinary seawater than penicillin out of mold" was an oft-quoted complaint of the period.

The Second World War, with its many casualties, created a tremendous need for the new wonder drug. However, availability of penicillin was limited until new methods for mass production were found. A researcher from the U.S. Department of Agriculture picked up a moldy cantaloupe in a Peoria,

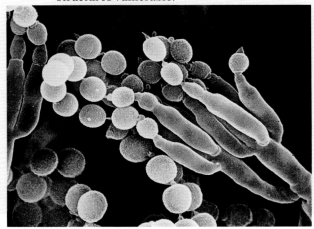

*Penicillin, derived from the mold* Penicillium *below, acts by interfering with the synthesis of a microorganism's cell wall, leaving the internal structures vulnerable.*

Illinois, market and found *Penicillium chrysogenum* on it, a mold that could produce about 200 times as much penicillin as the previous source. In 1943 only 29 pounds were produced; by the war's end, enough penicillin was available to treat 7 million patients. This was made possible by a new technique of growing the mold in huge tanks churned by paddles as large as a ship's propellers.

The impact of penicillin was truly impressive. Whereas, during World War I, the death rate from pneumonia in the U.S. Army totaled 18 percent, in World War II, it fell to less than 1 percent. In addition to pneumonia, blood poisoning, and strep throats, penicillin brought cures for such conditions as scarlet fever, diphtheria, syphilis, gonorrhea, meningitis, erysipelas, tonsillitis, mastoiditis, rheumatic fever, boils, and abscesses.

Some microorganisms have developed resistance to penicillins; a wide range of synthetic penicillins have been developed to counter this resistance, including oxacillin and methicillin.

Alexander Fleming, rescued from oblivion, was knighted in 1943, and two years later was awarded the Nobel Prize in Physiology or Medicine, as were Chain and Florey.

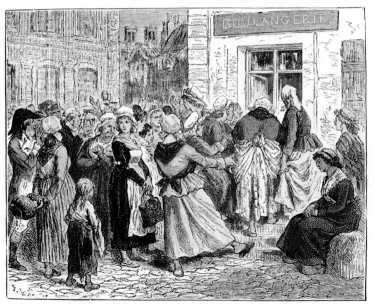

*The violent behavior of the mobs during the French Revolution may have been influenced more by hallucinations produced by fungus-infected bread than by anger over taxes.*

over a lifetime, you eat one peanut-butter sandwich every 10 days, the lifetime risk might be about seven cases of cancer per million consumers.

In some surveys, low levels of ochratoxin A have been found in as much as 3 percent of the wheat and 14 percent of the barley samples tested. Several European countries have set maximum legal limits for ochratoxin A; the United States and Canada have not. Trichothecenes, the culprit in the 1987 Kashmir outbreak referred to previously, occasionally turn up at low levels in breakfast cereals, breads, and baby foods.

### Fungi Madness

Ergot, derived from the fungus *Claviceps purpurea,* has been an important medical tool throughout the ages. Because it causes constriction of blood vessels, ergot was used for generations to control bleeding following childbirth, to speed labor, and even to induce abortion. Ergotism is a disease caused by eating rye infected with the fungus. One form of ergotism causes gangrene of the limbs; another form induces psychotic behavior. Ergot is a natural form of LSD, a mind-altering drug popular among counterculture groups in the 1960s. One historian attributes the rampages and mass looting in rural France in 1789 to the fungus-contaminated

rye bread that made up the bulk of peasants' diets. The accused "witches" of 17th-century Europe and New England may have been affected by ergotism. The disease is uncommon now in developed countries because of the carefully controlled conditions under which grains are processed and bread is baked.

According to Lloyd Bullerman, Ph.D., a University of Nebraska specialist in fungal contamination of food, interest has recently focused on a newly identified class of mycotoxins called fumonisins. These toxins, produced by the fungus *Fusarium moniliforme,* are thought to cause esophageal cancer. While fumonisins usually stay at low levels in contaminated grain, the process of fermenting moldy corn for beer enhances toxin production and therefore increases cancer risks.

### Fungal Parasites in Humans

Of the 300,000 species of existing fungi, only a few hundred cause disease (called mycoses) in humans, and usually only when the body's normal defense mechanisms are not working. The most common fungal infections (such as ringworm, athlete's foot, and jock itch) are caused by the 20 or so dermatophytes, which love to eat the hard, keratin-containing tissue of the skin, nails, and hair.

*The fungal infection tinea pedis causes the itchiness, soreness, and cracked, peeling skin more commonly known as athlete's foot.*

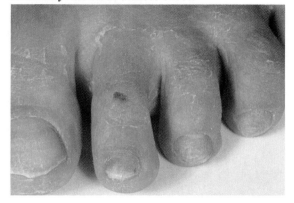

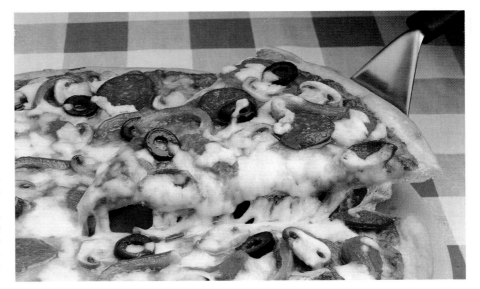

*Fungi greatly enhance pizza—yeast is used to make the pizza dough, the melted cheese was ripened and given its characteristic flavor by fungi, and the mushrooms on top add delicious flavor and texture.*

Most of these infections are easily recognized and treated with over-the-counter antifungal preparations.

A few types of fungi, such as commensal yeasts like *Candida albicans,* live happily on the surface of the skin or along the lining of the intestinal tract. They cause no harm as long as the balance between the host and the naturally occurring bacteria population is maintained. However, if the balance is upset, as by an antibiotic that kills off the normal bacteria, *Candida* can then cause infection of the mouth, skin, or vagina.

It is possible for fungi to invade and develop in the internal tissues of an otherwise healthy host. The principal infections in this group are histoplasmosis, blastomycosis, and coccidioidomycosis. These organisms are found in well-defined geographic regions such as the Southwest or the Ohio Valley. The majority of human infections are acquired by inhalation. Some fungi in the environment that ordinarily do not cause problems can create life-threatening disease in individuals who are immunocompromised, as from cancer treatment or AIDS.

### The Yeast Connection

So-called "clinical ecologists" have claimed that yeasts in the environment cause such widely varied symptoms as fatigue, irritability, muscle pain, short attention span, impotence, depression, and hyperactivity—just about everything that can ail you. To combat the growth of yeast in the body, antiyeast proponents recommend eliminating all sugar-containing foods from the diet, avoiding damp and moldy places, and using potent antifungal prescription drugs. The *Harvard Medical School Health Letter* has responded to these claims and recommendations by acknowledging that fungi can cause some allergic symptoms, such as nasal congestion and watery eyes. However, the *Health Letter* went on to state uncategorically that there is no more reason to think that yeasts are responsible for an epidemic of chronic disease in otherwise healthy people than there ever was to believe that "the Moon was made of green cheese."

## What to Do About Molds on Food

Nutritional-health experts give specific advice about avoiding mycotoxins:
• Molds just love bruises. Treat your produce gently.
• If hard or firm foods become moldy, cut out the mold and at least an inch of food around and under it.
• When a soft food develops mold (no matter how little), toss it out.
• Do not eat moldy or shriveled-up peanuts.
• Toss away the entire box of cornmeal when you see mold.

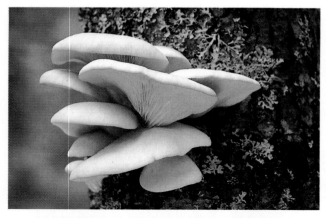

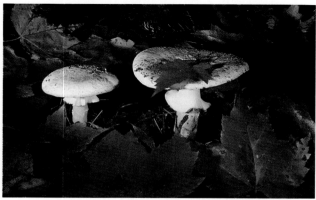

*Mushrooms are as varied in looks as they are in their effects on humankind. The oyster mushroom (Pleurotus ostreatus), top, is widely cultivated and makes excellent eating, while the poisonous Amanita virosa (above) can cause a painful, slow death if consumed. Turkey-tail fungi from the Polyporus family (below), on the other hand, are economically poisonous, causing wood rot on lumber.*

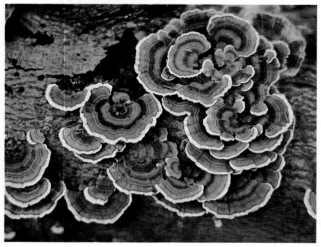

## The Ugly Fungi

Mushrooms are the most advanced groups of fungi and produce the largest fruiting bodies in the class Basidiomycetes. Although they contain some protein and minerals, mushrooms are composed largely of water and are of limited nutritional value. Mushroom poisoning is caused by the members of the *Amanita* genus. Especially dangerous are the "destroying angel" *(Amanita virosa)* and the "death cap" *(Amanita phalloides)*. The poisonous symptoms, often delayed for several hours after ingestion, consist of severe abdominal pain, vomiting, extreme nausea, diarrhea, salivation, sweating, excessive thirst, coma, and occasionally seizures. Extensive damage to the liver, kidneys, and central nervous system may also occur.

Members of the *Psilocybe* species of mushroom produce a hallucinogenic substance called psilocybin. For centuries, Mexican Indians have considered these mushrooms sacred and used them in their religious ceremonies. It was called *teonanácatl,* meaning "God's flesh," by the ancient Nahuatl Indians. Similar cults grew up around psilocybin and other psychedelic drugs in the U.S. during the 1960s under the leadership of Timothy Leary, then of Harvard University.

Of great interest among health-food aficionados is the *reishi,* a hard, wood-like mushroom used in the Orient for more than 1,000 years for its wonderful and extensive healing properties. Among countless other claims of its merits, *reishi* has been praised for lowering high blood pressure, strengthening the heart, combating insomnia, managing allergies and asthma, and even preventing and treating cancer.

There is reason to believe that many mushrooms have beneficial effects on health, although much more research is necessary to document the effects. According to Andrew Weil, M.D., author of *Natural Health Natural Medicine* (Houghton Mifflin, 1988), mushrooms may enhance cellular immunity, thereby increasing defenses against viral infections and cancer. Nevertheless, he cautions that many unsubstantiated claims are being made about mushroom products sold as dietary supplements, and, in some cases, these products are greatly overpriced.   ◇

# PROBLEMS "DOWN THERE"

*by Frank M. Szivos, Jr.*

John had lived with hemorrhoids for years. Embarrassed at having a condition afflict such an unmentionable area, John simply endured the occasional bleeding and transient pain in silence. When the discomfort grew intolerable, John relied on over-the-counter ointments and creams for temporary relief. A few times, John even considered consulting a doctor about his condition. But then, it always seemed, the hemorrhoids would calm down again, and John went about his life confident that nobody would learn his little secret. That is, until the company picnic.

That memorable afternoon, John and some associates were whizzing along in a golf cart toward the eighth hole. The hemorrhoids had been acting up a bit lately, John thought, but nothing out of the ordinary. Then, as John got out of the cart, he saw a truly alarming sight: blood smeared on the cart seat. The next sensation John felt was an odd dampness in his pants. He flushed, realizing that his white golf pants likely carried some bright-red stains.

John abruptly offered his apologies to his golfing partners and made a beeline for the clubhouse. From there, he called his doctor, who saw him right away. After a quick visual diagnosis, the doctor treated the hemorrhoids. One week later, John was back on the golf course. For the first time in years, he was experiencing

> *Experts say that at least half of all Americans will suffer from hemorrhoids at some time in their lives.*

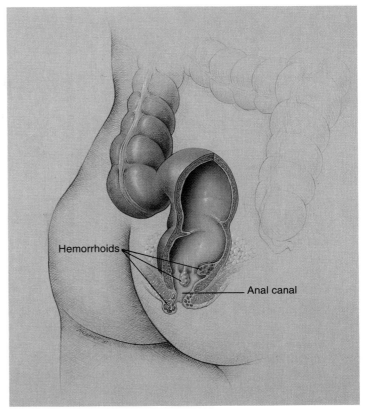

Hemorrhoids

Anal canal

*Hemorrhoids are cushions of tissue and veins that occur inside or outside the anal canal. When a hemorrhoid swells abnormally, it can cause pain, itching, burning, and bleeding.*

no pain "down there," nor did he worry about a sudden bout of bleeding. And before long, John threw out his considerable supply of special ointments and creams.

## A Common Problem

Like John, millions of Americans suffer hemorrhoids in silence. Hemorrhoids cause embarrassment. They prompt all sorts of crude jokes. But for the afflicted, hemorrhoids are no laughing matter. Hemorrhoids can cause considerable—and often acute—discomfort and pain. In severe cases, sitting can be nearly impossible. Sports are out of the question. And just the thought of a visit to the bathroom can take on a nightmarish quality.

It is understandable, of course, why most people resist discussing their hemorrhoids. What many sufferers don't understand, however, is just how common a condition hemorrhoids are: Fully one-half of all Americans older than 30 will suffer from hemorrhoids at one time or another. In fact, hemorrhoids are the most common problem of the anal canal.

## What Are Hemorrhoids?

Bluntly put, hemorrhoids are enlarged, bulging veins around the anus and lower rectum. Fortunately, hemorrhoids are rarely—if ever—life-threatening, and there is no relationship between hemorrhoids and cancer. Nonetheless, the incessant itching and pain can drive some people to distraction. All hemorrhoids are classified as either external or internal. All originally develop internally, but some swell below the dentate line (where the rectum and anus meet). They are considered external if they protrude permanently. People often have both internal and external hemorrhoids at the same time.

External hemorrhoids develop near the anus and are covered with highly sensitive skin that makes them the more painful of the two varieties. External hemorrhoids protrude and feel like hard, sensitive lumps. If they are small, they can go undetected; they become troublesome when they grow big enough to stretch the membrane of the vein

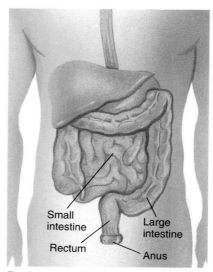

*During normal elimination, internal hemorrhoids help stool pass gently from the anal canal.*

Small intestine
Large intestine
Rectum
Anus

wall. As the hemorrhoids swell, the membrane becomes thinner and begins to bleed, especially when in contact with feces.

Sometimes an external hemorrhoid swells still further because a blood clot forms within it. The clot, or thrombosis, is extremely painful, although thankfully easy enough to treat. In a routine in-office procedure with only local anesthesia, a surgeon can lance the thrombosis and drain it. Relief is rapid.

Internal hemorrhoids develop within the anus beneath the lining of the rectum, an area that contains no pain-conducting tissue. During a bowel movement, painless bleeding can occur, especially if the hemorrhoid is forced to protrude externally during the activity. Fortunately, the hemorrhoid usually slips back inside the anal opening. In some cases the hemorrhoid can be manually returned to its "normal" position. Other times, however, the hemorrhoid becomes prolapsed—it protrudes from the opening and cannot be pushed back inside.

## Symptoms

Hemorrhoids have several common symptoms. Most of these symptoms can also arise from other, more-serious conditions. It is therefore advisable to be checked as soon as possible should any of the following symptoms arise:
• Itching or pain in the anal area.
• Sensitive lumps in the same region.
• The presence of blood on stools, on toilet paper, or in the toilet bowl after a bowel movement.
• The protrusion of a lumplike mass during or after a bowel movement.
  The American Society of Colon and Rectal Surgeons (ASCRS) urges anyone who experiences bleeding or pain in the anus or rectum to see a physician immediately. Simply because there's no correlation between cancer

*Though painless, an internal hemorrhoid may bleed. Sometimes a hemorrhoid protrudes, or prolapses, from the anus. A blood clot within a prolapsed hemorrhoid can cause much pain.*

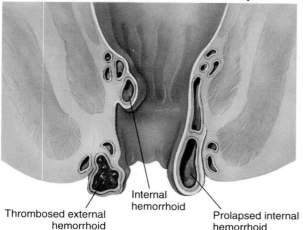

Thrombosed external hemorrhoid
Internal hemorrhoid
Prolapsed internal hemorrhoid

and hemorrhoids does *not* mean that cancer and hemorrhoids cannot co-exist. As Steven Hirshorn, M.D., a colon and rectal surgeon in Bridge-port, Connecticut, notes, "Thirty to 40 percent of my patients who come in the door thinking they have hemorrhoids *don't!*" Dr. Hirshorn adds that "Anal bleeding can indi-cate hundreds of condi-tions of the colon or rectum." Some of these conditions can be extremely serious.

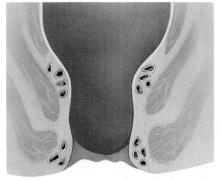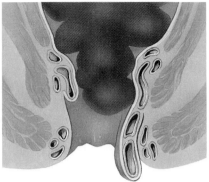

*Fiber-rich food forms soft stool which passes easily from the body (left). Without enough fiber, the stool becomes harder. The straining needed to eliminate such stool can cause hemorrhoids (right).*

## Causes

The exact cause of hemorrhoids is unknown, but doctors know that pressure plays a criti-cal role. In part, hemorrhoids could be the price humans must pay for standing upright and walking on two feet. Upright posture puts a great deal of pressure on the rectal veins, which can cause them to bulge. Since everyone has hemorrhoidal veins (there are three), anyone can develop the condition, says Albert Knapp, M.D., a clinical instructor in the department of medicine at New York Medical College in Valhalla, New York. "We all have hemorrhoidal veins, and when they get larger than normal, they're prone to clot-ting," Dr. Knapp says. "When that happens,

we call it hemorrhoids. When they block com-pletely, they can hurt badly." But the pres-sure, which can bring on hemorrhoids usually comes from one or a combination of the following causes:

• Aging. Years of pressure can force veins to protrude and swell.

• Chronic constipation or diarrhea. Both of these conditions can cause straining during bowel movements, which irritates swollen veins. Doctors say it's a fallacy that constipa-tion is a direct cause. When it occurs, consti-pation sets up the condition for hemorrhoids to develop.

• Pregnancy. Carrying a fetus applies tre-mendous force on the rectal veins.

• Heredity. It's unclear how much heredity plays a role, but hemorrhoids tend to run in families. Of course, everyone can develop hemorrhoids since we all have anal veins.

• Weakened bowel function due to an over-use of laxatives. This represents something of a Catch-22 syndrome. If you use laxatives, you're probably constipated, and if you're constipated, you likely strain during bowel movements.

• Excessive straining during a bowel move-ment. Forcing out stool applies intense pres-sure that can irritate hemorrhoids or cause them to prolapse.

• Spending long periods of time on the toilet. Sitting on the toilet, often while reading, puts sustained pressure on the anus area.

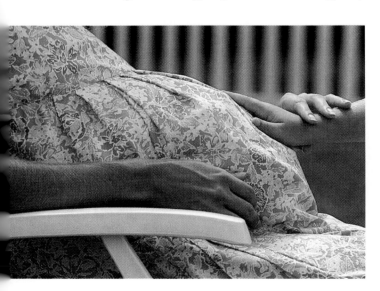

*The weight of a fetus exerts much pressure on the mother's rectal veins, a condition which makes pregnant women particularly prone to hemorrhoids.*

## Prevention

Since you can bring on hemorrhoids with such lifestyle habits as poor diet and irregular bowel routine, you can also prevent them by taking the proper precautions. Doctors recommend the following steps to avoid hemorrhoids:

• Add more fiber and roughage to your diet. Eat plenty of fruits and vegetables, and reduce your intake of high-fat and processed foods. Most doctors suggest a diet composed of 70 to 80 percent complex carbohydrates (fruits, vegetables, and breads) and about 20 percent fat. Foods high in fiber give the intestines the bulk and roughage needed to form softer stools, which are easier to pass without strain through the anal canal.

• Drink plenty of water, at least six to eight glasses a day, to soften stools and facilitate regular bowel movements.

• Develop better bowel habits. You should have a bowel movement at about the same time every day, and, if possible, you should try to set time aside for it. By establishing this pattern, the body will be ready to evacuate regularly, thus eliminating the straining that aggravates hemorrhoids. Listen to your body, which will signal you with a natural urge to defecate.

• Do not spend prolonged periods of time sitting on the toilet. This puts tremendous pressure on the anal region, and can irritate existing hemorrhoids or set up the conditions for developing new ones. While it may help pass the time, reading in the bathroom distracts you from the reason you're there in the first place, and serves only to extend the amount of time you spend on the toilet. Reserve your reading for a comfortable chair.

• Exercise on a regular basis. Good muscle tone promotes normal defecation. Many doctors agree that people with good muscle tone are less prone to hemorrhoids. Exercise, such as walking, will build up the abdominal, gluteal, and sphincter muscles used during defecation. Exercise also has the indirect benefit of encouraging you to drink more water.

• Be informed. People who know more about hemorrhoids tend to change their lifestyles to avoid the condition or to have existing hemorrhoids treated to avoid unnecessary pain and stress.

## Related Problems "Down There"

In addition to hemorrhoids, people can develop a whole range of other distressing and painful problems in the anal-rectal area. Among the more common problems are anal fissures—cracks or tears in the skin around the anal opening or in the canal. Unlike hemorrhoids, fissures can cause pains that come during defecation, or darting pains between bowel movements. The fissures normally require surgery to repair. Tenderness or aching, particularly around the anal opening, is another common condition that may indicate an abscess formation or a fistula—a kind of tunnel leading out of the anal canal that may harbor infections.

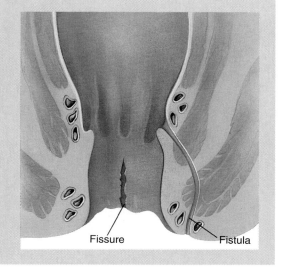

Fissure          Fistula

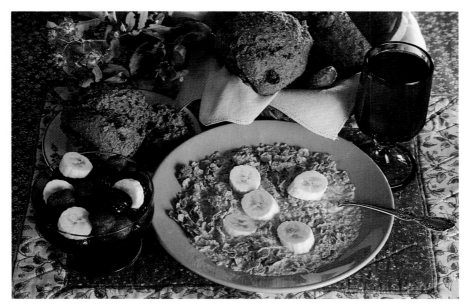

*A diet rich in fruit and fiber helps keep stool soft, lessening the need to strain in the bathroom, and thus reducing the likelihood of developing hemorrhoids. For people suffering with hemorrhoids, a bath several times a day can help alleviate the discomfort.*

## Treatments

Most hemorrhoids respond to medical treatment and never require surgery, according to Daniel Passeri, M.D., a surgeon at St. Vincent's Medical Center in Bridgeport, Connecticut.

"We treat most hemorrhoids medically," Passeri says. Doctors first recommend the taking of sitz baths several times daily. A sitz bath involves sitting in a tub filled with plain lukewarm water for about 15 minutes at a time. Doing this several times per day will usually bring some relief. Don't add to the bathwater anything that could cause irritation —such as bath oil, soap, Epsom salts, or bubble bath.

Another common treatment involves increasing the intake of fiber in the diet. Doctors lay some of the blame for hemorrhoids on the typical American diet, which is generally low in fiber. Natural high-fiber powders soften the stool by causing it to absorb more water, helping to minimize the need to strain during bowel movements. However, doctors warn against confusing fiber powders with laxatives, which work differently and can irritate hemorrhoids.

Lubricating the anal canal can also reduce friction. Over-the-counter creams and ointments are popular, but self-applied petroleum jelly works just as well and it's cheaper. Despite the claim of some manufacturers, no cream can make hemorrhoids disappear. Some companies add anesthetic agents, which bring "temporary relief," although

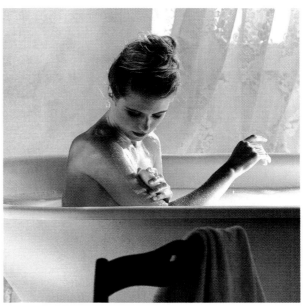

such products carry the risk of allergic reactions. Although less convenient, a hot sitz bath can bring just as much relief.

Unfortunately, some patients prefer to use creams instead of seeing a doctor. Occasionally these products offer some relief for milder cases. The more popular ones (Preparation H and Anusol) contain hydrocortisone, which actually helps shrink some hemorrhoids. Other creams contain astringents (belladonna, zinc compounds, tannic acid, or bismuth), supposedly to reduce the swelling by shrinking capillaries; any relief is temporary at best.

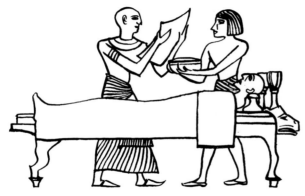

## Surgical Solutions

When the simpler treatments don't work, doctors have several options for treating hemorrhoids, most of which can be performed in the office. Improvements in medical technology and anesthesia have simplified procedures and shortened recovery time. "Treatments have not changed dramatically," says Samuel Labow, M.D., President of the American Society of Colon and Rectal Surgeons. "We have fancier ways of doing things, but we do the same thing. We either cook them, freeze them, or use [lasers]."

Ligation has given doctors an alternative to surgery. It involves stretching a minute rubber band over the hemorrhoid to choke off the protruding part, which eventually shrinks and falls off. This treatment dates back to Hippocrates, the ancient Greek physician, who used to tie thread around hemorrhoids to shrink them. Over the past two decades, ligation has become one of the most common medical treatments for hemorrhoids.

Doctors perform this procedure in the office without anesthesia. The patient feels only a slight pinch (when the rubber band is applied) and may experience some slight bleeding. With ligation the hemorrhoid and rubber band normally fall off within a few days, and the wound heals in a week or two. However, about 10 percent of patients who undergo ligation therapy develop hemorrhoids again.

Injection therapy involves injecting an internal hemorrhoid with solutions that cause scarring and shrinking of the hemorrhoid. This in-office treatment is ideal for patients who are bleeding heavily and may be in danger of anemia. Patients with coagulation (blood-clotting) problems or who are taking anticoagulants are also well suited for injection therapy, Dr. Labow says. There is a high recurrence rate with this procedure.

Surgery (hemorrhoidectomy) is still the best way to permanently remove hemorrhoids. Doctors choose the surgical option when clots repeatedly form in external hemorrhoids, ligation fails on an internal vein, the protruding hemorrhoid cannot be reduced, or when there is persistent bleeding. In a standard hemorrhoidectomy, the patient is placed under general anesthesia while the surgeon removes tissue that causes the bleeding and protrusion. Typically the procedure requires hospitalization for five to seven days, and home rest for up to 10 more days. Patients usually are prescribed painkillers for the first few days after the surgery; an anal pad may be necessary to absorb drainage.

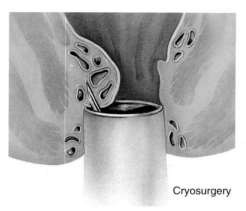

Cryosurgery

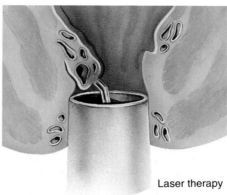

Laser therapy

*Doctors sometimes treat a hemorrhoid by freezing it with liquid nitrogen (far left); the hemorrhoid then falls off within a week or two. In laser therapy (near left), a laser beam treats the swollen tissue.*

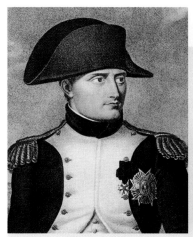
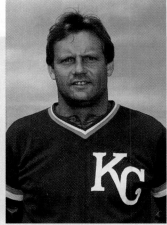
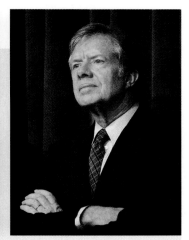

## Hemorrhoids Through History

Hemorrhoids are by no means a phenomenon of modern society. The ancient Egyptians suffered from them, and even developed a special ointment to treat them. The term "hemorrhoid" arose from the ancient Greek term meaning "blood flow." Way back then, classical Greek physicians were binding hemorrhoids with thread to choke them. In more recent times, Napoleon reportedly couldn't sit on his horse during the Battle of Waterloo thanks to an acute case of hemorrhoids.

When Jimmy Carter's hemorrhoids flared up during the 1978 holiday season, the president received a heartfelt letter from an Egyptian that read: "This illness should have been inflicted on an unjust leader rather than you, O Carter." In 1985 third baseman George Brett had an untimely siege of hemorrhoids—just as his team, the Kansas City Royals, made it to the World Series. Brett was forced to miss two games for surgery, but he went on to play eight more seasons.

Laser instruments are also used to remove hemorrhoids, although they don't offer any distinct advantage over standard surgical techniques, according to the ASCRS. Laser surgery on hemorrhoids is usually performed on an outpatient basis, however, and therefore requires no hospitalization. The laser emits high-frequency light waves that the tissue absorbs as heat. In turn the heat coagulates the hemorrhoid into a shrunken stubble about the size of a peanut. Patients can resume their normal routine in about a week.

In another method of treatment—cryotherapy—a probe cooled by liquid nitrogen to $-132°$ F is used to freeze the tissue. The hemorrhoid sloughs off in a few days, an event followed by several weeks of malodorous discharge. This type of treatment was more popular 10 years ago than it is now.

Electric current represents still another means of treating hemorrhoids. Just as in laser surgery, a doctor uses a probe to burn off the end of the hemorrhoid. Instead of light, however, electrical current coagulates the problem vein. Doctors perform this painless office procedure on internal hemorrhoids. (The ASCRS does not recommend this method for external hemorrhoids, since it would be very painful.) Being a relatively new method, it is still too early to determine the full effectiveness of electric currents in treating hemorrhoids.

The pain and embarrassment of hemorrhoids are invariably far worse than any of the treatment options. "We often have to depend on word of mouth for people to come in to get their hemorrhoids checked," Dr. Labow says. "If they hear one bad story, then they're usually scared to death. We need more-positive role models. There's so much pain and suffering with hemorrhoids that's just not necessary." ◇

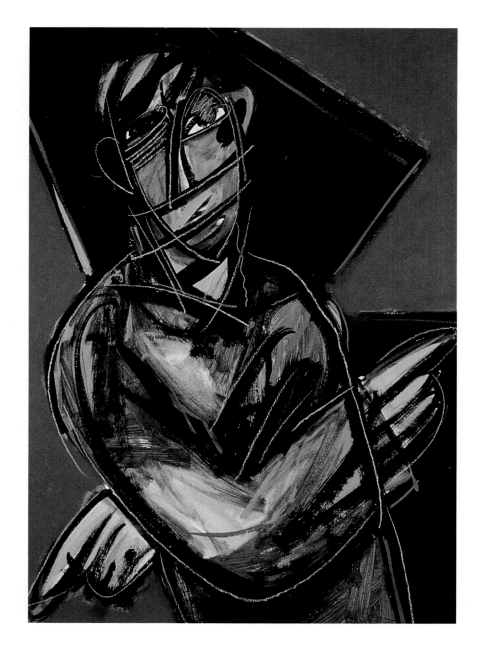

# TOURETTE SYNDROME

*by Janet C. Tate*

Maybe you once passed someone on the street who was muttering to herself, growling nonsensical sounds or obscenities, or perhaps even barking, and twitching involuntarily. Or maybe you remember a kid from school who not only could not sit still, but could not seem to keep from snorting and clearing his throat, blinking, or constantly jerking his head and shoulders. And maybe (like most of us probably would) you stared, scratched your head, and wondered: Is he crazy? Why doesn't he stop?

That is how Bruce Ochsman says he would react if he weren't aware that the woman on the street and the kid in the classroom probably have a complex neurological condition known as Tourette syndrome (TS), a disorder that afflicts 200,000 Americans and many more worldwide. And he would know, because he has it, too.

"You know that what you are doing seems very strange," says Ochsman, 36, a senior vice president for an investment firm in Washington, D.C. "I don't fault anybody for staring at me; it's just natural curiosity. I would stare, too."

### What Is It?
First formally described in 1825, and later named for Georges Gilles de la Tourette, the French physician who identified the condition, Tourette syndrome is a genetic disorder, and, "as with all genetic disorders, it leads to something not working right in the human body," says Gerald Erenberg, M.D., a pediatric neurologist and director of the Learning Assessment Clinic at the Cleveland Clinic Foundation in Cleveland, Ohio. In the case of TS, the patient experiences both physical and verbal tics—sudden, repeated, involuntary movements. "My Tourette's means I am moving constantly without wanting to," says Ochsman. "It means never being still, never being able to sit and relax and be calm."

Erenberg explains that the tics are most likely the result of a faulty monitoring mechanism within the brain. "We suspect that it is caused by a chemical imbalance involving the neurotransmitter dopamine, which helps code messages from one brain cell to the other," he says. "The theory is that an excess of dopamine leads to the inability of the nervous system to correctly inhibit certain processes. It may be that all of us would have ongoing muscle twitches and utterances if they were not filtered out by normal balance mechanisms."

Genetic studies show that TS is inherited as a dominant gene that causes a range of symptoms. A parent has about a 50 percent chance of passing on the genetic predisposition for TS to each of his or her children. The chances of a TS patient's offspring experiencing the disorder's symptoms are three to four times higher for a son than for a daughter.

(More males have TS than do females.) A TS carrier may pass a gene on to his or her offspring for a variation of the tic disorder. "For instance, I may have severe TS and have three kids, and one of them has TS, but in a barely noticeable form. Or I may have a barely noticeable form, but pass the gene on to a child who has it in a much more severe form than I do. Why that happens is unknown," says Erenberg.

The involuntary tics associated with TS can affect virtually any part of the body or any type of sounds, and no two TS patients will exhibit the same patterns or types of tics. Probably the most socially distressing vocal tic is *coprolalia,* or the uttering of obscenities —a vocal tic that, despite popular perception, occurs only in about 15 percent of TS cases. (Other common TS vocalizations are *palilalia,* which is repeating one's own words; *echolalia,* which is repeating the last sound heard; and sniffing, coughing, throat clearing, and barking.)

For up to 40 percent of TS patients, the tics are often preceded by a feeling of irritation, tickling, or a change in body temperature. An attempt by the TS patient to suppress the tics can create inner emotional tension, frequently described by TS patients as feeling like "a volcano about to erupt"—a tension that's momentarily released when the tic occurs.

"Many patients who have physical tics will say that the tic itself is preceded by a sensation of discomfort," notes Erenberg. "So with a head movement, for example, they actually get a sense of pressure building up in the neck muscles, which will then suddenly lead to the jerking of the head. This may even offer a moment of relief, but no more than a moment, and then the pressure and the tic return."

A TS patient's resulting emotional turmoil of anxiety, anger, stress, and fatigue can further exacerbate the tics. And as with any overuse of a muscle, the tics themselves can cause pain for the TS patient.

*A neurological disorder, Tourette syndrome afflicts some 200,000 Americans.*

## Diagnosis

The symptoms of Tourette syndrome show up first in childhood, usually between the ages of 5 and 11. "Mine started when I was 11," Ochsman recalls, "with snorting, exhaling hard, and, gradually, muscle tics and twitches. All the physicians kept telling me there was nothing wrong with me." Ochsman was finally diagnosed at age 19 by the psychiatrist who continues to treat him today. "Once I was diagnosed, it was wonderful," he says. "Just the fact that I finally had a name for it and no one could tell me that it was my fault anymore was a tremendous relief."

And indeed, it's not unusual for many years to elapse before TS patients know for sure what's wrong with them. Medical practitioners often miss the diagnosis for several reasons. For one thing, medical doctors may have a tendency to attribute the bizarre behavior associated with TS to psychological problems, and send the child or young adult on to a therapist. Even for more-astute observers, the misconception that coprolalia must be present to make a diagnosis of TS leads many to believe that its absence indicates the absence of the disorder.

Most important, TS has a very specific diagnosis; in order to pinpoint it, the patient's symptoms must be observed first-hand. This display doesn't always occur in the examining room; sometimes clinicians have to rely upon videotaped episodes. In fact, the Tourette Syndrome Association reports that up to 85 percent of correctly diagnosed TS cases are determined, not by doctors, but by perceptive family members or friends.

Here are clues an alert doctor looks for when diagnosing Tourette syndrome:
• Symptoms first develop before age 21.
• Symptoms have persisted for at least one year.
• A variety of involuntary physical tics are present.
• At least one vocal tic is expressed.
• The symptoms come and go.
• New symptoms gradually replace old ones.
• There is no other medical reason to explain the tics.

Tourette syndrome is what is known as a spectrum disorder—that is, its symptoms can occur in a variety of degrees. Each individual will also have a "waxing and waning" pattern: times when the tics are particularly severe, and times when they are not as prevalent. Particularly for children, the form of the tic is very changeable: "Your problem in March might be that you are blinking too much, but your problem in April may be that you are clearing your throat excessively," says Erenberg. For adults, any existing tic pattern will stabilize and probably become more consistent, although the severity of symptoms can still increase and decrease.

Another problem with identifying TS is that, especially in childhood, its symptoms are sometimes attributed to other conditions. For example, because eye blinking and other ocular movements are common among young people with TS, they are often sent first for an eye exam. Parents, teachers, and doctors may conclude that the restlessness, distractibility, and inability to control impulsive or compulsive behavior indicate attention-deficit hyperactivity disorder (ADHD) or learning disabilities.

While TS is not a disorder of the intellect or a direct cause of academic insufficiency, ADHD and learning disabilities are indeed frequent components of TS in children. "Among children who have tics, 65 percent will have ADHD problems as well," says Erenberg. "That complicates their social adjustment and potentially compromises their school performance." Thirty-five to 40 percent of TS children will have learning disabilities, and about the same number will suffer social difficulties because of their tics—an experience Ochsman still remembers vividly.

"My disorder created no academic problems," he says. "In fact, I did very well in school, probably because I was a loner and I like to read, because when I read, my tics go away. [Indeed, concentration on a demanding task, such as study or sports, alleviates the urge to tic in many TS patients.] But socially, it was just awful. I was stared at, joked about, made fun of, not invited places. I felt very uncomfortable in any kind of social situation because I was doing these strange things that everybody told me was my fault. I became a major-time loner."

It is not unusual for others to disbelieve that a TS patient's symptoms are truly involuntary. "The doctors kept telling my parents that I could stop it," says Ochsman. "They also told my parents I was psychologically damaged since I was the youngest of five kids, and I probably was not getting enough attention." Fortunately, experts find that 30 percent of the children who actually have TS will see a significant decrease in their symptoms by the time they are teenagers; another 30 to 40 percent will outgrow them altogether. The remaining affected individuals will carry their symptomology on into adulthood. There are several related disorders that can occur for some people. One of the most common is obsessive-compulsive behavior, in which the individual feels compelled to perform the same task or behavior over and over again, such as checking repeatedly to make sure doors are locked.

### Treatment

Tourette syndrome is not life-threatening, but there's no cure for it either. The majority of TS patients do not suffer from constant, severe tics. In fact, most cases are fairly mild and require no medication at all. But for TS patients whose symptoms are severe enough to interfere with their lives, treatments may include medications commonly used to treat obsessive-compulsive behaviors, such as clomipramine or pimozide. Doctors may also prescribe haloperidol, clonidine, fluphenazine, or clonazepam. Medications used for hyperactivity may actually increase the tics, so their use is controversial. For TS children with attention-deficit problems, doctors may sometimes instead suggest the use of tricyclic antidepressants. Because their symptoms tend to be worse, children with TS are medicated more often than are adults.

*Medication can help most—but by no means all —people who suffer from TS.*

As with other drugs, those prescribed for TS may have side effects. It is estimated that about half of the patients who use these medications experience varying degrees of side effects, which may include fatigue, weight gain, headache, insomnia, dizziness, photosensitivity, and dry mouth.

In any event, getting the right drugs in the right combinations at the right dosages with minimum interference from side effects can be a time-consuming, trial-and-error undertaking. Ochsman says he has been working on the right mix for more than a year. "On a scale of 1 to 10, my tics are like an 8," says Ochsman, who has tried various regimens with haloperidol, pimozide, and the antidepressant Prozac. "Since I have been on medication, they are more like a 2. I have had some weight gain, some lethargy, but this is the first time in 15 years I have not been moving every five seconds. I have not exactly got it down yet, but I am working on it."

It was once thought that the symptoms of TS lasted a lifetime. Now, though, case studies show that a minority of people experience significant improvement, and for a very few, even spontaneous remission, often without the benefit of any medication.

### Psychological Impact

While medication is not warranted in most cases of TS, it can provide tremendous relief for the patient whose tics are severe enough to prevent him or her from studying or paying attention to a task at work, or for whom the obsessive-compulsive component prevents enjoyment of activities.

"I do not go into crowded movie theaters; I do not go to plays. I am very uncomfortable in big crowds," says Ochsman. "If I go to restaurants, I like to sit against the wall, not out in the middle; if I go to a theater, I have to sit in the back row in an aisle seat. I know it is because of the socialization problems I had as a child. Even though we know that TS is a physiological ailment, psychological damage is done by it. I mean, it makes you very self-conscious. Even if you are not the center of attention, you still think you are."

But for the TS patient personally, the impact on his or her quality of life perhaps has less to do with the nature of the disorder itself than with society's reaction to and treatment of those affected. Says Erenberg: "A perfectly intelligent and sensitive human being who has obvious, bizarre tics will just be looked upon as different by most people in society, although in fact, in every other way, they're just like anyone else." ◇

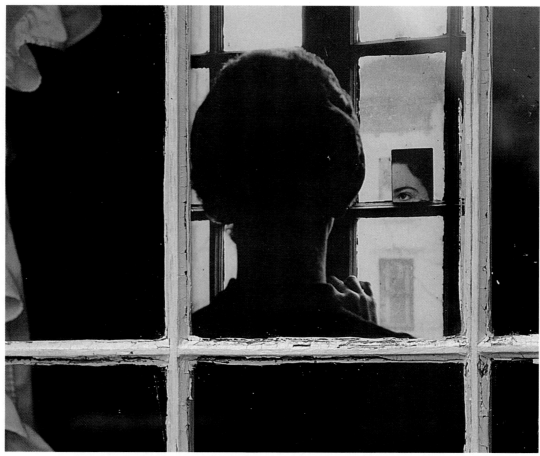

*In the United States, the number of women diagnosed as having AIDS is almost four times that of men. Minority women comprise nearly three-quarters of the diagnosed cases.*

# WOMEN AND AIDS

*by Marian Segal*

Infections with the human immunodeficiency virus (HIV), the virus that causes acquired immune deficiency syndrome (AIDS), are rising nearly four times as fast in women as in men. While AIDS cases among men rose 2.5 percent between 1991 and 1992, the increase among women during the same period was 9.8 percent. Among adults, men with AIDS outnumber women about 8 to 1; in adolescents the ratio is less than 3 men to 1 woman.

"Although in the United States, women currently represent a relatively small per- centage of persons with HIV, they are the most rapidly growing segment of the HIV-infected population in this country," says Janet Arrowsmith-Lowe, M.D., medical officer in the Food and Drug Administration's (FDA's) division of antiviral drugs, the Center for Drug Evaluation and Research.

The disease disproportionately affects minority women. Although black and Hispanic women make up only 21 percent of the country's female population, they account for 74 percent of women diagnosed with AIDS. This does not mean that a person is at risk simply because he or she is a member of a racial or ethnic minority group; rather, it reflects the larger minority population in communities with a high incidence of HIV infection.

In this country, most women who now have AIDS became infected with HIV by injecting illegal drugs. But the rate of infection through sexual transmission has also been rising dramatically. According to the national Centers for Disease Control and Prevention (CDC), cases diagnosed in 1992 marked the first time since the start of the epidemic that more women were infected through sex (50 percent) than through drug use (44 percent).

The CDC reports that "Many women in the United States are unaware they are at risk for HIV infection, and HIV-infected women often remain undiagnosed until the onset of AIDS or until a perinatally infected child [infected before or during birth] becomes ill."

### What You Don't Know Can Hurt You

"A woman may not know her sex partner uses or has used intravenous drugs or is bisexual or has had at-risk sex partners in the past," Arrowsmith-Lowe explains, "and as a result, doesn't seek testing or treatment. Symptoms that could serve as warning signals may go unheeded."

Delayed diagnosis affects survival. "In fact," says Randolph Wykoff, M.D., director of the FDA's Office of AIDS Coordination, "the late diagnosis in women contributed to reports in the past that women's survival time is shorter than men's. It's not. If a woman is diagnosed at the same point in the disease as a man, her survival is, on the average, the same. But most HIV-infected women are from poor populations with poor access to health care, whereas many men with HIV are more-affluent gay men from areas with better medical resources.

"Probably the biggest contribution that can be made to the survival of someone with HIV is to get them into early treatment, particularly to prevent PCP," says Wykoff. (PCP, or Pneumocystis carinii pneumonia, is a life-threatening infection commonly seen in people with AIDS.)

Based on experience with the gay-male population, it appears that education and awareness are important in stemming the tide of HIV infection. In the early years of the AIDS epidemic, gay men—who were then the hardest-hit group—organized and conducted an extensive education program that proved effective in bringing many gay men into clinics for testing and treatment.

"There hasn't been a commensurate education program for women or other men or for children who are potentially at risk for HIV," Arrowsmith-Lowe says, "although greater efforts have recently been targeted to these groups."

Government agencies are working together to step up prevention efforts, improve diagnostic and treatment services, and estab-

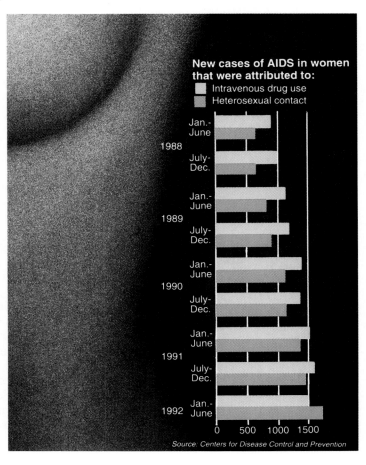

New cases of AIDS in women that were attributed to:
Intravenous drug use
Heterosexual contact

Source: Centers for Disease Control and Prevention

# Mother and Child—The HIV Connection

Most babies born to HIV-infected women escape the virus. According to the surgeon general's 1993 report on HIV infection and AIDS, about 1 in 4 of these infants, however, do become infected before or during birth. Scientists have been trying for some time to discover what influences whether or not a child will be infected with the disease.

"No one is certain when viral transmission occurs," says Janet Arrowsmith-Lowe, M.D., medical officer in the Food and Drug Administration's (FDA's) division of antiviral drugs, Center for Drug Evaluation and Research. "It may be during childbirth, when the placenta separates from the uterine wall and there may be some mixing of maternal and fetal blood, or as the child passes through the vaginal canal and is exposed to vaginal fluids. Or it may occur earlier in pregnancy, when there may be mixing of blood or passage of the virus across the placental wall." In any case, says Arrowsmith-Lowe, "All pregnant women—and especially those at risk of HIV—should seek early prenatal care."

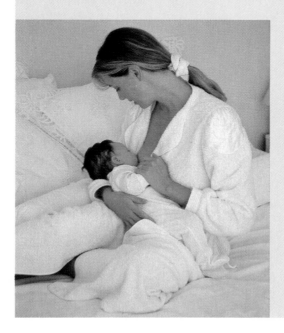

Apart from the timing of transmission, studies suggest that the likelihood of the child becoming infected may correlate with the mother's health during the pregnancy or birth. In the June 9, 1993, issue of the *Journal of the American Medical Association*, Michael E. St. Louis, M.D., and his colleagues report that a baby is more likely to become infected if the mother is in the very earliest stage of infection (when the virus is thought to be abundant) or in an advanced stage of disease, or if the membrane surrounding the placenta is inflamed. A child can also become infected after birth through the process of breast-feeding.

By 1994 an estimated 7,500 children in the United States will have developed AIDS from infection before or during birth or through breast-feeding. Not surprisingly, experts predict that as more women of childbearing age become infected with HIV, the number of infected children will also rise. A disturbing prospect under any circumstances, the significance of this projection is most poignant for minorities in New York City, where AIDS has already emerged as the leading cause of death in Hispanic children 1 to 4 years of age, and as the second-leading cause of death for African-American children of the same age group.

And those children fortunate enough to escape HIV infection still do not escape hardship. "As painful as it is to consider," says Arrowsmith-Lowe, "the facts as we see them now are that an uninfected child born to an infected mother will lose his or her mother before the child becomes a teenager."

According to the surgeon general's report, in the next decade, 125,000 or more children may become orphans because of AIDS, and such unfortunate children will need to be cared for by family members or other responsible adults, or placed in foster care.

lish community-based health-education and risk-reduction programs for diverse populations, including gay and bisexual men, prostitutes, intravenous drug users, heterosexuals with multiple sex partners, women at risk, homeless people, and youths in high-risk situations, such as runaways and youngsters in shelters or detention centers. In June 1993, President Clinton appointed Kristine M. Gebbie, a former Washington State health official, to coordinate federal-level efforts against AIDS.

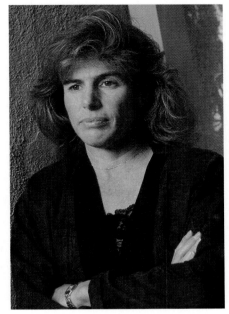

*Several HIV-positive women have emerged as advocates for people with AIDS. Elizabeth Glaser (above) works on behalf of HIV-infected children.*

type of cancer), toxoplasmosis, and others. As knowledge about HIV and AIDS has grown over the years, the CDC has expanded its definition to include additional AIDS-defining illnesses. In January 1993, the CDC added cervical cancer, pulmonary tuberculosis, and recurrent pneumonia to the list of AIDS-indicator illnesses in HIV-infected people.

The revised AIDS definition also includes all HIV-infected people with severe CD4-cell depletion (fewer than 200 CD4 cells per cubic millimeter). CD4 cells are critical immune-system cells that number from about 800 to 1,000 in a healthy person.

"According to the old definition," says Arrowsmith-Lowe, "if you had a very low CD4 count, but no AIDS-defining illness, technically you didn't have AIDS, and therefore couldn't qualify for assistance even if you felt sick. This CD4 cutoff should help those patients get assistance and medical care."

### New Drug Labels Provide Warning

To help increase awareness about the most common early indicator of HIV infection in women—recurrent vaginal candidiasis (yeast infections)—the FDA in October 1992 required manufacturers of over-the-counter drugs for such infections to include a new label warning on their products.

The warning states that frequent vaginal yeast infections (recurring within a two-month period), especially those that don't clear up easily with proper treatment, may be the result of serious medical conditions, including HIV infection, and advises women with these symptoms to see their doctors.

Other illnesses and infections in women that should prompt concern about possible HIV infection include pelvic inflammatory disease, cervical dysplasia (precancerous changes in the cervix), yeast infections of the mouth and throat, and any sexually transmitted disease, such as genital ulcers and warts, and herpes.

### AIDS Definition Revised

A doctor diagnoses AIDS when an HIV-infected person develops one of several infections or diseases specified by the CDC in its "AIDS surveillance case definition." These illnesses include PCP, Kaposi's sarcoma (a

### Treatment

"Recommendations for antiviral treatment with Retrovir [zidovudine, also known as azidothymidine, or AZT] or Videx [didanosine, or DDI] are the same for both sexes," says Arrowsmith-Lowe, "as are the guidelines for beginning preventive therapy against PCP when the person's CD4 count drops below 200 and stays there."

When people with HIV get an infection, they may be sicker and require more-aggressive treatment than do people who are not infected, because their immune systems may be weakened, Arrowsmith-Lowe says. For that reason, some doctors may prescribe oral antifungals for vaginal yeast infections in HIV-infected women.

Similarly, pelvic inflammatory disease (PID), syphilis, gonorrhea, and genital warts may be harder to treat in HIV-infected women. PID, which normally produces fever and pain, may go unnoticed in an HIV-infected woman because her body hasn't been able to mount the immune response that causes these symptoms. Therefore, her infection may worsen for quite some time before she gets medical help.

Syphilis, effectively treated with penicillin in an otherwise-healthy woman, may require higher doses or different drugs and may have a lower cure rate in an HIV-infected person. Genital warts, which are associated with cervical cancer and obstruction of the urinary bladder, may require laser surgery.

Cervical dysplasia, too, can lead to cervical cancer. In HIV-infected women, cervical dysplasia appears to be more common and may progress more quickly to cervical cancer than in noninfected women. For these reasons, Arrowsmith-Lowe says, the American College of Obstetrics and Gynecology and most practitioners recommend that women with HIV have Pap tests twice a year to make sure cancer is detected and treated early.

### Prevention

Armed with knowledge about risks and prevention, women can do much to protect themselves from HIV infection. According to the CDC, as of March 31, 1993, 49 percent of all reported cases of AIDS in adult and adolescent women were due to intravenous drug use, and another 35 percent resulted from sexual transmission. Transfusion of blood or blood products accounted for another 6 percent.

The risk from blood and blood products has been substantially reduced since 1985, when the FDA licensed the first HIV-I antibody test kit to test all transfused products, and since blood products used for hemophilia have been treated with cryoprecipitate.

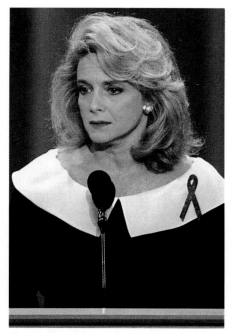

*At the Republican Convention in 1992, Mary Fisher (above) delivered an impassioned speech about the plight of those with AIDS.*

"The most important risks for women now," says Arrowsmith-Lowe, "are using injection drugs, having unprotected sex with someone who uses or has used injection drugs, and having unprotected sex with a man who has had sex with another man. Having multiple sex partners also increases risk of infection."

Of the women diagnosed with AIDS in 1992, nearly 60 percent of those infected through sexual transmission had sex partners who used injection drugs. Sex partners of most of the rest of the women were bisexual men.

### Safer Sex

"Anyone who is sexually active is at risk for HIV, and, basically, you have sex with anyone your partner ever had sex with," says Arrowsmith-Lowe. "Where AIDS is concerned, there is no such thing as completely safe sex. Neither you nor your partner may be aware of the risk factors your partner has been exposed to, so practicing safer sex can't be emphasized enough," she says.

In the United States, the odds of a woman becoming infected from a man are much greater than the reverse. In one recent study of 379 couples, researchers found a 1 percent rate of female-to-male transmission of HIV, compared with a 20 percent rate of male-to-female transmission.

"The surest way to protect yourself against HIV infection and other STDs is not to have sex at all, or to have sex only with one steady, uninfected partner," states the surgeon general's 1993 report on HIV infection and AIDS. For women who are not in such a relationship and engage in sex, Arrowsmith-Lowe advises the following:
• Your partner must wear a condom every time you have sex, whether it's vaginal, anal, or oral, and it must be used properly.

"By far the greatest failures with condom use have nothing to do with the product," says Arrowsmith-Lowe. "They're user failures—failure to use it at all, failure to use it correctly." Protection from syphilis, gonorrhea, chlamydia, herpes, and genital warts is important for preventing HIV infection as well, because sores from these diseases provide easier access for the virus to enter the bloodstream. Anyone with an STD should consider herself or himself at risk for HIV.
• Do not rely on other forms of contraception for full protection against HIV.

In April 1993, the FDA announced that birth-control pills, implantable contraceptives, injectable contraceptives such as Depo-Provera, IUDs, and natural-membrane condoms must carry labeling that states these products are intended to prevent pregnancy, but do not protect against HIV infection and other STDs.

The Reality Female Condom, made from polyurethane, may afford some protection against STDs, but it is not as effective as latex condoms for men. In approving the device in May 1993, the FDA required the labeling to indicate that for "highly effective protection" against STDs, it is important to use latex condoms for men. The male and female condoms cannot be used at the same time. If used together, both products will not stay in place.

In addition, there is no evidence that diaphragms, contraceptive sponges, or spermicides protect against HIV transmission.

### Drug Use

Any illegal drug use puts a person at risk for HIV. An HIV-infected person who shares needles can pass the virus to someone else through tiny amounts of blood that remain in the needle or syringe.

Women who use noninjection drugs, especially crack and other forms of cocaine, also increase their risk for HIV because they may engage in risky sexual activity. Drug and alcohol use may cause a person to be less careful about choice of sex partners or to neglect to use a condom.

The surgeon general's report advises that:
• If you use illegal drugs, try to get treatment to help you stop.

## AIDS Information Sources

**CDC National AIDS Hotline**
• English service
(7 days a week, 24 hours a day)
(1-800) 342-AIDS (2437)
• Spanish service
(7 days a week, 8:00 A.M. to
2:00 A.M. EST)
(1-800) 344-7432
• TDD service for the deaf
(Monday through Friday, 10:00 A.M. to
10:00 P.M. EST)
(1-800) 458-5231

**CDC National AIDS Clearinghouse**
(1-800) 243-7012
• English service
(1-800) 622-HELP (4357)
• Spanish service
(1-800) 66-Ayuda (662-9832)

**AIDS Clinical Trials Information Service (ACTIS)**
(1-800) 874-2572
• TTY-TDD
(1-800) 243-7012
• International
(1-301) 217-0023
• Fax
(1-301) 738-6616
(Monday through Friday, 9:00 A.M. to
7:00 P.M. Eastern time)

For a copy of the 1993 *Surgeon General's Report to the American Public on HIV Infection and AIDS,* call 1-800-342-AIDS.

• If you can't stop injecting illegal drugs, never share your equipment with anyone or reuse equipment used by someone else. HIV may be found in any equipment used to inject drugs, including needles, syringes, cotton, and "cookers" (containers used to mix and heat drugs for injection).
• Cleaning injection equipment decreases the potential for infection, but does not guarantee sterility or that all of the virus is killed. If you cannot stop injecting drugs, it's best to use only sterile needles and syringes.                    ◇

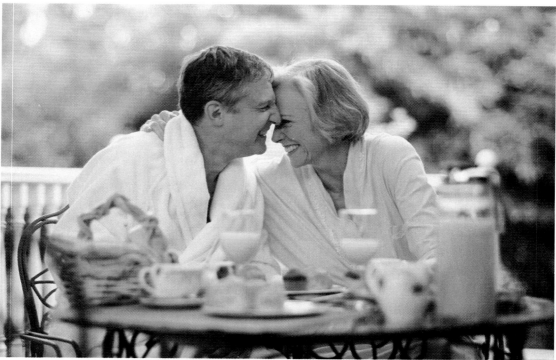

*Once shrouded in myth, menopause today is welcomed by more and more women as an enriching time of life. In the medical arena, menopause is fast becoming a leading women's health issue.*

# The Mystery of Menopause

*by Devera Pine*

As the Baby Boom generation ages, more and more American women are experiencing what was once euphemistically known as "the change of life"—menopause. Experts predict that some 40 million women will pass through menopause in the next 20 years. And as their numbers grow, these women are becoming increasingly vocal about both changing society's perception of postmenopausal women and about finding medical treatments for combating the negative physical effects of menopause.

Menopause affects different women in different ways. Ten percent of all women are lucky enough to pass through this time of life without any symptoms at all. For others, problems can range from occasional insomnia and irritability to frequent hot flashes, heart palpitations, and major mood swings. And while dated notions that view menopause negatively still exist, more and more women are welcoming this normal stage of life for the relief it gives them from monthly menstruation and from the possibility of pregnancy.

### An End to Ovulation

Technically, menopause occurs when the ovaries run out of eggs and lose their capacity to produce estrogen and progesterone. A woman is considered to have passed through menopause once her periods have completely stopped. Among American women the average age of menopause is 50.9 years. However, menopause is a gradual process —the ovaries don't simply cease to function overnight. "Women experience changes long before their ovaries run out of eggs," says Ellyn Modell, M.D., a reproductive endocrinologist in the department of obstetrics and gynecology at Maimonides Medical Center in Brooklyn, New York. In the stage known as *perimenopause,* which can begin up to 10 years before menopause, hormone levels begin to fluctuate, causing physiological changes. For many women the resulting discomforts bear a distinct resemblance to those of premenstrual syndrome (PMS): bloating, breast tenderness, and mood swings. Menstruation continues, but periods may be lighter or heavier than usual.

*Many women will spend more than a third of their lives in the postmenopausal years.*

There is some debate about the effect of menopause on mental health. It may be difficult to distinguish between psychological changes caused by menopause and those caused by other factors that menopausal women typically experience—the aging of their parents, the change in their families, and the aging of their own bodies. Nonetheless, perimenopause sometimes manifests itself very subtly through depression, difficulty concentrating, and headaches. "Given these symptoms," says Frederick Licciardi, M.D., assistant professor of obstetrics and gynecology at the Women's Health Services, New York University Medical Center, "most women are not aware that it's menopause." Licciardi suggests that women experiencing such symptoms should probably first visit their gynecologist, who can then recommend a neurologist or even a psychiatrist if the symptoms are not of menopausal origin.

### Classic Symptoms

As estrogen levels continue to drop, the classic symptoms of menopause emerge. Foremost among these are hot flashes, which in some women occur as frequently as once an hour, leaving them drenched in sweat. Scientists have not yet discovered the exact mechanism behind hot flashes. One theory suggests that the reduced levels of estrogen cause the brain's temperature-regulating center to release the neurotransmitter norepinephrine; norepinephrine, in turn, fools the body into "thinking" that it is overheated. As a result the body dissipates the nonexistent "extra" heat by dilating blood vessels near the surface of the skin, causing the face to flush, and through sweating. However, since the body's temperature was normal to begin with, other mechanisms soon signal that too much heat was dissipated. The result is shivering, to conserve body heat. This scenario of sweats and chills can last for up to 10 minutes per episode.

During the day, hot flashes can be both embarrassing and disruptive; at night, they can rouse a woman from a sound sleep. In

## The Women's Health Initiative

In an attempt to answer some of the questions about HRT, the National Institutes of Health (NIH) is now conducting the first large-scale, random clinical trials on the issue. The Women's Health Initiative, which began enrolling participants in September 1993, will evaluate whether HRT helps prevent heart disease and osteoporosis, and whether it increases the risk of breast cancer.

The study will be performed at 45 centers throughout the United States, looking at 55,000 to 60,000 postmenopausal women, ages 50 to 79, over the course of nine years. In addition to HRT studies, the Women's Health Initiative will examine the effects of a low-fat diet on preventing heart disease and breast and colon cancer, and the effects of calcium and vitamin D supplements on preventing such diseases as osteoporosis and colon cancer.

Finally, the NIH expects about 100,000 women to enroll in an observational study that will search for new risk factors and biological markers for diseases in women. In total, the Women's Health Initiative will study 150,000 to 160,000 women, take 14 years to complete, and cost more than $600 million.

extreme cases, hot flashes can lead to sleep deprivation, which in itself can make it difficult to deal with everyday stress, let alone the stress inherent in some women as they pass through menopause. Episodes of hot flashes can occur—with varying intensity—for up to five years as menopause progresses.

Changing estrogen levels can wreak havoc on the hundreds of tissues that have receptors for estrogen. Mucous membranes in the lining of the vagina may shrink and become dry, making intercourse painful, for instance; vaginal itching and infection may also occur. Breast size may decrease somewhat, and the skin may lose some of its elasticity.

Reduced estrogen levels also make the bladder and urethra more prone to irritations and infections. The muscles that control urination may weaken, resulting in frequent trips to the bathroom and perhaps stress incontinence—involuntary urination brought on by coughing, laughing, or other stimuli.

## Serious Changes

More significantly, the lack of estrogen production in postmenopausal women puts them at increased risk for many serious disorders. Estrogen helps bone absorb calcium from the bloodstream. As estrogen levels decline, bones begin to lose more calcium than they can absorb, and bone thinning occurs. In the first few years of menopause, this bone loss is accelerated, up to as much as 5 percent a year, says Licciardi. Such bone thinning, called osteoporosis, affects 4 out of 10 older women. White or Asian women, thin women, women who smoke or drink heavily, or those who have a

**The Menstrual Cycle**

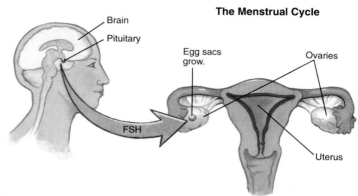

At the beginning of the menstrual cycle, follicle-stimulating hormone (FSH) is released, stimulating the growth of egg sacs, called follicles, which produce estrogen.

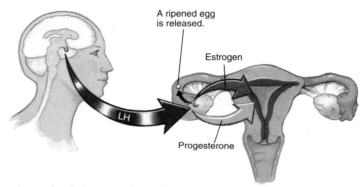

As estrogen levels increase, the uterine lining thickens, causing a surge of luteinizing hormone (LH). Increased levels of LH, in turn, trigger ovulation and a rise in progesterone. The uterine lining continues to thicken.

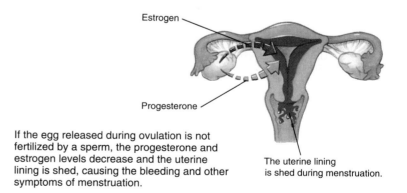

If the egg released during ovulation is not fertilized by a sperm, the progesterone and estrogen levels decrease and the uterine lining is shed, causing the bleeding and other symptoms of menstruation.

| Perimenopause | 12 months | Postmenopause |

▲
Menopause

family history of osteoporosis are at highest risk for developing this debilitating condition.

Unfortunately, the thinned bones of a woman with osteoporosis are more likely to fracture. In fact an estimated one-third of women over 50 endure some sort of osteoporosis-related spinal fracture. The condition called "dowager's hump" occurs from a loss of height due to thinned-out vertebrae that have collapsed. Thousands of women also sustain osteoporosis-related hip fractures. In elderly women, these injuries can ultimately have a fatal outcome, largely through such complications as pneumonia, blood clots, or urinary-tract infections.

Premenopausal estrogen levels indirectly protect against heart disease by helping to increase levels of HDL ("good") cholesterol in the bloodstream, while decreasing LDL ("bad") cholesterol. During menopause, therefore, a woman's blood-cholesterol level may gradually change even though her diet has remained the same. To make matters worse, some researchers now believe that estrogen may directly affect artery walls to prevent the deposit of fatty material known as plaque from forming there. Finally, estrogen may help stop coronary arteries from constricting—one of several reasons why premenopausal women have a lower incidence of high blood pressure than do men of equal age. By age 65, however, women are at higher risk. In fact, the postmenopausal woman is at a 30-times-higher risk of developing heart disease than is a woman who has yet to go through "the change."

It is an unfortunate fact of life, therefore, that once menopause has ended, women find themselves without the protective effect imparted by estrogen for so many years. Fortunately (at least for some women), the symptoms of menopause can be prevented or alleviated through hormone-replacement therapy (HRT)—the use of synthetic estrogen and progesterone.

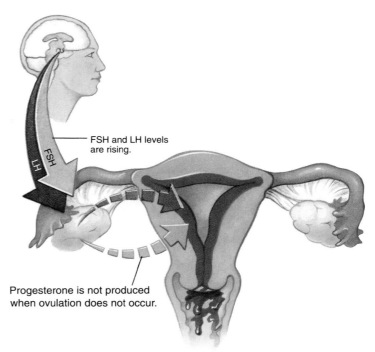

FSH and LH levels are rising.

Progesterone is not produced when ovulation does not occur.

Perimenopause begins as the body's egg supply runs out and less estrogen is produced, leading to irregular ovulation. The menstrual cycle may also become irregular and other symptoms, such as hot flashes, may develop.

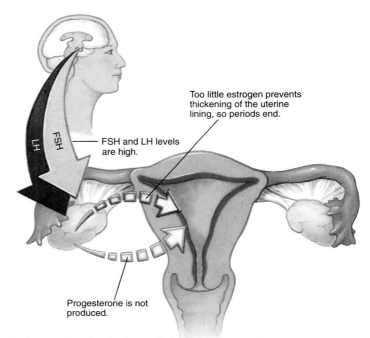

Too little estrogen prevents thickening of the uterine lining, so periods end.

FSH and LH levels are high.

Progesterone is not produced.

Twelve months after the last period, the body enters the postmenopause stage. Signs of change, such as hot flashes and night sweats, begin to subside. But long-term effects of estrogen loss, including osteoporosis and heart disease, may develop.

## The Hormone-Replacement Puzzle

Estrogen-replacement therapy first became popular in the 1940s, and then again in the 1960s, when the hormone was seen as the ticket to eternal youth. Synthetic estrogen then fell out of favor as scientists established a link between the hormone and both uterine and breast cancer. Today estrogen is back—this time combined with progesterone to help ward off cancer-producing effects. Still, the use of HRT remains clouded and controversial.

In the past the use of estrogen alone made women about seven times more likely to develop cancer of the uterine lining (endometrium). Today's HRT involves both lower doses of estrogen and the use of progestin, a synthetic form of progesterone. This combination of hormones, says Modell, virtually "wipes out the chance of getting cancer of the uterine lining."

As a result, many doctors now prescribe HRT to prevent symptoms that commonly occur with menopause, including vaginal dryness, urinary-tract symptoms, hot flashes, and excessive sweating. More important, HRT protects against the menopause-induced heightened risk of cardiovascular disease: In a 10-year study of 49,000 nurses, published in the *New England Journal of Medicine* in 1991, researchers found that compared to women who took no hormonal supplements, women on HRT had half the risk of heart attack and death from cardiovascular disease. (It should be noted that previous studies have produced contradictory results on the cardiovascular protection provided by hormone replacement. However, the 1991 study was larger than all previous research combined.)

HRT helps prevent osteoporosis as well. Women on hormone therapy have 40 percent

> *Postmenopausal women have a much heightened risk of developing heart disease.*

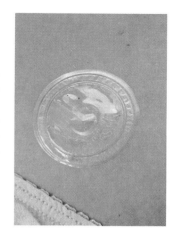

*Hormone-replacement therapy is administered by tablets or by skin patches (left). Both methods have been found equally effective in slowing the rate of bone loss, but many women find the skin patch more convenient.*

fewer hip fractures than do women not taking hormones.

Finally, there is some evidence that HRT can help ease menopause-related mood changes. In one study of 36 postmenopausal women, those on HRT were more optimistic, more confident, and less depressed than women who received a placebo. Other studies have shown that hormone replacement may improve cognitive function.

## A Link to Cancer?

Despite HRT's benefits, many women are reluctant to embark on this course of treatment because of the still-ambiguous link to cancer. It is not clear whether HRT increases the risk of getting breast cancer: Some studies show an increased risk; others do not. For example, in 1991 the Centers for Disease Control and Prevention (CDC) analyzed 16 studies and found that women who took only

*Menopausal women are especially vulnerable to the bone-thinning disease called osteoporosis. For many women, the bones in the spine begin to collapse, causing the spine to curve into what is known as a "dowager's hump."*

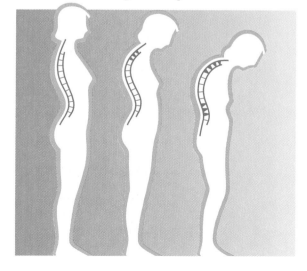

estrogen postmenopausally for 15 years had a 30 percent increase in the risk of getting breast cancer; women with a family history of breast cancer stood at greatest risk. Women who had taken estrogen for less than five years had no increased risk.

These findings are far from conclusive, however, since there has yet to be a large-scale study of breast cancer and HRT as it is prescribed today—a combination of estrogen and progesterone. Many of the earlier studies of hormone-replacement therapy also evaluated patients who used estrogen at higher doses than are typically prescribed by doctors today. Most experts agree that there is an urgent need to conduct more clinical studies. (See the sidebar on the Women's Health Initiative on page 57.)

For now, the decision to use HRT must be made on a case-by-case basis by a woman and her physician. Women who have had blood clots, unexplained vaginal bleeding, or a hormone-responsive cancer—a breast or uterine cancer that is estrogen sensitive—should not use HRT, says Modell. With proper monitoring, however, many doctors prescribe HRT to a woman with a family history of breast cancer. The reason? Many experts feel the protective effects of HRT far outweigh the possible increased risk of developing breast cancer. For example, a 50- to 94-year-old white woman has a 31 percent chance of dying from heart disease, and only a 2.8 percent chance of dying from breast cancer. "Our job is to tell women what the real risks are, and let them know that in most instances the protective effects outweigh any fears they may have," says Licciardi.

Since HRT has been found to reduce the risk of bone loss, women who are at high risk for osteoporosis are considered good candidates for HRT, as are those at high risk for cardiovascular disease. Moreover, women who, due to a hysterectomy, begin menopause before age 40 are generally prescribed hormone replacements.

*Despite its demonstrated protective benefits, HRT still remains controversial.*

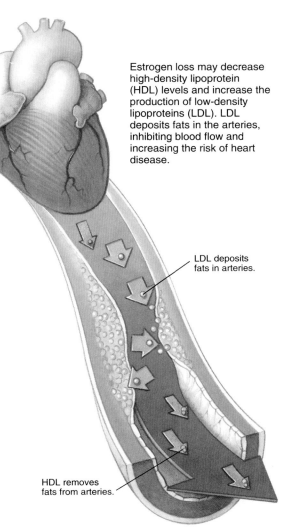

Estrogen loss may decrease high-density lipoprotein (HDL) levels and increase the production of low-density lipoproteins (LDL). LDL deposits fats in the arteries, inhibiting blood flow and increasing the risk of heart disease.

LDL deposits fats in arteries.

HDL removes fats from arteries.

## Other Considerations

Hormone-replacement therapy affects different women in different ways. For many women the return of a monthly period and premenstrual symptoms—bloating, breast tenderness, irritability, and the like—are particularly annoying side effects. Fortunately, many doctors now tinker with the timing and dosage of progesterone (which causes the lining of the uterus to slough off, producing a period). Instead of prescribing 25 days of estrogen therapy, 13 days of progesterone, and 7 days of no medication (the standard regimen), doctors prescribe a low daily dose of both estrogen and progesterone. Under the latter regimen, most women will bleed on and off for about three months, and then will not bleed again.

Curiously, some women find that certain brands of hormones work better for them

## Menopause for Men?

As they age, do men also go through the discomfort of a hot-flashing, mood-swinging hormonal flux? Not exactly, according to Wylie C. Hembree, M.D., associate professor of clinical medicine and clinical obstetrics and gynecology at the College of Physicians and Surgeons at Columbia University in New York City: "Although there are changes in sexual functioning that probably all men experience, it's inappropriate to use the word 'menopause.' "

The reason, explains Hembree, has to do with the unique hormonal design of the male and female reproductive systems. In women the growth of an egg-containing follicle and ovulation produce the hormones estrogen and progesterone. Once the ovaries no longer produce eggs, they also cease to produce these hormones (though most women still retain low levels of estrogen in their bodies). In men, on the other hand, the production of sperm and the production of male hormones such as testosterone are completely unrelated. As a result, unlike women, most men retain their ability to produce male hormones all through their lives.

However, some researchers believe that testosterone levels may gradually drop as much as 30 to 40 percent between the ages of 40 and 70. One controversial theory suggests that a drop in testosterone may result in increased body fat levels and decreased bone and muscle mass, virility, and fertility.

While there is still no direct evidence proving that lessening testosterone levels have these debilitating effects, age does change a man's sexual functioning. Age-related changes occur for various reasons. First, changes in the brain may slow down the secretion of the hormones that stimulate the production of testosterone. Moreover, other health problems—cardiovascular disease, high blood pressure, diabetes, kidney disease, alcoholism—can all damage the testicles and cause changes in sexual functioning.

Unlike HRT for women, researchers have been unable to find any scientific evidence that testosterone supplements would benefit most men. Moreover, the testosterone supplementation may cause heart disease and cancer, among other problems. Testosterone supplements, says Hembree, are only for the few cases in which sexual dysfunction is specifically related to low levels of testosterone.

---

than do others. "There are different estrogen compounds out there," says Modell. "You have to find someone who is willing to try them out." Licciardi agrees: "The dose can have an effect," he says. "Too much or too little can make the patient not feel well. We try to find the dose that's right for them, but it may take a few months or longer."

HRT is now available via either tablets or skin patches. However, it is not clear whether estrogen that enters the bloodstream directly through a skin patch provides protection against heart disease. Some experts speculate that estrogen must be taken orally so that it can pass through the digestive tract and affect the liver's production of cholesterol. The dose of estrogen generally given today is 0.625 milligram, compared to doses in the past of 1.25 to 2.5 milligrams. Birth-control pills, experts point out, now contain more estrogen than is used in HRT.

Given the confusion about HRT's long-term effects, it is not surprising that many women forgo hormone therapy. By some estimates, 35 percent of all women need HRT, and 60 percent could benefit from it. Yet only 15 percent of postmenopausal women use it. Moreover, many women—put off by having to take a daily medication and by getting a monthly period again—stop HRT in less than a year. Drug companies, meanwhile, are racing to develop more-acceptable hormone regimens to capture a market that already exceeds half a billion dollars.

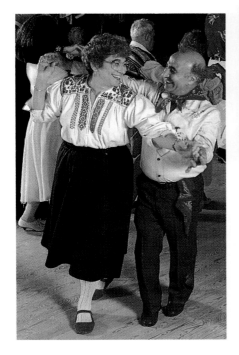

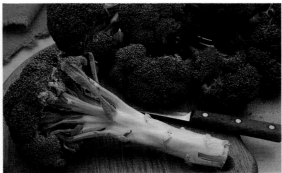

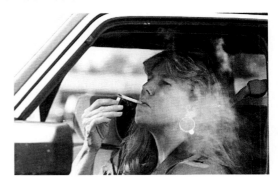

*Many women choose non-hormonal methods, including quitting smoking cigarettes, exercise, and good nutrition, to ease the symptoms of menopause and fend off osteoporosis and heart disease.*

## Nonhormonal Options

Fortunately, for those women unwilling to take synthetic hormones, there are some options for easing the symptoms of menopause. The following commonsense health measures, for instance, can help head off both osteoporosis and heart disease.

• Smokers should quit. Smokers are at greater risk for osteoporosis, heart disease, and stroke (among other diseases).

• Regular exercise keeps the cardiovascular system in shape and helps maintain a reasonable weight. And it doesn't take much to reap healthy benefits—one study of premenopausal, middle-aged women found that 20 minutes of exercise three times a week significantly lowered LDL cholesterol, raised HDL cholesterol, and took weight off. All three factors are related to the risk of heart disease. Surprisingly, most of the women in the study simply walked for exercise. Weight-bearing exercise such as bicycling also helps bones retain calcium.

• Diet also plays a part in maintaining health before and after menopause. A low-fat diet can head off heart disease; a diet high in calcium-rich foods such as dark-green leafy vegetables can help provide the calcium postmenopausal women need each day.

Postmenopausal women not on HRT need as much as 1,500 milligrams of calcium a day, according to the National Institutes of Health (NIH). Most experts recommend that women get as much of their daily calcium intake as possible through foods, not supplements.

Despite anecdotal reports that vitamin E and vitamin $B_6$ supplements ease hot flashes and other symptoms of menopause, no controlled studies exist that scientifically support these claims. Moreover, high doses of vitamins can cause health problems; megadoses of vitamin $B_6$, for instance, may produce neurological problems.

• The symptoms of vaginal dryness associated with menopause can be alleviated with vaginal lubricants such as K-Y Jelly. Regular sexual activity will keep natural moisture flowing and maintain pelvic muscle tone.

• Urinary incontinence can be helped with exercises to strengthen the muscles of the pelvic floor.

Finally, it helps to remember that menopause is not necessarily a negative event. Menopause, in which most women spend one-third of their lives, is, after all, not an ending, but the beginning of a new and potentially rewarding time of life.  ◇

# Housecalls

by George Valko, M.D.

**Q** *In earlier decades, there were warnings that people who took the hallucinogenic drug LSD did irreparable damage to their chromosomes. If this is true, it would seem as though children of former LSD users would have a high incidence of birth defects. Did this happen?*

**A** Much research took place in the 1960s and 1970s to test the theory that LSD would cause birth defects in offspring of users. As yet, we have no conclusive evidence that LSD causes the kind of permanent chromosomal damage that would result in such problems.

Whether mature sperm and eggs in users were impaired at the time of drug use is not clear, but eggs mature and bud monthly, and sperm is produced and turned over much more quickly. Even if LSD affects the stem cells that give rise to these gametes, it does not appear that the damage is sufficient to cause an increase in short- or long-term rates of birth defects in children of users.

---

**Q** *My sister has been diagnosed as having Lou Gehrig's disease. Do the symptoms of this condition ever go into remission? Is there a certain life expectancy associated with a Lou Gehrig's diagnosis? Any treatments?*

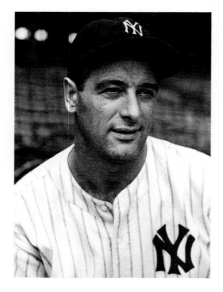

**A** Lou Gehrig's disease, or amyotrophic lateral sclerosis (ALS), is named for the famed "Iron Man" of the New York Yankees (left), who was diagnosed with the disease and later died from it. It is a motor-neuron (muscle) disease that produces progressive muscle weakness and paralysis of unknown cause.

Usually affecting people in or near their 40s or 50s, the disease takes a slow, unremitting course, and is usually fatal in two to five years. Only about 20 percent of patients are able to survive for more than five years. Treatments, purely supportive in nature, include pulmonary hygiene to stop secretions from building up and causing lung problems, and range-of-motion exercises to keep joints from stiffening.

There is no cure for this disease. But in 1993 scientists identified the defective gene that causes ALS. This discovery has sparked clinical trials of several well-known drugs that may retard the progress of this disease.

---

**Q** *I am six months pregnant, and was recently told I suffer from vaginal warts. Is my unborn baby endangered in any way? How did I get the warts in the first place?*

**A** In all likelihood, you contracted genital warts (or *condyloma acuminatum*) sexually. The human papillomavirus causes this condition.

You must see a doctor and have these genital warts treated before your child is born. They are not easy to treat, but your physician may be able to remove them successfully with laser surgery or a type of chemotherapy.

If the treatment proves inadequate, your doctor will probably recommend a cesarean section. Otherwise your child could contract the infection as he or she passes through the birth canal, and ultimately could develop the warts. The human papillomavirus has been known to occasionally infect a newborn's lungs or spread to other systems of the body, creating a potentially very serious condition.

---

**Q** *Is there any point to saving the last remaining smallpox viruses now that the disease has been eradicated? What were the typical symptoms of smallpox? Was the disease ever widespread in the U.S.?*

**A** The debate over what to do with the smallpox virus has been ongoing ever since the last known case of smallpox was found in Somalia in 1977. (Another case, in 1978, was due to a laboratory accident in England.) Since a worldwide vaccination program in the 1970s successfully wiped out smallpox, the virus has existed in—and been loaned out for research by—only two laboratories in the world: one in the United States and one in Russia. The two nations have maintained the virus for its scientific value, and perhaps for its potential use in germ warfare.

The end of the Cold War has again raised the question of what should be done with the virus. Permanently destroying any species of life, even something as small and "simple" as a virus, raises almost endless moral and scientific questions that are virtually impossible to resolve.

Typical symptoms of smallpox, or "variola," are fever, severe headaches, malaise, vomiting, and vascular and pustular eruptions. About 20 percent of sufferers die due to organ failure. The disease was epidemic in the United States until the 1920s, after which vaccinations exterminated it.

---

Q  *My baby recently contracted conjunctivitis at her day-care center. Her eyes swelled up so badly that she couldn't see, and ultimately she had to be hospitalized. Is conjunctivitis in a baby always so much more serious than in an adult? Should we expect any lasting aftereffects from the condition?*

A  Usually caused by a common virus, conjunctivitis is a reddening of the conjunctiva, the tissue-thin covering of the eyeball and inner eyelid. It can get so bad that the eye swells shut. Usually, though, it causes only the redness, itching, and discharge known as "pinkeye."

Inflammatory reactions in allergies can also cause conjunctivitis. More serious cases of conjunctivitis result from bacteria or herpes viruses, which can lead to scarring and impairment of vision or, in very serious, untreated cases, blindness. To prevent bacterial conjunctivitis, all newborns receive antibiotic eyedrops.

Conjunctivitis can be mild or serious in anyone, child or adult. It can also be highly contagious. Anyone with it should seek the care of a doctor. An ophthalmologist can determine if any scarring has taken place in your baby's conjunctiva.

---

Q  *Is it true that the appendix is a useless organ? Why does it seem as though anybody who gets appendicitis has the organ removed surgically? What happens if the appendix ruptures before surgery?*

A  The appendix does have a useful function. Like the glands in your neck and elsewhere (the ones that become swollen when you are sick), the appendix has lymphoid tissue in it, and so is part of the immune system, which helps the body fight disease. Specifically, the appendix is part of the gut-associated lymphoid tissue (GALT), which, like the rest of the lymph system, serves as a barrier to infection.

The appendix is nonetheless not indispensable, and if it becomes infected, it must come out before it ruptures. If the appendix does rupture before the patient gets to surgery, the danger comes, not from internal bleeding, but from a larger, more-life-threatening infection throughout the abdomen called peritonitis. Although this infection may not always develop right away, the patient with a ruptured appendix is treated in intensive care, and must still undergo surgery to clean the infection out of the abdomen.

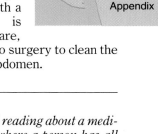
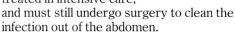
Ascending colon · Small intestine · Appendix

---

Q  *I seem to recall reading about a medical procedure where a person has all of his or her blood replaced with healthier blood. Is such a procedure ever done and for what reasons?*

A  The procedure is called exchange transfusion. Doctors take most of the patient's blood out, a little at a time, and replace it with the same amount of fresh blood. The procedure is usually done in babies who have poisoning by natural substances or by medications. Patients who have malaria, sickle-cell disease, or severe burns may also receive this treatment.

---

*Do you have a medical question?*
Send it to Editor, Health and Medicine Annual,
P.O. Box 90, Hawleyville, CT 06440-9990.

# Nutrition

**See also:**
Individual articles in the second half of this book, arranged in alphabetical order, for additional information.

Scientific research continues to demonstrate that the things people put in their mouths have a major influence on current and future health. And government groups are increasingly vocal in urging people to pay attention to this research. For instance, the importance of healthy eating habits received fresh emphasis during 1993 when the U.S. Department of Agriculture announced that it would now give nutrition equal status with farm concerns. High on the agenda was improving the quality of school lunches by increasing fruits and vegetables and reducing fat and salt. "A good school lunch or breakfast is just as important as a good schoolbook. You can't get what is in the book unless you energize the mind and body. We can't continue to deep-fry our children's health," stated Agriculture Secretary Mike Espy.

A report by the consumer group Public Voice for Food and Health Policy indicated that only 9 percent of children ages 6 to 11 consume the recommended five or more daily servings of fruit and vegetables; 57 percent eat less than one serving of fruit a day, and 32 percent eat less than one serving of vegetables a day. A survey by Mathematica Policy Research, Inc., of lunches served at 542 schools finds that 38 percent of the calories come from fat —significantly more than the 30 percent recommended maximum.

Many adult Americans also have bad eating habits. A survey conducted by Louis Harris & Associates found that only 53 percent of the people surveyed said they ate the recommended amounts of vegetables and other foods rich in fiber; only 51 percent avoided excess fats, and 46 percent avoided excess salt. These statistics are supported by records of food sales, which show that low-calorie and low-fat products have declined in popularity, while foods high in fat and salt are selling briskly.

Meanwhile, a study by researchers at Harvard University's School of Public Health shows that a diet rich in animal fats, especially from red meat, increases a man's risk of developing life-threatening prostate cancer by almost 80 percent. It appears that animal fats promote the growth of small prostate tumors, making them more likely to spread and become potentially lethal.

Margo Denke, M.D., associate professor of internal medicine at the University of Texas Southwestern Medical Center, finds that a diet fortified with calcium results in lower cholesterol levels. Another study, directed by Ian R. Reid, M.D., of the University of Auckland in New Zealand, finds that calcium supplements reduce bone loss in postmenopausal women by one-third to one-half. The women, who were getting about 750 milligrams of calcium a day in their diet, took an additional 1,000 milligrams daily.

There also is mounting evidence of the protective effects of vitamins. Particular attention has been given to vitamins C and E, as well as beta-carotene (a precursor of vitamin A). These compounds are antioxidants that appear to render harmless the toxic oxidants produced during normal cell activity. A five-year study of 29,584 Chinese adults shows that dietary vitamin and mineral supplements—particularly vitamin E, beta-carotene, and selenium—significantly reduce the risk of dying from cancer or stroke.

Exactly how much a person needs of various nutrients is the focus of intense research, notes Dr. Denke. "Research quantifying how much we need of certain vitamins and minerals is sorely lacking," she says. A growing number of health experts believe that the official recommended daily allowance (RDA) may be sufficient to prevent acute-deficiency diseases, but too low to help fight chronic ailments such as heart disease and cancer. For example, the vitamin E RDA is 30 units a day, but it is megadoses of 100 units or more daily that appear to combat heart disease and cancer.

However, the U.S. Food and Drug Administration (FDA) takes a dim view of marketers who make unsubstantiated health claims for their dietary supplements. At the end of 1993, the FDA released new labeling regulations that establish the same standards for dietary supplements as for foods, including prior approval for all health claims. Still, products containing folic acid (one of the B vitamins) can claim that they help prevent birth defects of the brain and spine, and calcium products can say they prevent osteoporosis. But additional scientific proof will be needed before the FDA will allow claims that antioxidants prevent cancer or heart disease.

*The message is clear: what people put in their mouths has a major influence on their health.*

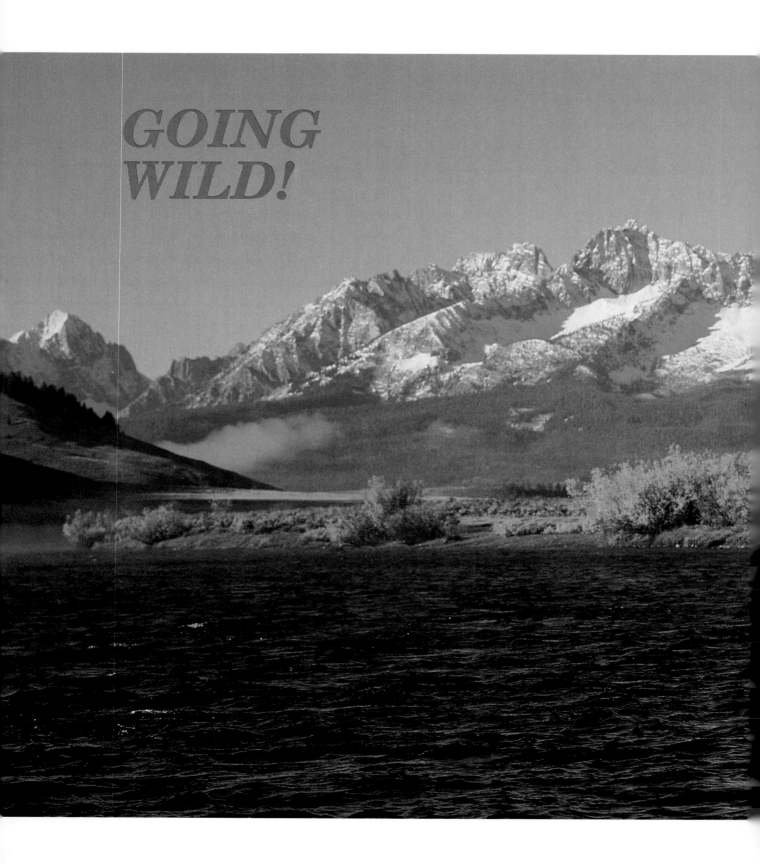

# GOING WILD!

# ...Game in
# the Kitchen

*by Sue Gebo, M.P.H., R.D.*

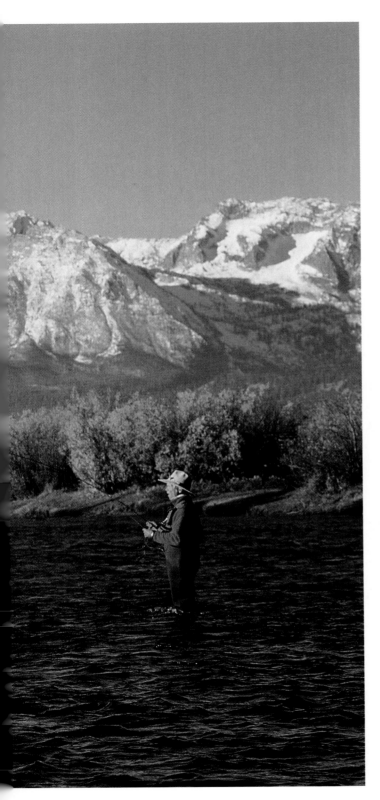

**W**hen the air turns crisp and flannel shirts become de rigueur, it's time for many an adventurous soul to dust off the orange vest and hit the woods and streams. Ironically, many of today's hunters belong to the generation that shunned golf, tennis, and other "Establishment" sports during the '60s and '70s. Then came the '90s, when some still-inexplicable event occurred that transformed the long-derided sports of hunting and fishing into the activities of choice for many of today's Renaissance men and women.

This phenomenon is all the more interesting in view of the fact that, aside from the occasional encounter with venison, quail, and rainbow trout in restaurants, most Americans remain absolutely clueless when it comes to wild game and fish. Even so, a growing segment of the population has developed an interest in hunting and fishing, a trend reflected by the upsurge in requests for hunting licenses. In 1991, 14 million hunting licenses were issued in the United States; by 1992 that figure had risen to 15.7 million. Recently nearly 70 million U.S. sport fishermen were counted in a single year. Perhaps it's the L. L. Bean/Eddie Bauer outdoorsy appeal that's hooking a whole new generation of hunters and fishermen. Perhaps it's the game of outsmarting the hunted. Or perhaps it's simply the pure

*When properly stored and prepared, game makes a tasty alternative to store-bought food.*

*Many people who engage in hunting and fishing do so in order to enjoy the solitude of the great outdoors, and only secondarily as a means of obtaining their next meal.*

joy of abandoning the civilized world for a time and plunging into a wilderness adventure, an excursion into the great outdoors where every sense is focused.

Whatever the motivation, tons of food are the result of the hunting and fishing revival. Recent figures estimate the total annual consumption of seven common varieties of wild game in the United States to be nearly 158 million pounds of dressed, boneless, skinless meat. Other varieties of wild game account for an estimated additional 25 million pounds per year. These quantities represent only wild game killed by licensed hunters, not game raised on game farms.

In addition, consumption of fish caught by licensed recreational fishermen in the United States is estimated at 1 billion pounds per year, representing over 20 percent of all fish caught in the United States. Thus, not only are hunting and fishing supplying recreational diversion, they are also offering up a bounty of fresh, high-protein food for those game enough to dress and cook it.

## Types of Game

Wild game is generally divided into five categories: (1) *Big game,* which includes deer, elk, moose, caribou, antelope, wild sheep, wild goats, as well as bears, cougars, and wolves; (2) *Waterfowl,* which includes ducks and geese; (3) *Upland game birds* (living at high elevations, away from the sea), such as wild turkeys, grouse, quail, mourning doves, chukar, partridge, and pheasant; (4) *Small game,* including squirrels, rabbits, and hares, as well as raccoons, opossums, muskrats, marmots, and beavers; and (5) *Varmints* or *vermin,* such as coyotes, weasels, bobcats, rats, mice, and other predatory and/or distasteful species that are not protected by game laws.

Sport fishermen, called anglers, are likely to catch a wide variety of edible aquatic species. Common varieties include whitefish, shad, smelts, lake trout, brook trout (including rainbow, cutthroat, and German brown), pike, perch, bass, crappies, and catfish.

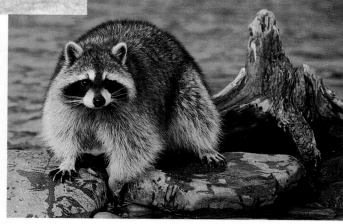

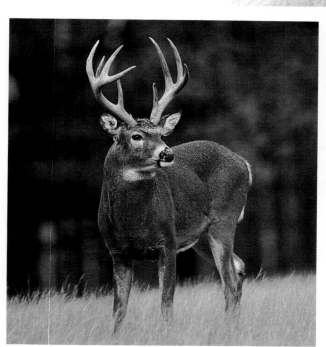

*The United States is home to a great variety of game animals. The whitetail deer (left) is the preferred source of venison. Pheasant (top) is considered a delicacy, while raccoon (above), although abundant in the United States, enjoys only limited popularity.*

## Game as Food

For the nutrition-minded, game provides high-quality protein, generally with less fat than domestic varieties of red meat and fowl. Because the game animal is more physically active than the ranched, bred, or caged creature, the meat is leaner but, more often than not, somewhat tougher.

The degree of toughness is dependent on a variety of factors. One is the age of the animal—in general, the older the game, the tougher the meat. Another factor is the animal's manner of death. When wild game is killed, the speed with which the creature dies influences toughness. An animal killed instantly by a clean shot will yield more tender meat than one that struggles or flees after shooting. This phenomenon is due to the flood of meat-toughening adrenaline released by an injured or frightened animal as it follows its natural instinct to escape.

Regardless of how the animal dies, aging the meat can reduce toughness. The enzymes present in the animal's tissue continue to work after death, breaking down connective tissue, thereby inducing tenderness.

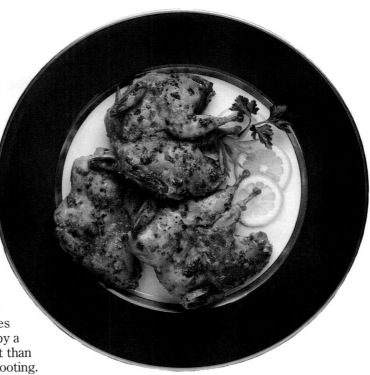

*Game food, like the plate of grilled red devil quail above, can make an elegant presentation on the dinner table.*

(More detail about the aging of game will be offered later.)

Because the diets of wild animals are not controlled like those of domestic animals, the flavor of each game animal varies; essentially, the flavor is dependent on the creature's available food sources. Strongly flavored berries, leaves, or other vegetation will influence the taste of the meat.

### Nutritional Value of Wild Game
(3-ounce portions)

| | Calories | Fat (g) | Cholesterol (mg) |
|---|---|---|---|
| Antelope (roasted) | 127 | 2.3 | 107 |
| Bear (simmered) | 220 | 11.4 | n/a |
| Beaver (roasted) | 180 | 5.9 | n/a |
| Bison (roasted) | 122 | 2.1 | 70 |
| Deer (roasted) | 134 | 2.7 | 95 |
| Duck, wild (breast, no skin) | 105 | 3.6 | n/a |
| Elk (roasted) | 124 | 1.6 | 62 |
| Goose (roasted, no skin) | 202 | 10.8 | 82 |
| Moose (roasted) | 114 | 0.8 | 66 |
| Quail | 123 | 4.2 | n/a |
| Rabbit (stewed) | 147 | 3.0 | 104 |
| Squirrel (roasted) | 147 | 4.0 | 103 |

From: N-Squared Computing. Nutritionist 3, Version 7.0. Silverton, Oregon: N-Squared Computing, 1991.
n/a = not available

### Estimated Annual Wild Game Consumption in U.S.*

| Animal | Pounds of Meat |
|---|---|
| White-tailed Deer | 105,000,000 |
| Mule Deer | 37,000,000 |
| Elk | 2,000,000 |
| Ducks | 4,725,000 |
| Geese | 3,750,000 |
| Turkey | 1,600,000 |
| Dove | 3,750,000 |
| TOTAL | 157,825,000 |

* Data provided by George Lapointe, International Association of Fish and Wildlife Agencies, from individual species data ranging from late 1980s through 1992.

## Big Game

*Venison* is by far the most common wild game consumed in the United States. While, to purists, venison means deer flesh, many hunters (and restaurants) consider the meat of elk, moose, caribou, and, occasionally, prong-horned antelope to be venison.

The white-tailed deer is the species of choice when it comes to venison. The renewed interest in hunting has also made this deer the most commonly killed species of wild game in the U.S. Somewhat less popular among hunters is the mule deer, a common species in the west.

Depending on the diet of the animal, deer may taste more or less like beef. Venison carries some of the flavors derived from the deer's diet. If a deer feeds primarily on cedar leaves, twigs, and berries, for example, a cedar taste will permeate the meat. In such cases the meat can be cooked with various seasonings to reduce the dominance of these flavors.

*Bears* are not a common U.S. food. Because bears are extremely large and heavy, removing their carcasses from the wilderness may prove an insurmountable task. Nevertheless, many recipes can be found for such delicacies as bear stew, bear roast, and bear steak.

Compared to other game, bear meat is quite fatty. The meat becomes rancid fairly easily and does not hold up well over long periods of freezing.

## Waterfowl

*Ducks.* Duck hunting has been a popular sport for centuries. The many varieties of ducks sought by hunters are generally divided into three groups: shallow-water, which feed on the surface of the water and in grainfields; deepwater, found in seas and bays, where they feed on crustaceans and aquatic vegetation; and fish-eating ducks, also known as mergansers.

Shallow-water ducks include the mallard, the black duck, the teal, the pintail, the baldpate, and the gadwall; deepwater ducks include the canvasback, the redhead, the scaup, and the ring-necked.

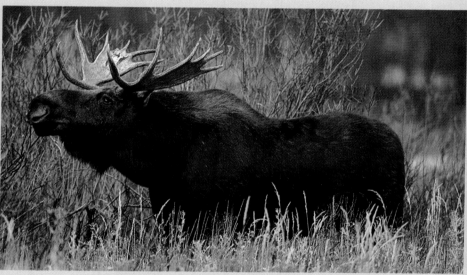

**Moose**

Fish-eating ducks are not prized as game food because their flesh and, in particular, their skin have an undesirable flavor. Unlike domesticated duck, wild duck tends to be quite lean.

*Geese.* The Canada goose is considered the choicest species for eating. Other desirable species include the blue goose, the white-fronted goose, and the snow goose. Geese are much larger than ducks; males (ganders) often reach a rather formidable weight of 26 pounds.

## Upland Game Birds

*Wild turkeys.* A member of the pheasant family, the wild turkey was once over-hunted to the point of scarcity. Wild-turkey populations have now recovered, making this bird once more a favorite of hunters. Generally reaching lengths of about 4 feet (males), the wild turkey has metallic green, bronze, or brownish plumage. It feeds on acorns, insects, berries, and seeds.

*Grouse.* Related to turkeys and quail, grouse are the ideal game bird: medium-sized and chickenlike. Ranging from 1 to 3 feet in length, grouse eat fruit, seeds, nuts, insects, leaves, bark, and buds. Grouse populations tend to be dense, and are all but impervious to heavy hunting pressure.

*Quail.* A member of the pheasant family, the quail includes a number of varieties of birds, including the partridge and the bobwhite, the latter being the most popular variety to hunters and farmers alike. Quail are brightly marked and crested. They average about 11 inches long, and devour many agricultural pests, which makes them (particularly the bobwhite) beneficial to farmers. To hunters, quail present both a challenging and a rewarding target. Perhaps most important, the quail has delicately flavored flesh.

*Mourning dove.* Actually a member of the pigeon family, the mourning dove is so named for its characteristic, sad-sounding song. The mourning dove is considered the most abundant and widespread game bird in North America, although it is a protected species in some states. It has a plump, compact body and small head. It feeds mainly on seeds and waste grains.

*Partridge.* Another seed eater, the partridge is a small to medium-sized member of the pheasant and quail family, generally reaching lengths of 6 to 18 inches. Popular varieties include the chukar and the gray partridge.

*Pheasant.* This medium-to-large bird is a popular bird for hunters. Its mildly flavored flesh is probably the result of its preferred diet of soybeans, corn, clover, wheat, and barley—much the same food as domesticated animals.

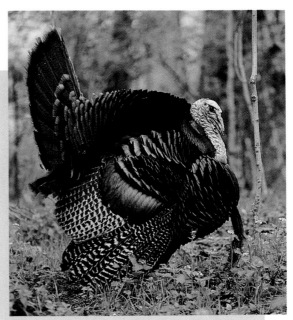

**Wild Turkey**

## Small Game

*Squirrels.* Squirrels were first hunted in the United States by early settlers; in fact, squirrel pie was a common menu item at the upscale eateries frequented by such personages as George Washington and Alexander Hamilton. Owing to their larger size, the fox squirrel and the gray squirrel are the varieties usually hunted. Squirrel meat is extremely lean and is often eaten fried.

*Rabbits and hares.* Cottontail rabbits and snowshoe hares are considered delicacies. Their light- to medium-colored flesh is tender. Rabbits are particularly desirable in early winter, when they are fat and their meat is very white.

*Raccoons.* A popular game food in the southern United States, the raccoon is quite abundant and is easy to field-dress.

*Opossums.* This marsupial has a diet ranging from other small game to insects and corn. The opossum is particularly desirable in the autumn, when it is larger and fatter than at other times of year.

*Muskrats.* A less common menu item than even the raccoon or the opossum, the muskrat is nonetheless eaten by some brave admirers. Enthusiasts prefer young muskrats, which are more tender than their elders.

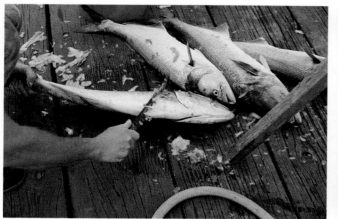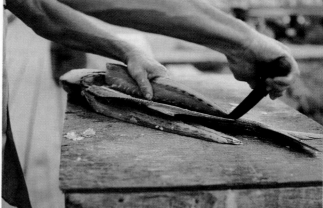

*Fishing is the most popular form of hunting in the United States. How well a fish dinner comes out depends upon the skill with which the fish is descaled (left) and filleted (right).*

## Dressing Game

Once the game has succumbed to shot or arrow, it's time to work fast. To ensure a wholesome and palatable product, experts recommend that big game, and many varieties of smaller game animals and birds, be field-dressed (gutted and bled) immediately after shooting. This allows rapid dissipation of the animal's body heat, thus eliminating a potential factor in spoilage.

The methods used to field-dress wild game are the subject of many books. There are, however, major points of caution common to all instructions on field-dressing:

• Maintain enough feathers or other identifying marks on the animal to meet state laws for species identification when reporting the take;

• Look for parasites, diseases, or other signs indicating an unwholesome product (these are species-specific);

• Prevent contamination of the meat with lichen, hair, unclean hands or equipment, or, more important, with the contents of the digestive tract or urinary tract of the animal;

• Prevent possible bacterial contamination of the meat by conditions where the temperature and/or humidity are too high or in which the meat gets wet.

After field-dressing, it is critical that all game animals be cooled to a temperature of 35° to 40° F as soon as possible. If this does not occur, the game will likely spoil.

Some species of wild game, especially rabbits, are likely to carry disease bacteria, usually killed during the cooking process. Because of this, it is wise to wear gloves

| Nutritional Value of Common Sport Fish (3-ounce portions) | | | |
|---|---|---|---|
| | Calories | Fat (g) | Cholesterol (mg) |
| Bluefish | 105 | 3.6 | 50 |
| Carp | 138 | 6.1 | 71 |
| Catfish | 132 | 4.8 | 65 |
| Eel | 201 | 12.7 | 137 |
| Pike | 96 | 0.8 | 43 |
| Ocean Perch | 103 | 1.8 | 46 |
| Perch | 100 | 1.0 | 98 |
| Pompano | 179 | 10.3 | 54 |
| Red Snapper | 109 | 1.5 | 40 |
| Rockfish | 103 | 1.7 | 37 |
| Sea Bass | 105 | 2.2 | 45 |
| Shad (baked w/marg & bacon) | 171 | 9.6 | 59 |
| Smelt | 105 | 2.6 | 77 |
| Sole | 99 | 1.3 | 58 |
| Trout, Rainbow | 128 | 3.7 | 62 |

From: N-Squared Computing. Nutritionist 3, version 7.0 (nutrient analysis software). Silverton, Oregon: N-Squared Computing, 1991.

during both the field-dressing and the butchering processes and, after storing, while handling before cooking.

## Aging

Many species of wild game are improved by aging. This allows the enzymes in the meat to tenderize it, yielding a more pleasing, mouthwatering product.

Successful aging of game is dependent on proper conditions: ideally an elevation of at least 5,000 feet (a condition not always readily met), a temperature of no more than 40° F, and adequate ventilation. At lower elevations the higher humidity hastens spoilage. Higher temperatures encourage bacterial growth, which makes the food inedible. With inadequate ventilation the animal will not cool properly, thus enhancing spoilage.

Experts recommend leaving the skin on most game while aging it; retaining the hide helps retain moisture and prevents the formation of a thick layer of darkened, dried meat that must be removed later.

Among big-game species, elk contains a large amount of connective tissue. It can thus be aged for longer than other big game—as long as 14 days for a bull elk, 7 to 10 days for a female. Antelope contains the least connective tissue; it should be aged no longer than 3 days. Bear may be aged for 3 days to a week; deer is best in 7 to 10 days.

Hanging the meat while aging achieves additional tenderness, since the tissues stretch. Meat can also be aged after skinning and quartering by wrapping the sections in cloth and placing them in the refrigerator.

If no aging is planned, delay butchering until the carcass is completely cooled and the muscles are no longer contracted—usually 24 hours.

### Freezing Wild Game

| Type of Meat | Wrapping Method | Maximum Storage Months |
|---|---|---|
| Big Game Roasts | Standard butcher wrap | 10 |
| Big Game Steaks | Standard butcher wrap | 8 |
| Big Game Ribs | Foil wrap | 5 |
| Big Game Organs | Standard butcher wrap | 4 |
|  | Water pack | 6 |
| Big Game Chunks | Freezer bag and paper | 6 |
| Big Game Burger | Freezer bag and paper | 4 |
| Cut-up Small Game | Standard butcher wrap | 8 |
|  | Water pack | 12 |
| Small Game Organs | Water pack | 10 |
| Whole Large Birds | Foil wrap | 5 |
| Whole Small Birds | Standard butcher wrap | 6 |
|  | Water pack | 12 |
| Cut-up Upland Birds | Standard butcher wrap | 8 |
|  | Water pack | 12 |
| Cut-up Water Fowl | Standard butcher wrap | 8 |
|  | Water pack | 12 |
| Bird Giblets | Water pack | 4 |
| Game Stock | Freezer containers | 4 |

## Butchering

When butchering, be sure to remove all traces of shot from the animal; these could become unwelcome additions to your roast or stew. It is also advisable to remove the tissue around the area where the animal was shot, as it may be tough.

Label all pieces with species, cut, estimated age of animal, and date. All of these bits of data will influence your choice when you open your freezer. Older animals, due to their tougher texture and stronger flavor, lend themselves only to particular dishes, so it is wise to flag them. Remember, even wild game has a limited freezer life.

## Storing

Freezing is the most common storage method for wild game. Wrap the game tightly in freezer bags, freezer paper, butcher paper, or foil. One advantageous freezing method is to water-pack the game. This involves freezing the game in a water-filled plastic bag. Through this process the game is protected from exposure to air, which can cause freezer burn.

## Regulation

Virtually all game served in restaurants is produced on game farms, where the health and nutrition of the animal can be carefully monitored to ensure a wholesome product. In many states, it is illegal to sell hunted wild game to restaurants and grocery stores or to donate it to soup kitchens; state laws govern such matters. If in doubt, it pays to check with your state game agency.

The Food and Drug Administration (FDA) deals only with game that is transported between states, and then only if the game is adulterated or spoiled.

The U.S. Department of Agriculture (USDA) controls meat and poultry safety in the United States. It is responsible for inspecting farm-raised game animals if the animals or their products are transported over state lines. If the animals and their products remain in-state, then state laws and inspectors have jurisdiction. Many state laws require that any game used in commercial facilities be inspected by a licensed inspector before slaughter.  ◇

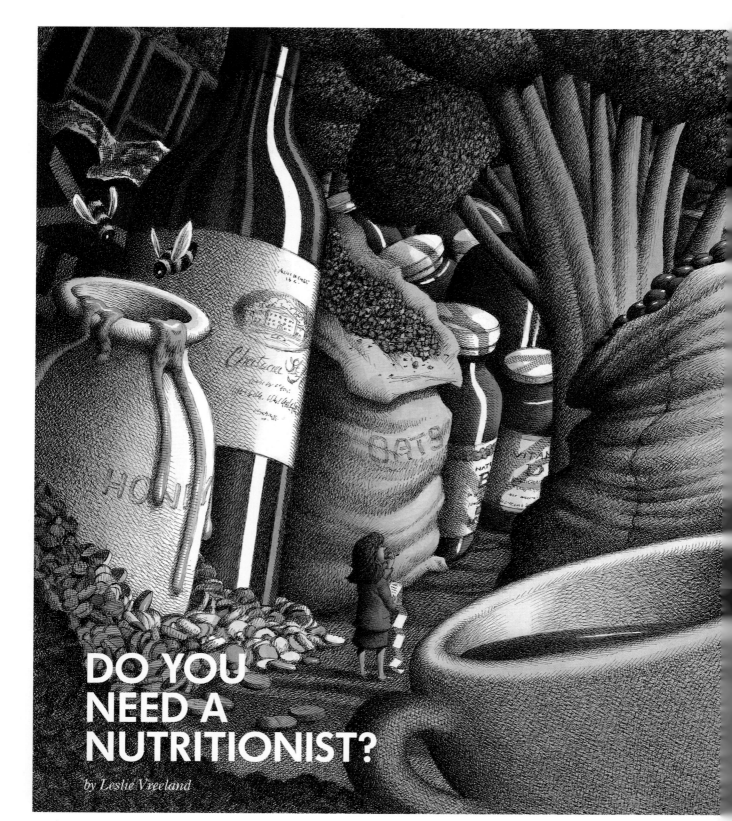

# DO YOU NEED A NUTRITIONIST?

*by Leslie Vreeland*

About two years ago, Pamela Berry, 29, who works in the human-resources department at Reebok in Boston, Massachusetts, signed up for a six-week, company-sponsored course in healthful eating. "I was overweight and sick of yo-yo dieting," says Berry. The nutritionist who taught the class helped her lose weight, most of which she's since kept off. Berry also learned to eat only when truly hungry, rather than when bored or depressed, and to splurge occasionally on sweets without feeling guilty. "The program was well worth the money," says Berry. "It changed the way I think about food."

It used to be that eating right was just a matter of common sense. But these days, many Americans feel they need in-depth knowledge of nutrition, not only to help them shed pounds, but also to keep up with the mounting scientific evidence that certain foods may cause or help prevent disease. Some look to the media for this information, others to their doctors. And more and more consumers are turning to nutritionists for dietary guidance.

Before you jump on the bandwagon, however, be warned: Because nutritionists aren't nearly as well regulated as physicians, psychologists, and other health professionals, there are lots of unqualified ones out there. They may make you believe you have a health problem when you don't; they may try to convince you that all your health problems are related to your diet; or they may even make you sicker. So make sure you choose a nutritionist carefully.

While picking a good nutritionist is essential, make sure you have a valid reason for seeing one in the first place. Who can benefit from dietary advice? If you have high blood pressure or high cholesterol, a nutritionist can tell you how to cut the sodium, fat, and cholesterol out of your diet. If you're genetically predisposed to illnesses such as cancer and osteoporosis, you might see a nutritionist to find out how to lower your risk by changing your eating habits. Or if you're a frustrated yo-yo dieter,

*More than ever, Americans are turning to nutritionists for guidance in planning their diets.*

a nutritionist can tailor a weight-loss plan to your needs. Finally, if you don't have any specific health problems, but do have a nagging desire to improve your diet, a nutritionist can give you practical advice on how to accomplish that goal.

**How Nutritionists Can't Help**
Unfortunately, many misguided people seek a nutritionist's advice with unrealistic expectations—from curing arthritis to boosting immunity. Don't expect a nutritionist to be able to treat the following conditions:

**Allergies.** Many people ascribe a host of health problems to suspected food allergens, but very few Americans actually have food allergies, says Victor Herbert, M.D., a professor of medicine and director of the nutrition center at Mount Sinai School of Medicine in New York City. In any case, if you think you're allergic to a certain food (or anything else), you should see a doctor who is a board-certified allergist, not a nutritionist.

Other people mistakenly believe that certain foods exacerbate allergies to other things, such as pollen, and they think a nutritionist can help them pinpoint the offending food. "That's pure hogwash," says H. James Wedner, M.D., chief of clinical allergy and immunology at Washington University School of Medicine in St. Louis, Missouri. There is no evidence suggesting that food is playing an aggravating role in allergic symptoms. And according to the National Institute of Allergy and Infectious Diseases, there have been no clinical studies showing that food can alleviate allergies either.

**Arthritis.** "We see many patients who claim that diet helps alleviate arthritis pain," says Cody Wasner, M.D., a rheumatologist and chairman of the unproven-treatments committee of the National Arthritis Foundation. "But there's no scientific evidence that it does. Arthritis comes and goes, and when it's worse, we're tempted to blame whatever we've been eating at the time."

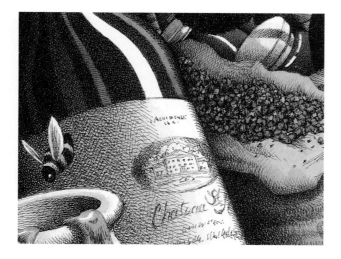

A nutritionist put Ron Weiner, a 50-year-old arthritis sufferer who lives in Great Neck, New York, on a "rotation" diet, which meant he had to eat different foods each day of the week. The nutritionist also prescribed 43 high-potency vitamin and mineral supplements a day. After three weeks, says Weiner, "I was vomiting, the room was spinning, and I never felt so bad in my life." He went off the diet and stopped taking the supplements; three days later, he felt fine. He never saw the nutritionist again.

**A Weak Immune System.** Some nutritionists recommend drinking acidophilus (a bacterium found in some yogurts) granules dissolved in lukewarm water to boost the immune system. "That sounds wonderfully seductive, but it's totally bogus," says Wasner. "Anyone who says diet can influence your immune system is moving in uncharted, unproven waters."

**Fatigue.** "If you feel worn-out or just want to feel 'better,' you should see your physician, not a nutritionist, because you might have a medical problem," warns Richard Rivlin, M.D., head of the clinical-nutrition research unit at Memorial Sloan-Kettering Cancer Center and New York Hospital in New York City.

**Hyperactivity.** Parents who believe certain foods—especially those high in sugar—cause hyperactivity in their children often seek a nutritionist's guidance. But scientists are skeptical that diet makes a difference. Studies show that sugar and artificial additives affect an extremely small number of children. If your child seems hyperactive, take him to your pediatrician.

If you think you have a good reason to seek dietary counseling, your next step may be to get a checkup from your doctor. Many conditions for which nutritional advice is needed, such as high blood pressure and osteoporosis, should be diagnosed by a physician, says Stephen Barrett, M.D., a board member of the National Council Against Health Fraud (NCAHF) in Loma Linda, California. Even if you don't have a specific health problem, you might want to let your physician know that you'll be seeing a nutritionist.

Your doctor may not, however, be a very good source of nutrition advice. "People are going to doctors for dietary guidance, but many of them, including my own, don't know a thing about nutrition," says Stephen Schiaffino, executive officer of the American Society for Clinical Nutrition in Bethesda, Maryland. According to Schiaffino, only about 30 of the 126 medical schools in the United States have programs in clinical nutrition. Also steer clear of psychiatrists, psychologists, chiropractors, and other health professionals who dispense nutrition advice without sufficient training in the field.

*People who think they're allergic to certain foods should see a doctor, not a nutritionist.*

### Choosing a Nutritionist

Your best bet is to see a registered dietitian (R.D.), a title established by the American Dietetic Association (ADA), or someone with a master's degree or doctorate who has training and experience in clinical nutrition, says Johanna Dwyer, M.D., director of the Frances Stern Nutrition Center at New England Medical Center in Boston, Massachusetts. To become an R.D., applicants must complete an ADA-approved program at an accredited university; they must also perform 900 hours of supervised training and pass an exam. R.D.s also take continuing-education classes to keep up with new developments in the field. To find an R.D. in your area, ask your physician for a recommendation, or call

## Can You Afford a Nutritionist?

The cost of one-on-one nutrition counseling depends on whom you see and where you live: Fees range from $50 to more than $200 an hour. How often you go also varies greatly. Some nutritionists, such as Boston-based registered dietitian (R.D.) Nancy Clark, meet with clients infrequently. "Initially, I see my patients two or three times," she says. "Then they check in anywhere from twice a month to once a year." On the other hand, one non-R.D. nutritionist said her clients are "well on their way to good eating" after about 14 sessions —at which point they will have spent about $1,300, excluding the cost of vitamin supplements. Expenses are covered by health insurance only when there's a serious medical problem—if, say, a physician sends a cancer patient to a nutritionist because the patient needs help maintaining weight.

the ADA at 800-366-1655. To verify a nutritionist's R.D. credentials, call 312-899-0040.

Physicians and Ph.D.s who are certified by the American Board of Nutrition (ABN) in Bethesda are also recommended, says Barrett. Once you've found a qualified nutritionist, make sure he or she doesn't just hand you a stack of impersonal pamphlets, but is willing to tailor his or her advice to your needs —otherwise, you may never put all that sound advice into practice.

Warns Mount Sinai's Herbert: "Thousands of so-called nutritionists have phony credentials and are promoters of nutritional fraud." The problem is, there are few regulatory checks on nutritionists' training or the advice they give. In most states, anyone can declare himself (or herself) a nutritionist, hang out a shingle, and start peddling advice. Only 17 states* (plus the District of Columbia and Puerto Rico) require dietary advisers to be "licensed," which means they have to meet requirements similar to those set forth by the

ADA for R.D.s. Licensing is supposedly the strictest form of regulation on dietary advice, but states' requirements for licensure vary, as does the extent to which states enforce the law. Nine other states** require nutritionists who call themselves "certified" to meet certain professional standards (these vary from state to state). But certification is voluntary, and noncertified nutritionists are free to practice, too. In California, nutritionists may be "registered"—which is less restrictive than "licensed" or "certified"—but nonregistered nutritionists may also practice. In the remaining states, nutritionists aren't regulated at all.

Given how poorly they're policed, it's no surprise that some nutritionists get their qualifications from correspondence schools. To prove how easy it is to get a certificate from these schools, Herbert got one for both his cat, Charlie Herbert, and his poodle, Sassafras Herbert.

Consumers who receive advice that actually harms their health have little recourse. They can sue for malpractice, but that route is expensive and its outcome uncertain. In states where nutritionists are required to be licensed, the authorities may revoke the nutritionist's right to practice. (To find out which government agency, if any, oversees nutritionists in your state, call the ADA's Office of Government Affairs at 202-371-0500.) But according to William Jarvis, M.D., president of the NCAHF and a professor of public health and preventive medicine at Loma Linda University School of Medicine in California, "if you try to go after a bad nutritionist, you're unlikely to get much satisfaction." It all adds up to this: Choose a nutritionist carefully at the outset, and you'll save yourself pounds of cure later on. ◇

---

*These states require nutritionists to be licensed before they can practice: Alabama, Arkansas, Florida, Illinois, Iowa, Kansas, Louisiana, Maine, Maryland, Montana, New Mexico, North Carolina, North Dakota, Ohio, Oklahoma, Rhode Island, and Tennessee.

**These states require nutritionists who call themselves "certified" to meet certain professional standards before they can practice: Georgia, Kentucky, Mississippi, Nebraska, New York, Oregon, Texas, Utah, and Washington.

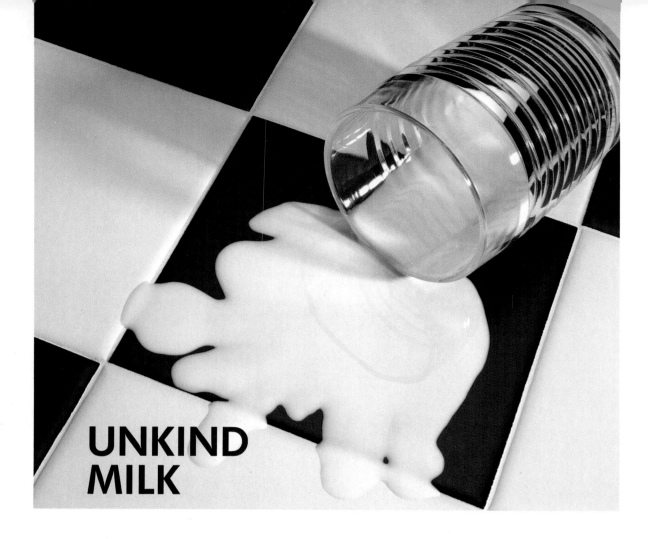

# UNKIND MILK

*by Colleen Sauber*

For some people, "Come on, I'll treat you to an ice cream cone" has an ominous ring. The problem is that ice cream, like most dairy products, is rich in *lactose,* a large milk sugar not usable by the body until that sugar has been cleaved in two. For about four out of five white Americans, an enzyme called *lactase* neatly accomplishes this task. For the rest an encounter with a scoop of

*The lactase-deficient have difficulty digesting milk and other foods containing lactose. Such people might even become distressed after eating a peanut butter cookie.*

Cherry Garcia ice cream can mean hours of abdominal cramping, gas, and diarrhea.

When people don't have enough lactase to split the lactose into its component sugars, glucose and galactose, the intact molecule travels through the stomach and small intestine to reach the colon. There bacteria ferment it into a brew of small fatty acids, hydrogen, carbon dioxide, and methane. The unfortunate person's gut retains water and sodium, which, in combination with the carbon dioxide and other gases, produces the disorder's characteristic miseries.

## It's in the Genes

At birth, humans and other mammals manufacture lactase in the lining of the small intestine. This enzyme enables babies to digest their mothers' milk, and less lactose is produced once the babies are weaned and switch to a more adult diet. Throughout much of the world, lactase levels in humans begin to decline between the ages of 2 and 7. By the time most people are teenagers or young adults, they make about 10 percent as much lactase as they did in their infancy. Levels of the enzyme then stabilize for the remainder of their lives.

This gradual fall in lactase levels is perfectly normal. It doesn't interfere with the body's ability to use the proteins, vitamins, and other essential nutrients found in dairy products. Nor does it constitute an allergy to milk proteins, which is a different problem.

About 10,000 years ago, according to scientists' best guess, a genetic mutation occurred among the populations of northern and central Europe that had learned to herd dairy animals and thus had come to depend upon milk products for much of their diet. This new development allowed about 80 percent of these people and their descendants to produce ample amounts of lactase into adulthood, making them an exception to the human rule. Lactose intolerance is a very common condition among other ethnic groups; for example, milk disagrees with about 50 percent of all adult Hispanics, and with at least 75 percent of people of African, Asian, or Native American descent.

Some people have trouble digesting lactose, not because they were genetically programmed to stop producing lactase, but because some other disease or event has damaged the small intestine's lining, where the enzyme is normally made. This *secondary lactase deficiency* may be caused by parasitic infection or by illnesses including viral gastroenteritis, Crohn's disease, or celiac disease. Secondary lactase deficiency may also be part of a broader malabsorption syndrome brought on by therapeutic measures—for example, surgery, radiation, or treatment with medications such as broad-spectrum antibiotics, colchicine (used for gout), or the antiarrhythmia drug quinidine. Once the initial condition has cleared up or the treatment has ended, the person's small intestine may regain its normal ability to produce adequate amounts of lactase.

## Testing the Tract

Opinions differ on whether lactose intolerance is a problem that warrants an official workup by a physician. Do-it-yourself diagnosis is neither difficult nor uncommon: A person can drink a glass or two of skim milk in the morning, on an empty stomach, and then monitor symptoms for two to four hours. If bloating, gas, and diarrhea occur, lactase deficiency is probably to blame.

When physicians suspect lactose intolerance, they often use one of two tests to confirm the diagnosis. In the *breath hydrogen test,* a person who has fasted overnight consumes 50 grams of lactose mixed with water (this is the amount in about a quart of milk). Over the next two to four hours, the person exhales into a container at intervals, and technicians measure the amount of hydrogen in the expired air. Whereas normal digestion does not produce measurable amounts of this gas, fermentation of lactose yields an ample supply.

A slightly more invasive assay, the *lactose-tolerance test,* also begins with ingesting 50 grams of lactose. A technician draws blood several times over the next one to two hours, and monitors serum-glucose levels. Glucose rises if the individual has enough lactase to

*About 20 percent of Americans experience great distress if they eat foods rich in lactose.*

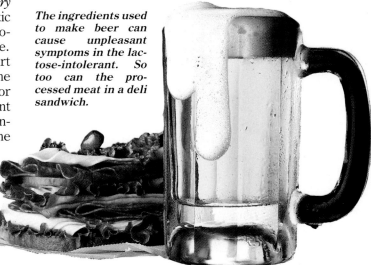

*The ingredients used to make beer can cause unpleasant symptoms in the lactose-intolerant. So too can the processed meat in a deli sandwich.*

break lactose into its component sugars; a static glucose level signifies an enzyme deficiency.

Low lactase is almost always confirmed using one of these methods. Only rarely will physicians use a more expensive and invasive test, an intestinal biopsy, to rule out other explanations. "I biopsy only when it's a case such as someone 35 to 40 years old who develops lactose intolerance, never having had it before," says Theodore Bayless, M.D., director of clinical gastroenterology at Johns Hopkins Hospital in Baltimore, Maryland.

Another option is to measure acidity and glucose levels in stool, but most physicians don't put much stock in this approach because it is less accurate than methods that test breath or blood.

### Manageable, but No Magic
Once lactase deficiency has been diagnosed, just what is required to manage it varies according to how much of the enzyme a person makes. Many people find that by exercising certain cautions, they can continue to enjoy milk products. They minimize symptoms by consuming small amounts of such foods at different times of day (instead of chugging two glasses of milk at a single sitting), always eating something else along with dairy

products, substituting certain low-lactose foods for lactose-rich ones, and using lactase drops or tablets.

The amount of lactose consumed at one time makes a big difference. When tested following an overnight fast, about 25 percent of lactose-intolerant people develop symptoms after drinking one glass of milk, 50 percent suffer after two glasses, and 75 percent will be downright miserable if they gulp down a whole quart.

Most people don't have any desire to drink the entire carton. And for the majority, having one glass of milk (about 12.5 grams of

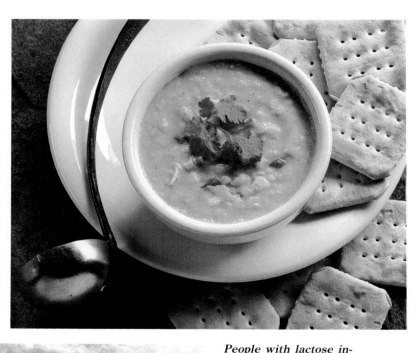

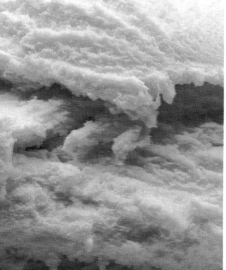

*People with lactose intolerance should beware of creamy-looking soups. Bread and bread-coated meat and poultry have been known to trigger a reaction in people sensitive to lactose.*

lactose) along with a meal will produce little or no discomfort. The other foodstuffs consumed during the meal indirectly promote digestion of lactose by slowing its passage through the small intestine, giving the lactase on hand more time to act. "Digestion of a glass of milk is three times better with a meal than when taken alone," says researcher Dennis A. Savaiano, Ph.D., professor of food science and nutrition at the University of Minnesota.

Even tiny amounts of lactose can be the undoing of people whose bodies produce little or no lactase. They can be made miserable by the hidden presence of whey, casein, milk solids, and other lactose-containing derivatives of milk that are often added to drugs and nondairy foods. These people should scrutinize food labels and check with the pharmacist about lactose in medications.

### Choose Your Poison

Many people who would be in agony after drinking milk or putting sour cream on a baked potato find that they can tolerate other dairy products much better. Among these are naturally aged hard cheeses such as Swiss or cheddar, which contain hardly any lactose. The trade-off is that more than half the calories in these cheeses come from fats.

*Even a tiny amount of lactose can trigger a reaction in sensitive people.*

For health-conscious people, low-fat or nonfat yogurt offers a better alternative. Yogurt manufacture requires the addition of bacterial cultures that produce beta galactosidase, an enzyme that breaks down 30 to 40 percent of the lactose present prior to fermentation. If these cultures are alive when the yogurt is eaten, the enzymes they contribute to the digestive tract can help break down lactose consumed at the same time.

All yogurts are not created equal, however: Some are heated after fermentation, which kills the beneficial bacteria; others contain added milk solids, which can trigger symptoms instead of preventing them. The only way to be sure is to read labels carefully.

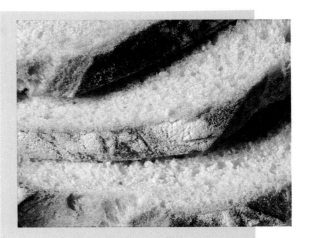

## Hidden Offenders

Check labels carefully to determine whether products contain milk or milk by-products such as sodium caseinate, whey, nonfat dry milk solids, or lactalbumin. Lactose is found in medications and in a wide range of seemingly unlikely foods. In addition to obvious villains like ice cream and cream sauces, potential offenders include the following foods:

**Beverages:** cordials, liqueurs, beer, instant coffee, breakfast drinks; drinks prepared with malted-milk powder, chocolate, or cocoa.

**Grain products:** bread, cereal, crackers, pancakes, waffles, packaged baking mixes.

**Desserts:** cake, cookies, piecrust, pie filling, custard, pudding, sherbet, frozen yogurt, butterscotch, caramels, chocolate candies, toffee.

**Meats and fish:** breaded fish, poultry, or meats; processed meats (kosher meats contain no milk products).

**Vegetables:** frozen vegetables with sauce, instant potatoes.

**Miscellaneous:** artificial sweeteners, gravy, margarine, molasses, dietetic and diabetic products, salad dressings, soups, spice blends, prescription and over-the-counter medications such as oral contraceptives and antacids.

The best bet is to look for the "Live and Active Cultures" seal affixed to products that contain at least 10 million live bacteria per gram at the time of sale.

### Mother's Little Helpers

Lactose-reduced milks and lactase supplements increase the cost of dairy foods, in some cases doubling the price, and in others adding only a few cents per serving. But the cost notwithstanding, many people who are troubled by intolerance find these products are well worth the money, especially considering the unpleasant alternative.

Many grocery stores now carry lactase-treated nonfat and low-fat milks that contain 70 percent less lactose than does regular milk. Studies indicate that such milk is as effective as yogurt in preventing symptoms of intolerance.

Many people also use lactase supplements —nonprescription liquids or pills that contain bacterial or yeast beta galactosidase. Mixing lactase drops with milk can cut its lactose level by 70 to 97 percent, which is a greater

*Foods especially formulated with low levels of lactose as well as nonprescription lactase supplements help many people avoid unpleasant symptoms when they consume dairy foods.*

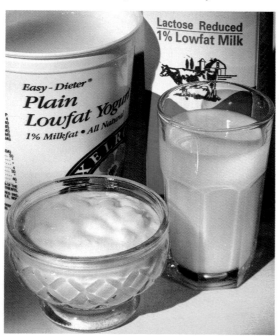

reduction than most adults need to prevent indigestion. This method isn't always convenient, though, since the milk must sit for 24 hours before being consumed. Tablets are designed for use immediately before eating dairy products.

Such aids aren't necessary for everyone who is short of lactase. One study reports that when it comes to promoting lactose digestion, the microbial lactase in yogurt is superior to that in commercial enzyme supplements.

### Bugs in Training?

Certain bacteria that normally flourish in the colon produce enzymes that can break down the hard-to-absorb lactose, and some scientists believe that a systematic feeding program can boost their ability to do this. If they are given lactose routinely, the colonic bacteria "learn" to digest it. According to Dr. Savaiano, "Bacterial lactase increases sixfold if people eat lactose, and it decreases sixfold if they do not." He hypothesizes that if milk is consumed daily and the amount is gradually increased, these bacteria will increase their ability to thrive in a lactose-rich environment and to break this large molecule into smaller, less troublesome sugars.

There is no clear proof that this happens, Dr. Bayless says, but it is reasonable to think that slowly increasing the amount of milk people drink could improve their ability to digest lactose. Lactase-deficient individuals who want to give this a try could start by drinking a small glass of milk with one meal each day. They would probably feel at least some discomfort at first, but that likely would lessen with time.

Most physicians don't want to see people with lactose intolerance give up dairy products entirely. Besides supplying protein and vitamins, dairy foods provide about 75 percent of the calcium in the American diet. Calcium is especially important for women during pregnancy and lactation—and after menopause, when the risk for developing osteoporosis rises.

Lactose-intolerant people who eliminate dairy foods must manage their eating habits carefully to compensate for the lack of calcium and other essential nutrients. ◇

# ACCENT ON ANTIOXIDANTS

*by Maria Guglielmino, M.S., R.D.*

In the ever-continuing quest for the fountain of youth, health-conscious adults and nutrition experts alike are hailing the antioxidant nutrients—vitamins E and C and beta-carotene—as antidotes to the ravaging effects of cellular aging. Acting as benevolent crusaders, antioxidants fight to neutralize free radicals, the biological terrorists implicated in such chronic degenerative disorders as cancer and heart disease. While scientific proof of the preventive or curative potential of antioxidants is just now becoming available, debate still rages concerning the best way to consume enough of these nutrients to experience their potential benefits.

### The Price We Pay for Breathing

The body converts about 5 percent of inhaled oxygen into free radicals. A free radical is a molecule with an unpaired electron, a condition that gives the molecule an electrical charge. In an attempt to neutralize its electric charge, a free radical constantly tries to steal an electron away from, or give up its own electron to, a nearby molecule, such as a protein. Often a free radical will set off a domino effect as nearby molecules continue to steal and donate electrons. As a result, formerly stable compounds become "oxidized"; that is, they become highly volatile radicals that can damage any neighboring molecule.

This process of oxidation can be destructive in the human body—cell walls can be damaged or DNA may be altered, for instance—causing mutations that may lead to cancer. Research has found a link between free-radical damage and chronic diseases associated with aging, including heart disease, cancer, cataracts, adult-onset diabetes, and Parkinson's disease. Free-radical damage may even be at the heart of the degenerative changes that occur in the aging process.

Oxygen also reacts with certain metals, such as iron and copper, to form free radicals. A recent Finnish study found that men with high levels of ferritin (an iron-storing protein) were more likely to experience heart attacks. The study results suggest that low-density lipoprotein (LDL), the so-called "bad" cholesterol, becomes oxidized when it reacts with iron and oxygen. It is this oxidized form of LDL that appears to cause the plaque to form in the arteries, a condition that can lead to heart attacks. Other recent studies support the theory that it is only oxidized LDL that initiates the atherosclerotic process, or hardening of the arteries, that leads to coronary-artery disease.

### A Necessary Evil

While free radicals have earned a bad reputation in the media, the truth is that we could not live without them. As by-products of normal metabolism, free radicals are essential for certain functions, such as fighting off infection or breaking down food. Moreover, the human body has many protective mechanisms that normally check free-radical destruction in cells.

A multitude of different enzymes in the body function as antioxidants, neutralizing free radicals before they can cause damage. Superoxide dismutase, for example, sponges up dangerous superoxide radicals and metabolizes them into hydrogen peroxide. The body's arsenal against free radicals is reinforced by the antioxidant vitamins. Soluble in water, vitamin C merges with free radicals so that they are eventually excreted in the urine. Vitamin E and beta-carotene work in the fatty cellular membranes, soaking up free radicals, thus preventing damage to the cell walls.

*Antioxidant nutrients like vitamins C and E and beta carotene act as antidotes to the ravaging effects of cellular aging.*

Unfortunately, the body's protective mechanisms become overwhelmed by aging, as well as by certain habits and environmental conditions that increase the body's production of free radicals. Exposure to cigarette smoke, sunlight, X rays, cosmic radiation from air travel, ozone, and environmental pollutants heightens the output of free radicals, causing what is called oxidative stress. Even exercise increases oxidative stress, although individuals who exercise regularly become very efficient at neutralizing free

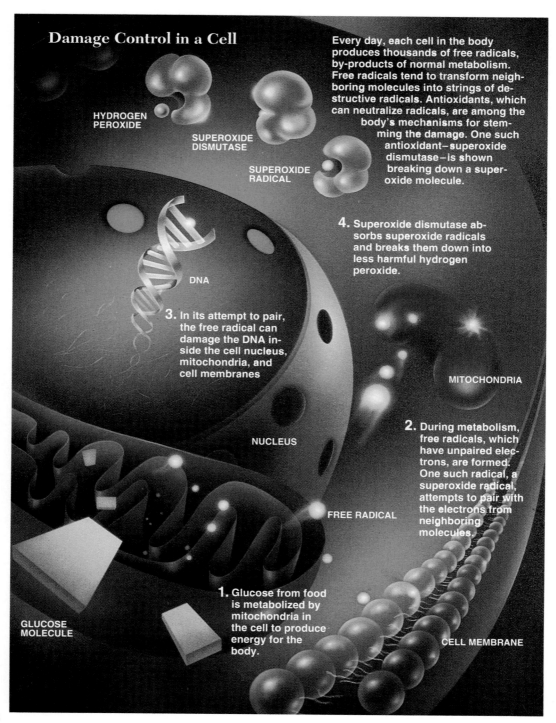

**Damage Control in a Cell**

Every day, each cell in the body produces thousands of free radicals, by-products of normal metabolism. Free radicals tend to transform neighboring molecules into strings of destructive radicals. Antioxidants, which can neutralize radicals, are among the body's mechanisms for stemming the damage. One such antioxidant—superoxide dismutase—is shown breaking down a superoxide molecule.

HYDROGEN PEROXIDE

SUPEROXIDE DISMUTASE

SUPEROXIDE RADICAL

**4.** Superoxide dismutase absorbs superoxide radicals and breaks them down into less harmful hydrogen peroxide.

DNA

**3.** In its attempt to pair, the free radical can damage the DNA inside the cell nucleus, mitochondria, and cell membranes

MITOCHONDRIA

NUCLEUS

**2.** During metabolism, free radicals, which have unpaired electrons, are formed. One such radical, a superoxide radical, attempts to pair with the electrons from neighboring molecules.

FREE RADICAL

**1.** Glucose from food is metabolized by mitochondria in the cell to produce energy for the body.

GLUCOSE MOLECULE

CELL MEMBRANE

radicals. In contrast, weekend warriors may just be increasing oxidative damage, since they are not fit enough to counteract the extra free radicals produced during exercise.

### The Supplemental Question

Many experts are convinced that excessive free-radical damage can be counteracted by consuming foods high in antioxidants, such as leafy green vegetables, carrots, and citrus fruits. Others recommend that vitamin supplements are necessary to augment the antioxidant vitamins in food.

"The weight of the scientific evidence substantiates that diets that are high in fruits and vegetables are associated with a reduced risk for cancer and heart disease," says Catherine Woteki, Ph.D., director of the Food and Nutrition Board of the National Academy of Sciences (NAS). "My recommendation and the recommendation of the Food and Nutrition Board's publication, *Diet and Health,* is to eat a diet that contains five servings or more of fruits and vegetables per day." Though fruits and vegetables are not rich sources of vitamin E, Dr. Woteki does not recommend supplementing with vitamin E.

Dr. Woteki and other nutrition experts have legitimate concerns about supplementation. For one, it is likely that some people will rely on taking vitamins rather than eating fruits and vegetables. In so doing, they will miss out on other vitamins and minerals, fiber, phytochemicals, and other carotenoids, all of which have health benefits. In addition, interactions of antioxidant nutrients with drugs and with other nutrients need to be examined more closely. Some believe that more research needs to be conducted before effective doses can be determined.

Advocates for supplementation argue that antioxidant supplements should be taken as added insurance in addition to a healthful diet. Says Jeffrey Blumberg, Ph.D., associate director of the U.S. Department of Agriculture's Human Nutrition Research Center on Aging at Tufts University in Boston: "I think that rational supplementation represents a proactive, positive health behavior that we can encourage people to engage in." He warns that "supplements are not magic bullets. You can't take supplements and still eat

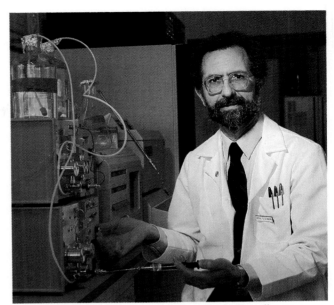

*Vitamin supplements are not "magic bullets." Dr. Jeffrey Blumberg (above) warns that vitamin supplements do little good for an individual who subsists on a high-fat, low-fiber diet.*

a high-fat, low-fiber diet and think that supplements will do you good."

Those in agreement with Dr. Blumberg point out that, while it would be ideal if Americans ate five to nine servings of fruits and vegetables per day, the reality is that only 9 percent of the population is eating even five servings. Supplements might help people who are not committed to improving their diets, and as added insurance for those who already eat a high-fiber, low-fat diet.

Despite this controversy, many Americans are already taking supplements of the antioxidants, choosing not to wait for a definitive recommendation from the NAS, the federal institution that sets the recommended dietary allowances (RDAs) for nutrients. Consumers seem to be flocking in droves to pharmacies and health-food stores for antioxidant supplements. In the United States, 1992 sales of vitamin E alone were over $338 million. Hoping to ride this wave, pharmaceutical companies are manufacturing single capsules that provide beta-carotene, vitamin C, and vitamin E—the "big three" antioxidants.

### Beta-Carotene

Beta-carotene, a compound naturally occurring in dark-green leafy vegetables and deep-orange fruits and vegetables, is converted by the body into vitamin A as needed. While megadoses of vitamin A are toxic and

# Food Sources of the Antioxidants

| FOOD | SERVING | | BETA CAROTENE (milligrams) |
|---|---|---|---|
| Sweet potatoes | ½ | cup mashed | 14 |
| Sweet potatoes | 1 | medium baked | 10 |
| Spinach | 1 | cup cooked | 10 |
| Collard greens | 1 | cup cooked | 7 |
| Carrots | 1 | medium, raw | 6 |
| Kale | 1 | cup cooked | 6 |
| Apricots | 10 | dried | 6 |
| Peaches | 5 | halves, dried | 6 |
| Canteloupe | 1 | cup pieces | 5 |
| Apricots | 3 | medium, fresh | 4 |
| Mustard greens | 1 | cup cooked | 4 |
| Pumpkin | ½ | cup cooked, mashed | 4 |
| Beet greens | 1 | cup cooked | 4 |
| Winter squash | ½ | cup cooked, mashed | 3 |
| Broccoli | 1 | cup cooked | 2 |
| Parsley | ½ | cup, chopped | 1.6 |
| Mango | ½ | medium | 1.3 |
| Romaine lettuce | 1 | cup, shredded | 1 |

| FOOD | SERVING | | VITAMIN C (milligrams) |
|---|---|---|---|
| Chili peppers (green or red) | 1 | pepper | 109 |
| Strawberries | 1 | cup | 85 |
| Orange, navel | 1 | medium | 80 |
| Kiwifruit | 1 | medium | 75 |
| Orange juice | 6 | ounces | 72 |
| Canteloupe | 1 | cup pieces | 68 |
| Green pepper, raw | ½ | cup | 64 |
| Broccoli, boiled | ½ | cup | 49 |
| Brussels sprouts, boiled | ½ | cup | 48 |
| Grapefruit, white | ½ | medium | 39 |
| Kumquats, raw | 5 | medium | 35 |
| Cauliflower, boiled | ½ | cup | 34 |
| Sweet potato, boiled | ½ | cup, mashed | 28 |
| Parsley, raw | ½ | cup, chopped | 27 |
| Tangerine | 1 | medium | 26 |
| Honeydew melon | ¼ | small | 23 |
| Tomato, raw | 1 | medium | 22 |
| Potato, white, baked, without skin | 1 | medium | 20 |
| Cabbage, boiled | ½ | cup | 18 |

| FOOD | SERVING | | VITAMIN E (international units) |
|---|---|---|---|
| Total wheat cereal | 1 | ounce | 45 |
| Product 19 | 1 | ounce | 45 |
| Wheat germ oil | 1 | tablespoon | 39 |
| Sunflower seeds | ¼ | cup | 24 |
| Filberts | ¼ | cup | 12 |
| Wheat germ, toasted | ¼ | cup | 11 |
| Nutrigrain wheat cereal | 1 | ounce | 11 |
| Abalone | 3 | ounces | 10 |
| Sunflower oil | 1 | tablespoon | 10 |
| Sweet potato, baked | 1 | medium | 8 |
| Safflower oil | 1 | tablespoon | 7 |
| Mayonnaise | 1 | tablespoon | 6 |
| Margarine spread, light | 1 | tablespoon | 5 |
| Avocado | 1 | medium | 4 |
| Escargots | 6 | | 4 |
| Turkey liver | 3 | ounces | 4 |
| Corn oil | 1 | tablespoon | 4 |
| Peanuts | ¼ | cup | 4 |

can lead to liver damage and other medical problems, high intakes of beta-carotene are not harmful. Studies have linked diets rich in beta-carotene with a reduced risk of stroke, heart attacks, and cataracts. A growing body of evidence indicates that beta-carotene may also boost the immune system, possibly by enhancing the number of natural killer cells that fight disease.

During the past decade, epidemiological studies have associated a high intake of foods that are rich sources of beta-carotene with a lowered risk of lung cancer, oral cancers, gastrointestinal cancer, and cervical cancer. In clinical trials, researchers at the University of Arizona Cancer Center in Tucson found that 30 milligrams (mg) of supplemental beta-carotene given daily for three to six months significantly reduced precancerous mouth lesions in 70 percent of the subjects.

Although the mechanism is not completely understood, researchers believe that beta-carotene and the other antioxidant vitamins prevent LDL cholesterol from being oxidized, thus averting plaque formation in the arteries. Results from the Harvard Nurses' Health Study, which followed over 87,000 female nurses, reveal that women who consumed more than 15 to 20 mg of beta-carotene per day lowered their risk of stroke by 40 percent, and of heart attacks by 22 percent, compared with those subjects who ate less than 6 mg per day.

Currently, there is no established RDA for beta-carotene. Results of ongoing clinical studies may help nutrition scientists determine how much beta-carotene is needed daily for protective effects. According to Dr. Blumberg, preliminary research has shown that intakes of beta-carotene from diet, or from supplements of between 6 and 30 mg, provide beneficial effects. By eating three to five servings of vegetables and two to four servings of fruits per day, it is possible to obtain these levels of beta-carotene—as long as the foods that are chosen are rich in beta-carotene, such as sweet potatoes, carrots, or spinach. Relying on food sources rather than supplements has the added benefit of adding fiber, other carotenoids, and a host of other nutrients that may work together with antioxidant vitamins to fight disease.

## Vitamin C

Current research indicates that vitamin C may very well be a preventative for certain debilitating diseases. Chemically known as ascorbic acid, vitamin C is normally present in the eye in large quantities in direct proportion to how much is consumed. As a result, vitamin C holds promise for preventing cataracts, the leading cause of blindness in the elderly. Vitamin C fights oxidative damage, especially that caused by exposure to ultraviolet light, thus preventing the changes in proteins that are the hallmarks of cataract development. Allen Taylor, Ph.D., director of the Laboratory for Nutrition and Vision Research at the USDA Human Nutrition Research Center at Tufts University, found that guinea pigs fed supplemental vitamin C had less lens damage from ultraviolet light than animals fed diets without supplementation. Dr. Taylor found similar results in humans when they receive 2 grams of supplemental vitamin C per day. The National Institutes of Health (NIH) has begun a long-term study on cataract formation in humans to corroborate these findings.

There is also mounting evidence that vitamin C guards against cancer. A 1992 review of nearly 100 studies by Gladys Block, Ph.D., professor of nutrition at the University of California at Berkeley, reveals a strong association between vitamin C intake and reduced risk for cancers of the stomach, throat, mouth, and pancreas. Vitamin C appears to inhibit formation of nitrosamine, a powerful carcinogen, in the stomach. Dr. Block's review reveals that vitamin C also provides some protection against cancers of the lung, cervix, rectum, and breast.

Ascorbic acid's antioxidant properties work in the heart as well, lowering the risk for hardening of the arteries. Research suggests that high blood levels of vitamin C block free radicals, preventing oxidative damage to LDL cholesterol and raising levels of HDL, the "good" cholesterol that carries cholesterol to the liver for excretion. A major study of over 11,000 adults published in *Epidemiology* reveals a significant association between high intakes of vitamin C from diet and/or supplements and a reduction in cardiovascular mortality.

The current RDA for vitamin C is 60 mg for nonsmokers and at least 100 mg per day for smokers, who typically have low blood levels of this vitamin.

Current research indicates, however, that the present RDA is not sufficient for disease prevention. According to Dr. Blumberg, preliminary research indicates that daily intakes of 250 to 1,000 milligrams of vitamin C are needed to provide protective effects against diseases. It is possible that the RDA for vitamin C may be increased, depending upon the Food and Nutrition Board's decision on the fate of the RDAs, due sometime in 1994.

In the meantime the best prescription for obtaining vitamin C's disease-preventing properties is to eat a minimum of five fruits and vegetables per day. Good sources include citrus fruits and juices, cantaloupe, strawberries, peppers, and broccoli. Just one medium orange and 1 cup of broccoli provide approximately 180 mg of vitamin C.

### Vitamin E

Hailed by food faddists for years as a panacea for a variety of problems, vitamin E has recently gained recognition in the scientific community as its powerful antioxidant properties have become increasingly apparent. Research indicates that vitamin E reduces the risk of cancer, may prevent heart attacks and cataracts, and lessens the symptoms of Parkinson's disease. Moreover, vitamin E helps fight disease progression by strengthening the immune system.

An *American Journal of Epidemiology* study reveals that the risk for oral cancer was reduced by 50 percent in individuals who took vitamin E supplements compared to those who did not. However, since many of the subjects took other vitamin supplements in addition to vitamin E, the investigators acknowledged that the protective effect may have resulted from a combination of vitamins. The results of another recent investigation published in the *Journal of the National Cancer Institute* in December 1993 revealed that vitamin E reduced the risk of esophageal and oral cancer.

Like vitamin C, vitamin E can prevent formation of nitrosamines in the stomach. Since this vitamin is fat-soluble, it can still do the job even when nitrites or nitrates enter the stomach in high-fat foods. Vitamin E's ability to strengthen immunity provides additional armor against carcinogens.

Two large *New England Journal of Medicine* studies have added convincing evidence that vitamin E guards against heart disease. Harvard researchers following 87,000 female nurses in one investigation and 45,000 male health professionals in another found that daily supplements of 100 international units (I.U.) or more of vitamin E taken for at least two years was correlated with a 40 percent reduction in coronary-artery disease.

Most of the research with vitamin E has shown beneficial effects with 100 to 1,200 I.U. daily. While the RDA for vitamin E is 30 I.U., Dr. Blumberg recommends daily levels between 100 to 400 I.U. Most Americans do not meet the RDA for vitamin E, averaging less than 10 I.U. per day when they rely on food alone. Unlike vitamin C and beta-carotene, it is almost impossible to take in protective levels of vitamin E without taking in significant quantities of fat and calories. Most of the richest sources of vitamin E are high-fat foods such as vegetable oils, wheat germ, and nuts.

*Research suggests that vitamin C may help prevent cataracts, guard against cancer, and lower the risk of developing hardening of the arteries.*

People have been taking vitamin E supplements for years without any observable side effects. There have been anecdotal reports of problems, such as nausea and headaches, among individuals taking large doses (around 800 I.U. per day). Individuals choosing to take supplemental vitamin E before waiting for public-health recommendations should be cautious. Moderate supplementation, 100 I.U. per day, appears to be safe. However, people who take anticoagulants should not take high doses of supplemental vitamin E, since it could cause bleeding. Until well-controlled studies are conducted with people taking vitamin E over long periods, it is impossible to predict whether large doses are safe for everyone.◇

# Caffeine: The Hidden Ingredient

*by Alice Naude*

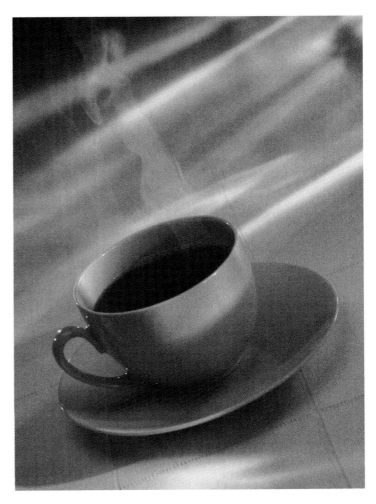

Coffee drinking has evolved into something of a cultural institution in the United States, and indeed all over the world. Millions of people routinely start their day with a cup of coffee, end dinner with a cup of coffee, and have a few cups in between. Part of the pleasure of a cup of coffee is the little "pick-me-up" it gives its drinker, a little burst of energy that leaves a person feeling better after the coffee than before. That little lift comes from caffeine, a mild stimulant that occurs naturally in coffee. In recent years, however, caffeine has come under fire as having potentially harmful effects on health. And though as yet no health risks from caffeine have been irrefutably proven, the negative publicity surrounding caffeine has created something of a siege mentality among diehard coffee drinkers, who see their favorite repast as a final outpost of self-indulgence, especially now that alcohol, cigarettes, fats, and sugars are all but proscribed in the name of good health.

As is the case with many substances that *might* be harmful, many people would rather just avoid caffeine than risk developing a health problem months or years down the road. This tendency has opened up new markets for products that are decaffeinated or caffeine-free. Today almost every restaurant in the United States offers decaffeinated coffee (and tea), and many upscale establishments even have decaf espresso and cappuccino on their menus. But life without caffeine entails more than just decaf coffee and tea. Americans consume an enormous amount of caffeine, often without even knowing it. Many soft drinks, over-the-counter painkillers, and diet aids, and even chocolate contain caffeine in varying concentrations. Many people panic just realizing how much caffeine they incidentally consume in the course of a day or week. This panic is usually unfounded, given that nothing about caffeine is explicitly harmful.

## Caffeine and the Body

At one time or another, caffeine has been associated with cancer, heart disease, birth defects, and a number of other serious disorders. Despite these persistent rumors,

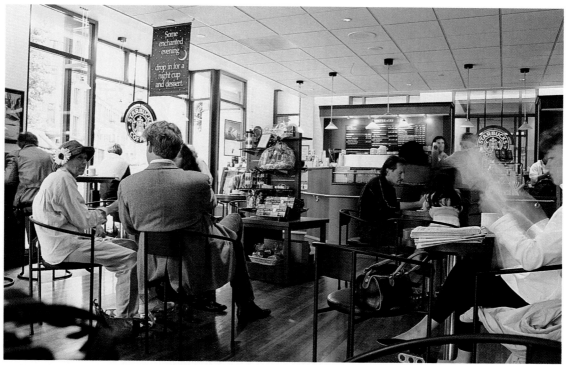

*Almost all restaurants—including the trendy coffee bars (above) that have sprung up around the country—now feature a selection of decaffeinated beverages on their menus.*

countless scientific studies have produced no conclusive links between caffeine and disease. In fact, the scientific community agrees more or less that moderate caffeine intake doesn't pose any health risks whatsoever.

One thing that the studies have proved is that caffeine has psychoactive properties—it affects the central nervous system, and can alter behavior in a variety of different ways. Some people have a high tolerance for caffeine, while others feel pronounced effects just from a half a cup of coffee, which contains only about 30 milligrams (mg) of caffeine.

Almost all people experience a "lift" from caffeine. Caffeine apparently produces this stimulatory effect by blocking the action of adenosine, a neurotransmitter that generally contributes to behavioral slowing. But behavioral effects themselves have yet to be clearly demonstrated, according to Jack James, Ph.D., chairman of the department of behavioral sciences at La Trobe University in Victoria, Australia, who has published *Caffeine and Health* (Academic Press, 1991), considered by many to be the definitive work on caffeine research.

Depending on the amount of caffeine consumed and an individual's sensitivity to it, caffeine may increase heart rate and metabolism. It can also promote the secretion of stomach acid, which may aggravate peptic ulcers. And, as almost anyone will tell you, caffeine steps up the production of urine. Psychomotor effects have been more difficult to identify. "The most consistent effect demonstrated," says Dr. James, "is hand steadiness."

Roland Griffiths, Ph.D., professor of psychiatry and neuroscience at Johns Hopkins University in Baltimore, Maryland, asserts that "even relatively low doses of caffeine are psychoactive and can change mood and behavior." Symptoms can occur at levels as low as 20 to 60 mg, he says—the equivalent of a small cup of brewed coffee, a 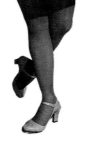 can of caffeinated soda, or one dose of a caffeine-containing analgesic.

Individuals who ingest large amounts of caffeine, on the order of 750 mg per day, or the caffeine equivalent of seven cups of coffee, may experience what is termed "caffeinism." Signs of caffeinism include nervousness, anxiety, irritability, muscle twitching, jitteriness, and insomnia.

Surprisingly, many people experience these effects from a much lower intake of caffeine—as low as 150 to 250 mg. This is roughly the same range of caffeine intake suggested for "moderate" consumption.

People who drink coffee regularly tend to develop a tolerance for it and notice its side effects less. The Coffee Science Source notes that coffee does not produce the addictive behavior typical of alcohol or opiates. Nonetheless, caffeine is addictive, and people who suddenly deprive themselves of it may experience uncomfortable withdrawal symptoms (primarily headaches). Indeed, giving up caffeine may rank as its biggest drawback. "Caffeine consumption poses few probems for most individuals but quitting caffeine abruptly is likely to produce some level

## Cutting Down Without Cutting Out

While there is no evidence that caffeine is hazardous to your health, if you think it is the cause of your insomnia, nervousness, or jitteriness, there are some simple and relatively painless ways to cut down on caffeine intake.

In the case of coffee and tea, the amount of caffeine ingested varies considerably according to how you prepare your brew. Boiled coffee has the highest caffeine content, while a drip-method coffee maker will generally give you higher caffeine content than a percolator. Instant coffee contains about half the caffeine of brewed coffee, and decaffeinated coffee has no more than 2 to 5 mg per serving.

Tea generally contains between one-third and one-half the caffeine of regular coffee. But it, too, will vary depending on how you prepare it. A long steep will mean more caffeine in the pot. Generally a five-minute soak yields about two times the caffeine of a one-minute brew.

When it comes to soft drinks, the best way to avoid caffeine is to read the labels. It's a sure bet that all colas have caffeine, unless you go for the decaffeinated versions. But a surprisingly large number of fruit- and citrus-type sodas also have caffeine. Generally, however, all ginger ales, club sodas, tonic waters, and root beers are caffeine-free.

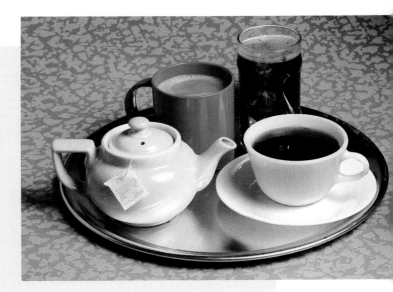

Chocolate-drink mixes will vary from 1 to 20 mg of caffeine in a glass. Pure cocoa and chocolate syrup will be on the higher end of the scale, while instant chocolate drinks like Quik offer less.

If caffeine is a problem, but giving up chocolate is not your style, simply try to avoid dark chocolate. Hershey's Special Dark has the highest caffeine content of any chocolate bar sold in the United States. Milk-chocolate bars have about one-third of the caffeine, and chocolate-covered caramel or wafer bars have even less.

As with soft drinks, the best rule to follow for analgesic products is to read the label. Caffeine-free formulations of all standard analgesics are available. And if there's caffeine in the product, the list of ingredients must say so.

of withdrawal in most people," says Geoff Mumford, Ph.D., a caffeine researcher from Johns Hopkins.

According to a recent study authored by Dr. Griffiths, clear evidence of withdrawal symptoms can occur when an individual terminates caffeine intake of as low as 100 mg per day, the level consumed daily by the great majority of the population.

One segment of the population that caffeine researchers are particularly concerned about is children. American children ingest much caffeine from soft drinks. It is reasoned that because of a child's lower body weight, the physiological impact could be more significant in kids than it is in adults.

A study sponsored by the National Institute of Mental Health (NIMH) in the mid-1980s tested this theory on boys between the ages of 8 and 13. The researchers found that anywhere from two to seven cans of soda caused the boys to be jittery and experience insomnia. Based on this and other studies, the Center for Science in the Public Interest recommends children avoid caffeine. The Food and Drug Administration (FDA), however, does not make a specific recommendation for children, suggesting only that pregnant women avoid caffeine.

### Surprising Sources

Keeping away from soda may well be better advice than kicking the caffeine habit. While a single serving of a soft drink contains only 36 to 40 mg of caffeine (about one-third the amount in a cup of coffee), soft-drink consumption is becoming more pervasive than coffee drinking. In fact, coffee consumption has been cut in half since the 1940s, while soft-drink consumption is soaring.

The soft-drink industry is by far the largest consumer of raw caffeine (caffeine that has been extracted from coffee beans and/or caffeine produced synthetically). Many people think caffeinated soft drinks are confined to cola beverages such as Coke, Pepsi, and Dr. Pepper. But more than two-thirds of the soft drinks consumed in the United States contain added caffeine. A 1981 study by *Consumer Reports* found that of the 10 best-selling soft drinks, only two, 7-Up and Sprite, contained no caffeine.

Caffeine is even added to citrus-type soft drinks like Sunkist and Mountain Dew. Mountain Dew contains one of the highest caffeine levels of any soft drink on the market —about 52 mg per 12-ounce can. The prize, however, goes to Jolt, which clocks in at a mighty 71.2 mg per 12-ounce serving.

The FDA sanctions caffeine's use in beverages as a flavor additive. But caffeine clearly provides a stimulant effect at dietary doses. A 1980 study commissioned by the Federal Trade Commission (FTC) even speculated that beverage manufacturers might be inclined to add caffeine to their formulations for its mildly addictive qualities. This issue remains at the core of the debate between consumer groups and industry over the use of caffeine in soft drinks.

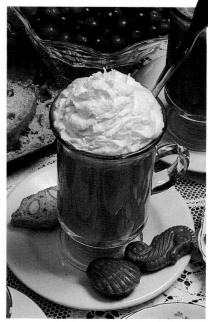

*Chocolate's calories are more worrisome than its caffeine.*

Another dietary source of caffeine for children and adults alike is chocolate. But if this seems a cruel addition to the ever-growing list of nutritional taboos, it may come as some relief to know that chocolate ranks as the mildest source of "hidden" caffeine. Depending on the kind of chocolate, caffeine content can be as low as 6 mg per ounce, or 9 mg per bar. Cocoa and chocolate milk have even less caffeine, between 2 to 8 mg per glass or cup.

The highest level of caffeine in chocolate is found in dark, or sweet, chocolate: about 31 mg per ounce. Stanley Tarka, Ph.D., senior director of food science and nutrition at Hershey Foods Corporation, points out that this kind of chocolate is not widely consumed in the U.S. "The predominant chocolate is milk chocolate," he says. In fact, most chocolate Americans eat is of the milk variety.

The caffeine content of a chocolate-chip cookie or a brownie will vary depending upon how the item is prepared, although, in most cases, it is minimal. Because baking chocolate is dark chocolate, a brownie may contain more caffeine than a cookie made with milk-chocolate chips. Desserts prepared with cocoa or chocolate syrup will have an even lower caffeine content.

Dr. Tarka says, "Even though baking chocolate contains a higher level of caffeine, the symptoms it will produce are minor." This generally means that unless a person is highly reactive to caffeine, there is no reason to give up chocolate. In any case, adults often keep an eye on their chocolate consumption because of its calorie content. It is relatively easy for parents to control their children's caffeine-from-chocolate intake.

While they may know about chocolate, many people don't know that over-the-counter (OTC) drugs frequently contain caffeine. Most people are aware that stimulant tablets like Vivarin and No Doz are almost pure caffeine—one two-tablet dose of No Doz contains a whopping 200 mg. But what is not so apparent is that weight-control aids like Dexatrim and Dietac contain just as much of the stimulant.

Caffeine is also an active ingredient in many nonprescription analgesics, including some formulations of aspirin and acetaminophen. "With OTC products," says Dr. Griffiths, "you must read the label. It's possible

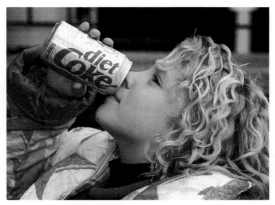

*More than two-thirds of the soft drinks consumed in the U.S. contain manufacturer-added caffeine.*

to get as much as 65 mg of caffeine per tablet." While previously this level of caffeine was not thought to change behavior, he says, more-recent studies reveal "symptoms of caffeine withdrawal can occur at an intake of 100 mg per day— the equivalent of only a few analgesic tablets." Consequently, people who repeatedly use an analgesic containing caffeine for headaches may develop headaches as part of withdrawal symptoms.

"No one is really able to say exactly how caffeine works in conjunction with analgesia," says Debbie Lumpkins, a microbiologist for the FDA's division of OTC drugs. "One theory is that caffeine's stimulant effect generally makes people feel better. Another is that caffeine influences endorphins, the body's natural painkillers."

Recently an advisory committee to the agency's OTC division ruled that there was no clear demonstration that caffeine enhances the action of acetaminophen. Despite this ruling, caffeine probably will not be taken out of other acetaminophen products in the near future.

*Caffeine is considered an active ingredient in many over-the-counter analgesics. Often the caffeine content is surprisingly high.*

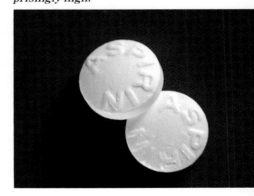

## What to Do?

It remains up to consumers to be knowledgeable about the caffeine they ingest. All major brands of analgesics have a caffeine-free formula, and if caffeine is added to any medications, it must be listed with other ingredients. Because everyone reacts differently to caffeine, no one can really tell you how much is too much. It's up to you to find out.  ◇

# What's Cooking in Cookware?

*by Janet C. Tate*

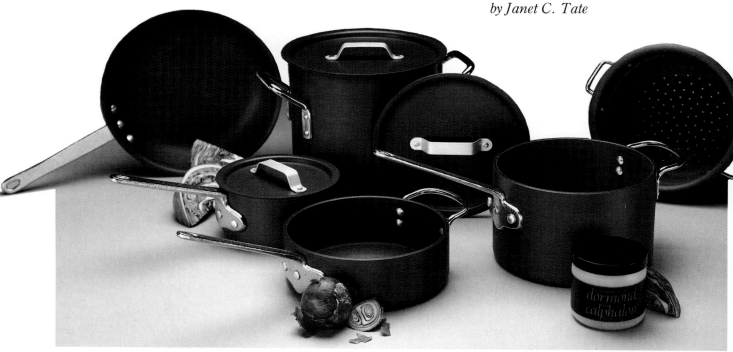

**Many people worry that toxic substances leach from their pots and pans into their food. Some cookware, like Calphalon (above), is manufactured in such a way as to prevent leaching.**

Karen received a beautiful lead-crystal baby bottle as a baby-shower gift. She would love to use it—but she is afraid about the possibility of lead leaching from the bottle into her baby's juice. Is her fear a realistic one?

Ada, age 56, was recently diagnosed with Alzheimer's disease. In addition to grappling with her disease, Ada's husband and children are wondering what role—if any—the aluminum in Ada's soft-drink cans and in her cookware played in her illness. Is there an aluminum connection to Alzheimer's?

When Jason and Paula returned from their honeymoon in Acapulco, Mexico, they brought back a set of brightly colored glazed-ceramic coffee mugs. They have no way of knowing if the mugs were properly fired so as to render them free of lead contamination, and thus safe for daily use. (The same might be said for any of the numerous electric cooking pots they received as wedding gifts.) How can they know for sure?

And finally, Marie's grandmother, a bred-in-the-bone Southern cook, always maintained that her family benefited in more ways than they knew from the fried chicken, corn bread, and black-eyed peas she serves up in her cast-iron stewpots and skillets. She claims her cookware adds iron to the diet. Is she right?

## Trace Elements

As we become more aware of elements in our surroundings that may affect our health, we are starting to pay more attention not only to larger factors—clean air and water (or the lack thereof), for example, and the foods we eat—but also to the very items we use to prepare and serve food in: glasses, serving dishes, and cookware.

The main source of concern involves the possible leaching of certain metals into foods from cookware. Spurred by news reports and disparate studies that seem to indicate there is reason for alarm, many of us have started to question the safety of aluminum pots and pans, glazed-ceramic pottery, lead-crystal stemware, and even our stainless-steel and cast-iron cookware. But is there really any reason to fear our Farberware?

It should be noted, of course, that the human body requires trace amounts of some essential minerals—zinc, iron, copper, and manganese, to name a few—in order to survive. "There is a whole host of mineral elements that we need in small amounts, but that we don't need in large amounts," observes Forrest Nielsen, Ph.D., director of the Grand Forks Human Nutrition Research Center's Agricultural Research Service in North Dakota. "It is when they appear in the human diet in the larger amounts that there may be cause for concern."

But how much is too much? And how can you protect yourself from getting more than you need, not to mention possibly toxic levels of those you don't need? Here is a look at the most common forms of cookware and dishes and their potential for causing any harm.

## Cookware Overview

**Ceramicware and Crystalware.** Both your breakfast cereal bowl and your fanciest lead-crystal stemware are potential sources of lead. This ubiquitous metal is found in our drinking water (mainly via lead-soldered pipes), the air we breathe (courtesy of automobile exhaust and other industrial emissions), and the paint in buildings and homes we inhabit. Even so, lead poisoning is not usually a problem for adults; for children, however, it can be deadly. Because a child's system is not mature enough to safely absorb the metal, the ingestion or inhalation of lead by a child affects the production of hemoglobin and certain essential enzymes in the brain and nervous system. Excessive lead in the bloodstream can lead to nervous-system disorders,

behavior and learning disabilities—even death.

Acidic liquids, such as orange juice or wine, can leach lead from lead-crystal glasses and decanters in a matter of minutes. The substance does not even have to be particularly acidic to pick up lead: in a 1991 study conducted by Columbia University's Joseph H. Gaziano, Ph.D., and Conrad Blum, M.D., crystal baby bottles containing apple juice, water, and formula attained lead levels considered dangerous for infants within a matter of four hours. Of particular concern is the indefinite storage of foods and liquids in crystal containers; the Food and Drug Administration (FDA) recommends against that practice, especially if you are pregnant or in your childbearing years.

*Are the very items in which we prepare and serve food a source of unwanted substances?*

Most glazes on oven-fired ceramic dishes have some lead in them. (By the way, enamel- or ceramic-coated cookware is different; there is no lead involved in these coatings.) Ceramicware brought home from other countries could also have been colored with pigments containing cadmium, which can be a factor in high blood pressure, or even arsenic. Since 1971 the FDA has had regulations governing the acceptable amounts of lead in ceramic glazes for dishes sold and used in the United States. "But if you are thinking about using something glazed from overseas, I would think twice about it," says Nielsen. "Although our federal laws try to prevent this, some will slip through."

It is possible to come across improperly fired pottery and mugs abroad, and at home from local amateur potters and craftspersons. To tell if your crockery is O.K. to use, try at-home lead-testing kits or take your dishes to a commercial laboratory for testing.

*Orange juice, wine, and other acidic liquids can leach lead from lead-crystal glassware in a matter of minutes. Do not store food in crystal containers.*

**Aluminum Cookware.** Long prized for its superior heat conductivity and distribution, aluminum has also come under fire since the 1970s as a possible cause of Alzheimer's disease, a degenerative disorder associated with aging that can affect memory, judgment, and behavior. According to the latest thinking, aluminum does seem to accumulate in the brains of Alzheimer's sufferers; whether the aluminum levels lead to the disease or the disease permits the aluminum buildup is still debatable. "[Research] has more or less disproved the idea that aluminum causes Alzheimer's disease," says Nielsen. "And, in fact, some of these accumulations may even have been contaminants. There is no question that the brain-cell membranes of people with Alzheimer's disease do change, and there is a tendency for certain elements to accumulate. One of these might be aluminum if people were taking in high amounts, but in terms of cookware being a predisposing factor toward this, it is quite remote." Nielsen points out that we ingest a lot more aluminum from other sources than we would probably ever obtain from using aluminum cookware. "One good-sized potato, especially if you eat the skin, probably has more aluminum in it than you would get from cooking a basket of tomatoes in an aluminum pot," Nielsen says. "And many aluminum-containing products, such as a baking-powder biscuit or a buffered aspirin, will give you a good dose of aluminum. The amount you would get from cookware just pales beside those types of intake."

As with some other forms of cookware, foods that are particularly acidic or salty, such as tomato sauce or sauerkraut, do tend to release the aluminum from cookware. One alternative is to consider anodized aluminum pots and pans, such as those manufactured under the brand name Calphalon. This type of cookware has had its aluminum oxide film electrochemically thickened, a process that the manufacturer claims seals the aluminum and prevents its leaching into foods.

**Stainless Steel.** Second only to aluminum in popularity, stainless-steel cookware is actually an alloy of iron and other metals, including nickel and chromium, which accounts for the substance's "stainless," or spot-resistant, quality. Chromium and iron are not only harmless, but are actually desirable in the diet; the jury is still out on nickel. Although it is thought to be essential in trace amounts, nickel's biochemical role has not been established. For those allergic to, for example, the nickel-

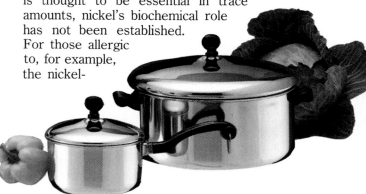

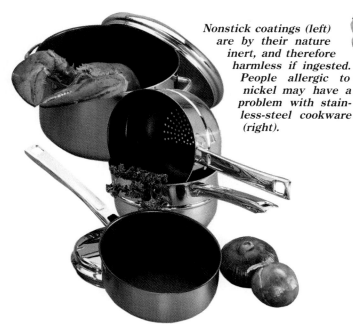

*Nonstick coatings (left) are by their nature inert, and therefore harmless if ingested. People allergic to nickel may have a problem with stainless-steel cookware (right).*

plated back of a wristwatch, contact with stainless-steel cookware can also have an effect. "Some people are sensitive to nickel, because nickel—as well as chromium—can cause dermatitis," Nielsen observes. "The preparation of acidic foods in stainless steel could release a little bit of nickel, so for those people who are nickel-sensitive, it might be best if they did not cook with it." Nonetheless, the FDA does not consider the presence of nickel in cookware to represent a real source of concern, especially given the fact that stainless steel's leaching ability apparently diminishes as the cookware ages.

**Copper.** The Cadillac of cookware, copper pots and pans look gorgeous, conduct heat like nothing else, and cost more than a few pretty pennies. But highly prized as it is, copper can not stand alone; it is usually lined with tin or stainless steel, since otherwise the metal can dissolve into some foods easily and cause nausea, vomiting, and diarrhea.

**Microwavable and plastic containers.** With leftovers, it may be the ultimate in convenience to use the same plastic container both for refrigerator storage and for microwave reheating. But some studies show that chemicals can leach from some microwave-oven plastic containers into foods with high fat or sugar content. The best bet may be to fork the leftovers onto a serving platter or dinner plate before reheating.

**Nonstick coatings.** In the 1960s a revolutionary nonstick cookware coating called Teflon liberated cooks everywhere from the drudgery of having to scour or soak food-encrusted skillets. But as even the gentlest wooden-spoon wielder can testify, the nonstick proof may end up in your pudding if you scrape the bottom of the pan too hard. Are those little flecks of coating floating in your food harmful? "Nonstick coatings, like Teflon, are about the most inert substances you can get," says Nielsen. "Even if they were to peel off and you were to eat them, you would get nothing from it. They are highly protective against getting any kind of bad substances into food." The FDA agrees, noting from their research that any ingested particles would remain unchanged and pass harmlessly through your system. The resins can decompose if heated for long periods at high cooking temperatures, but studies have shown no harmful effects from either this or from any fumes given off when the cookware is overheated.

**Cast-iron skillets.** Grandma was right: food cooked up in her cast-iron skillet not only tastes better, it can actually be better nutritionally. This is one type of cookware in which metal leaching is apparently O.K. Cast iron is inexpensive, it conducts heat evenly, and it will contribute iron to your diet.

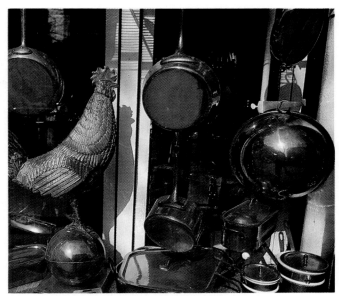

*People who eat food into which copper has leached risk illness. Fortunately, the stainless-steel lining in most copperware prevents such leaching.*

There is, of course, a very remote possibility of getting too much of a good thing. "There has always been a concern about the old iron skillet imparting too much iron in the diet," Nielsen says. "Perhaps, in the old days, that is how people got a lot of the iron in their diet. Most of the time, it is probably of benefit and not harmful at all." But particularly now that many American kids down a cartoon-shaped, iron-fortified vitamin pill with their breakfast, it is possible for children under the age of 5 to get too much iron. "But even that generally is not considered much of a concern in terms of cookware," Nielsen says. "I do not know that you could get enough iron into the diet from a skillet to be toxic. Young children have less tolerance for available iron than do older people, but I have never heard of any child being poisoned by it, so I do not think it is anything of life-threatening concern."

**The Final Analysis**
In general, there is really no reason to worry about your pots and pans harming you. The amounts most of us take in from cookware are negligible. And anyway, if our food contains a little bit of iron, magnesium, zinc, copper, manganese, or chromium from our cookware and dishes, the amount we get probably is more beneficial than harmful. ◇

# Housecalls

by Mona Sutnick, Ed.D., R.D.

**Q** *My dentist has suggested that if I must chew gum, I should chew only the sugarless variety. Unfortunately, sugar-free gum seems to produce intestinal distress for me, and, on a few occasions, diarrhea. Should I just quit chewing gum altogether?*

**A** The type of artificial sweeteners contained in sugarless gum causes digestive distress in some people. The sweeteners are called "sugar alcohols," a class that includes sorbitol, mannitol, and others. They are distinct from peptide sweeteners, such as aspartame. On the list of ingredients, you can recognize them because their names always end in "ol."

Sugar-alcohol sweeteners are not digested or absorbed in the body. As a result, they can stay in the intestine and draw in water, causing digestive distress and diarrhea.

Although most people have no problem with these sweeteners in small amounts, many will experience symptoms if they ingest large amounts. It's a question of individual tolerance.

Sugar-alcohol sweeteners are also present in diet preserves and syrups, sugarfree hard candies, certain toothpastes, and other products. Look for them on the label, and moderate your intake if they cause you problems.

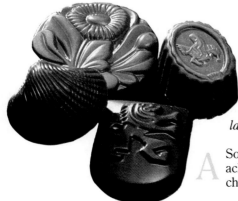

**Q** *My husband is a chocolate freak. Unfortunately, after he eats chocolate, he often develops a headache. Is there a proven relationship between eating chocolate and getting headaches?*

**A** Some people do suffer headaches as a result of eating chocolate. The reaction comes from phenylethylamine, a natural protein metabolite in chocolate, structurally related to a neurotransmitter. Tyramine, a similar substance present in red wine, chicken liver, certain cheeses, and other foods, also causes headaches in some individuals. For most people, these foods are not a problem. If your husband thinks that chocolate is the source of his headaches, he should try cutting it out of his diet to see if the headaches go away. Then he should reintroduce chocolate at least one more time to see if the headaches return—before he reduces or eliminates it altogether. Your husband might consider consulting a physician who specializes in allergies, to help guide him through the elimination diet.

---

**Q** *Is it possible to drink too much water? Also, is there a significant difference between tap water and springwater? I prefer the taste of springwater to that of water that comes out of my tap.*

**A** It's possible to drink too much water, but not easy. You would have to drink vast quantities to be in danger of harming yourself (10 quarts or more, in a day of normal activity). Otherwise, unless you are on some sort of diet where you are consuming water at the expense of balanced nutrition and needed calories, the only thing you'll have to worry about is lots of trips to the rest room. Not drinking *enough* water and suffering dehydration is a far more common problem.

The answer to the tap-water/springwater conundrum is that it depends on where your tap water and springwater originate. Recent data show that many municipal water supplies are not meeting Environmental Protection Agency (EPA) standards for healthfulness. On the other hand, most public water does not appear to have caused health problems. Water from wells or springs is not necessarily better, because it can be subject to contaminants as well. In rural areas, for example, agricultural runoff can be a factor in water quality.

On the other hand, municipalities and most springwater companies test their water, and you can request results. Alternatively, you can have the water tested yourself or purchase a filtering device.

Keep in mind that the temperature of water affects its taste; to compare two different sources of water for taste, they must be at the same temperature.

---

Q *My wife tends to eat only two meals a day, usually skipping lunch. She insists that her eating habits help her keep her weight under control. Is what she's doing considered wise by nutritionists?*

A No, it is not. Surveys show that people who eat more regularly do better nutritionally.

Data do not support the idea that skipping meals is a good way to lose weight. Concentrating most of her food intake in one or two meals probably doesn't change the number of calories your wife takes in by the end of the day. Those who skip meals altogether are also more likely to snack, and snack foods are often high in calories and low in nutrition.

The other issue is that your wife is going a long time without refueling her body. Something as simple as yogurt or a sandwich at lunch would probably provide her more energy during the day.

Because of our lifestyles, many of us find dinner the only meal where we can relax or visit with family. The emphasis on this meal tends to increase its size. Although it is probably better to put the larger meal earlier in the day, the idea that calories consumed before bedtime are more likely to be stored as fat is a myth. Nevertheless, one's energies are best served by a hearty breakfast and by remembering that it's just as easy in the evening to have a light meal.

---

Q *A few years ago, vitamin E was all the rage. What is the current thinking about vitamin E? Is it worth taking vitamin E supplements?*

A Vitamin E's popularity is surging again, thanks to scientific evidence that it may help to prevent certain conditions such as cancer and heart disease. The attention has spilled over to a group of nutrients collectively referred to as "antioxidants" (see "Accent on Antioxidants," page 85), which include vitamin C and beta-carotene as well as vitamin E.

The American Dietetic Association and other official groups have yet to embrace any across-the-board recommendation on taking antioxidant supplements, but they are watching the new findings carefully. Their primary recommendation is still to get your nutrients from eating a healthful diet that includes plenty of fresh fruits and vegetables, and whole grains.

However, the doses of vitamin E found beneficial in some research are almost impossible to get through the diet. You would have to consume enormous quantities of vegetable oil, wheat germ, or other vitamin E-rich foods to get the supposedly therapeutic dose present in supplements. In recent years the negative effects of taking large doses of certain vitamins (including another antioxidant, vitamin A) have received deserved publicity, and people are much more cautious about supplements. However, doses of up to 800 milligrams per day of vitamin E have not been shown to have toxic effects. (Larger amounts can interfere with the function of other nutrients.) Sales of vitamin E—and antioxidant supplements that combine vitamins E and C and beta-carotene— have increased dramatically.

---

Q *I love asparagus. The strange thing is, after I eat asparagus, my urine has a very pungent, rather unpleasant odor. Is this just me, or does asparagus have this effect on everybody?*

A Most likely, two sulfur-containing compounds in asparagus cause this reaction. Just a few spears of asparagus can create this odor in the urine in a short time. Research is not conclusive on whether all people, or just most people, experience this phenomenon, but, as you've noticed, if you're one of them, you can't miss it.

---

*Do you have a nutrition question?* Send it to Editor, Health and Medicine Annual, P.O. Box 90, Hawleyville, CT 06440-9990.

# Fitness and Health

**See also:**
Individual articles in the second half of this book, arranged in alphabetical order, for additional information.

Evidence of the benefits of keeping fit continues to accumulate. A proper diet, regular exercise, and sufficient sleep make people healthier both physically and mentally by helping to build bones, fight heart disease, lower the risk of chronic diseases such as diabetes, and by brightening one's mental outlook. Staying fit saves money, too. According to the Centers for Disease Control and Prevention (CDC), businesses that provide exercise programs for employees significantly lower their medical-insurance claims; they save as much as $7 for each $1 invested in the exercise programs.

Any type of regular physical exercise is beneficial. Some people prefer vigorous activities, such as jogging, tennis, and cross-country skiing. But less strenuous activities, such as brisk walking, can be equally beneficial. What is critical, experts agree, is getting at least 20 minutes of continuous aerobic activity three to five days a week.

Conversely, lack of regular exercise can be deadly. According to former U.S. Representative Tom McMillen, co-chairman of the President's Council on Physical Fitness and Sports, some 250,000 deaths each year are attributable to inactivity. Doctors at Deaconess Hospital in Boston, Massachusetts, report that people who are out of shape greatly increase their risk of a heart attack when they engage in strenuous activity—whether it's a sport or a mundane activity such as carrying furniture or shoveling snow. Among people who exercise less than once a week, strenuous activity increases the risk of a heart attack by 107 times. For people who exercise once or twice a week, the risk is 19 times higher. For people who exercise three or four times a week, the risk is nine times higher.

According to the CDC, about 60 percent of Americans over age 10 are physically inactive. A survey released in 1993 by Louis Harris & Associates found that in 1992 only 33 percent of Americans engaged in strenuous exercise at least three days a week—as compared to 34 percent in 1983. The same survey provides other negative news, too: the percentage of overweight Americans increased, people were sleeping less, and fewer people were trying to eat healthy diets.

In general, sedentary people know they should exercise more, but "knowing" and "doing" are not the same: such people show few signs that they'll cease to be "couch potatoes." The President's Council on Physical Fitness and Sports surveyed 1,019 sedentary Americans; 64 percent said they would like to exercise more, but didn't have the time. However, the great majority of these people watched television for three or more hours a week, indicating that they did indeed have time.

It's never too late to begin exercising, but the sooner one starts, the greater the benefits, concludes a study of 10,269 male graduates of Harvard University. The study found that men who took up moderately vigorous sports when they were 45 to 54 years old lived an average of 10 months longer than men who remained sedentary. Among men 55 to 64, exercise added an average of nine months to their lives; for those 65 to 74, it added six months; and for men 75 to 84, it added two months. The researchers note that in addition to living longer, people who keep in shape also tend to live better.

One of the most serious problems among older Americans is falling. "The problem is startling," says Mark Grabi-ner, director of the Clinical Biomechanics and Rehabilitation Program at the Cleveland Clinic Foundation. "More than one-third of all people older than 75 fall. People who fall once are more predisposed to falling multiple times again." Research shows that some of the risk factors contributing to falls and fall-related injuries can be modified. An Australian study reported that gentle aerobic exercise emphasizing balance and flexibility improved women's strength, reaction time, and balance—all factors in preventing falls.

Women eager to keep fit may want to watch their waist-hip ratio. According to a study of 41,837 women aged 50 to 69 directed by Aaron R. Folsom, M.D., at the University of Minnesota School of Public Health, the bigger the waist in comparison to the hips, the greater the risk of death—regardless of the person's weight. Aaron says that a woman's waist should be less than 80 percent the circumference of her hips (for men, the waist should be less than 95 percent of the hips).

*People who stay in shape have fewer aches, pains, chronic diseases, and other physical problems.*

# MARTIAL *Arts*

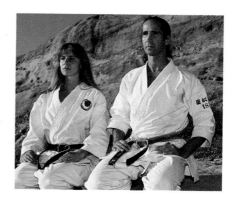

*by Barbara Alden Wilson*

artial-arts classes aren't just for Bruce Lee or Steven Seagal wannabes. Just take a look inside a reputable *dojo,* or studio, and you'll likely see plenty of women, as well as men and kids, working on their form while getting physically fit and mentally balanced. And they're having fun in the process.

According to the U.S.A. Karate Federation, karate—just one form of martial arts popular today—provides the second-most aerobic benefit of all kinds of exercise, coming just behind cross-country skiing as an effective workout. "It's also sound as far as what it asks the body to do," says Katherine Jones, *sensei* (instructor) and spokesperson for the Washington Karate Association in Seattle. "It won't wear you down physically. I certainly can't say that about what years of ballet did to my body."

Challenging aerobic exercise isn't the only benefit provided by the martial arts. A wide variety of disciplines offers everything from athletic combat techniques to slower, yoga-like moves designed to heighten one's sense of inner peace. The following are some of the more popular forms of martial arts:

### Tae Kwon Do

Tae Kwon Do (pronounced "tie kwahn doe"), directly translated, means "art of open hand and bare foot"; it is the single most popular martial art in the United States. Since becoming an Olympic sport in 1988, Tae Kwon Do continues to attract about half of the roughly 5 million martial-arts students in the United States. Hollywood's glamorization of the sport hasn't hurt class enrollment. Hype from Chuck Norris movies, the tamer but more mainstream *Karate Kid* movies, and the

Teenage Mutant Ninja Turtles sent kids clamoring for lessons in Tae Kwon Do and other martial arts. But like all martial arts, the first rule of Tae Kwon Do is discipline. "Parents considering sending their child to a martial-arts class need to understand that it's not going to be playtime," Jones warns. "If your child wants to take any martial-arts class just because they like the Ninja Turtles, signing them up might not be such a good idea. But kids who see the other kids in class excel-

*Devotees of the martial arts derive much more than aerobic benefits from their workouts. Most enthusiasts find that they gain a new sense of discipline through the martial arts.*

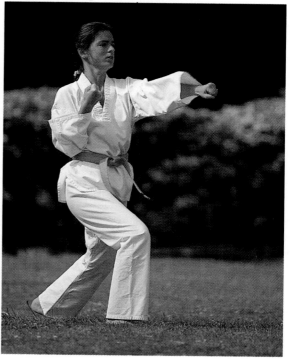

ling, and those who really want to learn, actually *like* the discipline of it."

Adults tend to focus more on Tae Kwon Do's body benefits: a leaner, more muscular, more flexible physique. Done correctly, the 2,000-year-old Korean martial art has all the elements of a full anaerobic and aerobic workout—toning all major muscle groups and improving balance and coordination. Classes focus on perfecting the moves of the art while maintaining a calm, but alert, state of mind.

A typical 90-minute class begins with 20 to 25 minutes of warm-up exercises followed by drills in basic punching, blocking, and kicking. Students may then practice combinations of moves, the pace of which increases according to a student's skill level. The class may conclude with either rehearsed or free sparring. Whatever a student's abilities, classes tend to be composed of nonstop motion. Aggressive participants may burn up to 20 calories a minute; the average student burns 10. That's about twice the calories the average person burns walking 3.5 miles per hour.

Many schools of Tae Kwon Do also teach breathing and meditation techniques, which are meant to contribute to an aura of tranquillity and rejuvenation. Instructors emphasize mental awareness and self-discipline, particularly with new students.

At a Tae Kwon Do studio, or *do-jang,* Eastern tradition demands that the mood be formal and respectful. Instructors are addressed as "sir." Students bow upon entering and departing, and when addressing a black belt. This discipline generally fosters a sense of camaraderie among participants. But students should never put up with treatment that makes them uncomfortable, Jones warns. A reputable school —whether it offers classes in Tae Kwon Do or some other form of martial arts— will not cross the line between demanding respect from students and demeaning them.

*A man who has attained mastery of an art reveals it in his every action—*

Samurai proverb

Most people involved in the martial arts take classes at a studio, or dojo. Typically, students wear special clothes and address instructors and more-advanced students respectfully.

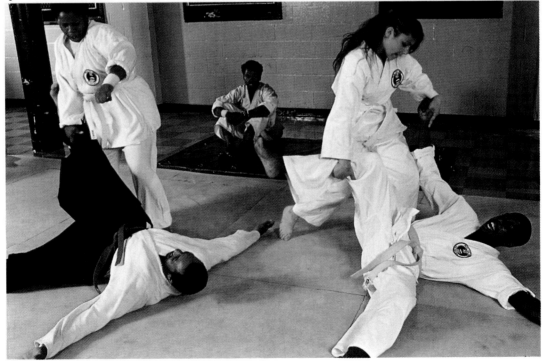

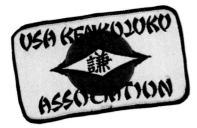

*Each martial-arts studio has its own special symbol, often worn as a patch.*

"You should not be *made* to do things in class that make you feel uneasy," Jones says. "Honor, respect, and duty are practiced every day, and you should expect to act accordingly in class. But verbal beatings and mumbo jumbo about 'philosophy' should never be a part of training."

Once you start taking Tae Kwon Do classes, you'll need a minimum of two to three classes a week to become proficient. If you want to reach competitive status, you'll probably need to increase your class attendance to four or five times a week.

### Karate

Karate, which is actually an umbrella term for more than 1,000 hard, external fighting styles, is the Japanese counterpart to Tae Kwon Do. It differs from the kick-dominated

their less-developed upper-body strength by concentrating on lower-body moves. Whatever a student's gender, the art of karate is the same: to learn how to kill or maim one's opponent by kicking or punching major acupuncture points, such as the solar plexus, head, and collarbone.

Kata (pronounced KAH-ta), the forms of karate that are perfected in class, is the heart of martial arts, according to the U.S.A. Karate Federation. "When you perfect these forms, you learn the art and integrity of karate," Jones explains. "The Kata is the development of self. It is the 'art' of martial arts. To remove Kata from martial-arts training is to remove the art of being a warrior." The disciplined protocol in karate class calls for bowing to the instructor upon entry and exit, as well as paying respectful attention while class is in session. "The attitude is much like chivalry in Western culture," Jones notes.

Like Tae Kwon Do, karate can contribute to aerobic endurance, muscle tone, flexibil-

*Karate students work to perfect techniques of defense and attack, called Kata. In the form of Kata known as Heian #4, a student prepares to deliver a side kick (near right) to an imagined enemy attacking from the side; he executes the side kick with his right foot, simultaneously delivering a back-fist strike (second from left). Then, with his hand extended to the head of his imagined attacker (facing page left), the student shifts to a forward stance, striking out his elbow toward the attacker's head (far right).*

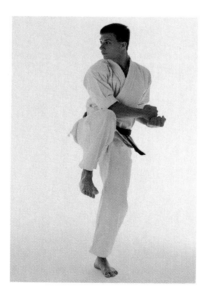

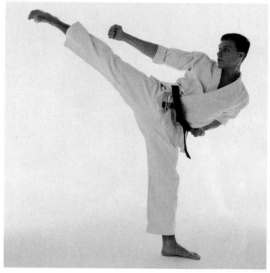

Tae Kwon Do, however, in that fighting styles emphasize hand and foot techniques equally. These techniques were originally designed for the male body, when Chinese monks began practicing them to uphold strict meditation practices in the 6th century. Today women in karate can compensate for

ity, balance, and coordination. It may also help relieve stress and build self-confidence and discipline. In a beginner class, the warm-up may include 100 sit-ups and 30 push-ups. "You don't necessarily have to be in top-notch shape to join a class," says Jones, "but if you're grossly overweight, you'd do well to lose some weight and get your doctor's permission before you sign up." To gain a basic level of proficiency within a year, expect to attend three classes per week.

### Aikido

Roughly translated as "a way of fitting in," aikido (eye-KEE-doe) stresses becoming compatible on both a mental and physical level with the force or movements of an opponent. Aikido was developed in Japan in the 12th century, and introduced into the United States in the early 1950s. This martial art involves more than 2,000 interrelated throws, locks, nerve-point attacks, and strikes. Because there are "hard" and "soft" schools of traditional aikido, the basic techniques that beginners are taught may be called by different names depending on who is teaching them.

The major differences between these two schools are in their training methods. The soft approach emphasizes exaggerated movements, and concentrates on theoretical attack situations. In a sense the attack is choreographed, with the "attacker" executing a prearranged strike so that the "victim" can move in a set pattern and successfully spar with his or her opponent. The foundation of the soft-school philosophy is the *ki* (kee) principle, the belief that a competitor's concentration is centered at a point just above the navel, providing a spiritual source of strength necessary to execute aikido movements and techniques properly.

The hard approach to aikido, on the other hand, relies more on teaching students to duplicate a set pattern for each movement or technique, as demonstrated by the instructor. In some hard schools, force is substituted for the natural flow of movement and execution. Attack situations in these classes tend to be more re-

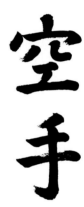

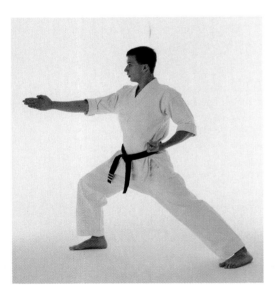

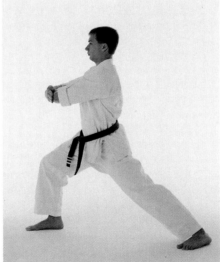

*The Japanese characters above spell* kara te *(karate), meaning "empty hand," a term that refers to the unarmed form of self-defense practiced by the Okinawans.*

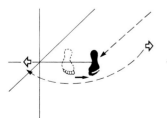
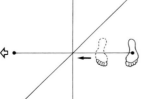
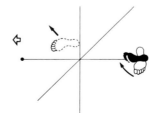
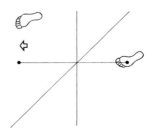

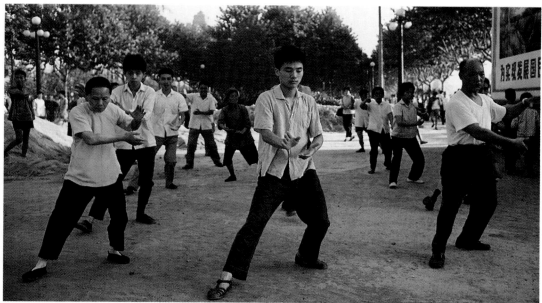

*All of the major forms of martial arts arose in Asia. In China (above), people of all ages practice Tai Chi Chuan, the martial art that most closely approximates yoga.*

alistic than in the soft lessons. Hard schools also originated the use of the *atemi* (ah-TEH-mee), or strike, as a diversionary tactic against one's opponent. (Some soft schools have incorporated this also, but students wear hand protectors rather than using their bare hands.)

Aikido can provide just as much of an aerobic workout as Tae Kwon Do or karate. To become proficient, aikido students should expect to attend a minimum of two sessions, each two hours long, per week. Because aikido is best performed by two people working out together, solo workouts at home do little to help a student's advancement.

A judo-type uniform—a white, robelike jacket wrapped with an *obi,* or fabric belt, and ankle-length pants—called a *dogi* (DOE-jhee), is the generally accepted garb for aikido practice. Another common choice of clothing among aikido scholars is the navy-blue or black *hakama,* similar to a skirt. This is worn by both women and men after they have attained a certain level of skill, depending on the protocol of the dojo. The hakama is generally reserved for special events, however, and is not considered a regular practice uniform.

### Tai Chi Chuan

Also known as Tai Chi (tie chee), Tai Chi Chuan has been called the martial arts' equivalent of yoga. According to Douglas Lee in his book *Tai Chi Chuan* (Ohara Publications, Burbank, California, 1986), the three main similarities between yoga and Tai Chi Chuan are their basic principle of enlightenment through meditation; the fact that they both stress breathing techniques based around the psychic navel center; and the fact that they both emphasize softness, pliability, and total relaxation as essential to attaining *satori,* or sudden enlightenment.

There are also more subtle ways in which Tai Chi Chuan differs from yoga. For example, while yoga uses breathing techniques to create good biorhythms (the body's physiological cycles, such as sleeping and waking), Tai Chi Chuan implements flowing body movements to accomplish that goal. The belief in Tai Chi Chuan is that good breathing will automatically follow. Yoga, Lee writes, is an internal activity that creates external

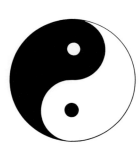

The Yin-Yang Symbol

*Bruce Lee once said, "The less effort, the faster and more powerful you will be."*

serenity. Tai Chi Chuan, however, is external activity that creates internal tranquillity.

Tai Chi Chuan is the martial art based on the concept of *yin* and *yang*. Most people are familiar with the yin-yang symbol—a circle divided by a serpentine line into two equal parts, one white and one black. The yin, the black area of the circle, represents anything in the female, passive, soft, negative, or night part of the universe. The white yang represents the opposite: male, active, hard, positive, or day realm of the universe. The curved line between the two represents the flow and eventual synthesis of one area into the other. The black spot in the white area and the white spot in the black area symbolize that everything includes its own opposite. Nothing, in other words, can be so completely itself that it doesn't contain some of its opposite. The circle surrounding the yin

## What to Look For

Once you've decided which type of martial art you'd like to pursue, visit a few dojos. Be sure to be there while a class or two is in session. The U.S.A. Karate Federation suggests the following list of things to look for in a school:
• How long has the dojo been in business? While not all new schools are suspect, the longer the school has been around, the less chance there is that it is a fly-by-night operation that will take your money and run.
• Is anyone at the dojo promising instant success from their program? Is a "black belt" guaranteed after a specific number of weeks? If so, they are not telling the truth; look elsewhere.
• Is the dojo licensed? Not all unlicensed studios are bad; however, attending class at a licensed dojo guarantees that it keeps up with what is going on in the martial-arts educational field and is committed to maintaining a safe learning environment.
• Is the dojo clean, with a professional atmosphere?
• Does the dojo have an open-door policy, in which parents may walk in and observe a class at any time?
• While class is in session, is each student at least somewhat capable? Is the class active and interesting? If not, or if only a few students seem to get up and show off while the others barely participate at all, move on to another dojo.
• What are the instructors' qualifications? Every instructor should be certified in

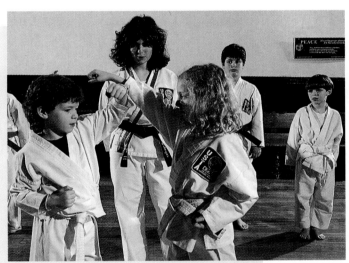

*Parents should learn as much as possible about the operation of a martial-arts studio before they enroll a child in classes.*

CPR. If the class is for your child, the instructors should also be sanctioned by American Coaches Effectiveness Program (ACEP), an Olympic Committee–sanctioned program.
• Are the instructors educated to a level you feel comfortable with? Don't be shy about asking whether they have a college degree.
• Are the instructors articulate? If they try to impress you with a lot of jargon and little factual information, don't sign up for the class.
• What is the injury rate at the dojo? Get a specific answer.

Above all, trust your instincts. Even if a dojo measures up on paper, you may have an uneasy feeling about it. That is as good a reason as any to keep looking.

# Building Confidence in Kids Who Need It Most

More and more, physicians and counselors who work with children with learning disabilities are directing their clients' parents to sign the kids up at a reputable martial-arts studio. The reason? Martial-arts classes provide an additional type of "therapy" that has been effective in helping learning-disabled students make tremendous strides in the physical, mental, and emotional areas of their lives.

Martial arts provide an ideal atmosphere for building confidence in children who have trouble keeping up in the real world. For one thing, size and natural ability do not matter when it comes to mastering karate, Tae Kwon Do, or any other martial art. The same cannot be said of traditional schoolyard sports such as basketball and softball. Children who are not naturally coordinated or have difficulty comprehending the rules of a game find the slow, decisive learning process of Kata far less intimidating than the mechanics of other sports. Martial arts' use of constant repetition with advancement in small increments also appeals to kids with learning disabilities.

Not only do children gain a strong feeling of competence from such classes, but their ability to follow directions, their comprehension, and their skills for coping with frustration improve as well in the respectful, disciplined environment of a dojo.

"We have seen an awful lot of happy kids and happy parents as a result of the medical community beginning to recognize the benefits of karate lessons for the learning-disabled," says Katherine Jones, instructor at the Washington Karate Association.

and yang is their common bond—the whole that contains and produces both parts. This whole is Tai Chi.

Despite its emphasis on the meditative, Tai Chi Chuan is also a physical martial art. But unlike the "hard" styles of Tae Kwon Do and karate, Tai Chi Chuan is an "internal," or "soft," art that uses throwing and grappling rather than kicking and punching. It is an excellent martial-arts choice for men and women recovering from sports injuries or for women suffering from osteoporosis. That's because —like most weight-bearing exercises—it increases bone mass as well as flexibility.

There are 108 moves in the most common yang style of Tai Chi Chuan. Memorizing these moves takes about three months. Perfecting them enough to gain health and martial-arts benefits can take three years or more of weekly classes along with daily half-hour practice sessions.

Clothing isn't an issue in Tai Chi Chuan classes, as long as it's comfortable. Loose-fitting pants and a T-shirt or sweatshirt are favored if you don't want to invest in a traditional dogi or similar garb, which can cost up to $100. As in virtually all martial-arts disciplines, participants go barefoot, and no other equipment is needed.

## Not for Self-Defense

Although the martial arts are often termed the "self-defense" arts of sports, the truth of the matter is that most martial-arts studios do not focus on the kind of self-defense that will be of much help on the street—nor should they espouse that you'll be able to protect yourself once you master a martial art. Most martial-arts schools train using toe-to-toe combat in controlled situations, such as in a class or in an organized competition. The martial arts are not necessarily meant for use to defend oneself in a predatory situation, such as when a woman is grabbed from behind and knocked down in an attempted rape.

There are self-defense courses that incorporate martial-arts strategies as part of a total program, but to expect to be able to fight off an attacker based on what you learn in a martial-arts class would be foolish.  ◇

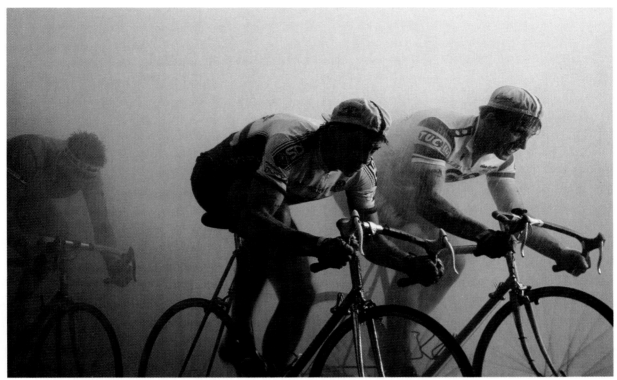

*Exercising outdoors can be fun. But weather conditions should always govern the extent and intensity of any activity. When we go outside and ignore the weather, our bodies pay the price.*

# Weathering Your Workout

*by Gode Davis*

Todd Smith expected to wheeze on that December morning. For six weeks in 1976, stalled high pressure above Salt Lake City's bowl-shaped valley had trapped moist, frigid air near the ground, producing ice fog. Ultimately the fog turned into a grayish-brown, ozone-plagued smog, blotting out the Sun.

"Just a 2-mile jog today," Smith told his wife, Sarah, as he bounded toward the door, his graceful strides exuding peak-condition vigor. Sarah was a jogger, too, but she had coughed so much after the previous day's jog that she'd decided to forgo a repeat experience. "It's awful out there," she said. Before going a half-mile, Todd discovered just how awful. Wheezing and gasping, Todd's strides degenerated into a jerky slow motion that stopped altogether when he collapsed. "They

rushed me to the hospital, and even afterwards, I couldn't stop coughing for months," Smith says.

Smith's adverse experience resulted from exercising outdoors when he should have taken his workout indoors. Jogging in smog is about as sensible as riding a bicycle for a half-mile in the teeth of a bitter cold wind chill —naked. What Smith didn't realize was that weather conditions should always govern the extent and intensity of outdoor activities. When we go outside and ignore the weather, our bodies pay the price.

## Exercise Weather

Attuning our bodies to the weather begins with a given—a nearly constant body temperature. Healthy human beings maintain an average "comfort zone" core temperature of around 96° F. This normal temperature fluctuates less than 1° F through the course of each day, with low temperatures occurring in the morning hours after midnight, and high temperatures occurring in the late afternoon —a trend almost parallel to the daily swing of air temperatures.

Human bodies maintain this constant temperature by producing a constant flow of heat energy. How much energy do we need to keep us in the comfort zone? It depends upon both air temperature and exercise intensity. At rest the body pours out the energy equivalent of a 100-watt light bulb per hour. In 50° F air temperature, a sports spectator sitting outdoors wearing running shorts or other light clothing will not generate enough energy to feel comfortable.

Exercise changes everything. During intense exercise, muscle activity increases internal heat production 15 to 20 times over resting levels. So when a 170-pound champion athlete runs a marathon (26.2 miles or 42 kilometers), he expends over 1,300 calories each hour for a little over two hours. The resulting heat production from this intense workout makes the spectator's chilly day of 50° F seem pretty hot to the runner. In fact, if the mechanisms balancing the athlete's body temperature failed, his body temperature would soar by some 7° to 9° F—to a lethal level. A 170-pound person walking at 4 miles per hour while wearing light clothing expends as much as 360 calories per hour of heat energy—just enough energy to make temperatures between 40° and 60° F seem like ideal "exercise weather," especially if dry conditions and little wind resistance prevail.

Perfect exercise weather is seldom a given. Due to the vagaries of storm tracks, seasons, and local effects like air quality and sea breezes, weather conditions are often less than ideal for outdoor exercise. Extremes of heat and cold or stormy weather will wreak havoc upon exercise regimes— unless precautions are taken to get the most exercise out of the worst weather.

## Hot Weather

The human body has a brilliant mechanism for regulating internal temperature. When a person's blood temperature rises above 98.6° F, the hypothalamus, a tiny control center in the brain, sends signals that trigger the heart to pump more blood and to dilate the blood vessels, particularly those close to the skin. Excess heat from the blood is thus diffused through the skin into the cooler atmosphere. At the same time, water pours

*Heat radiating from a basketball court or concrete can raise the body's "thermostat" dangerously. Athletes need to acclimatize to hot, humid weather.*

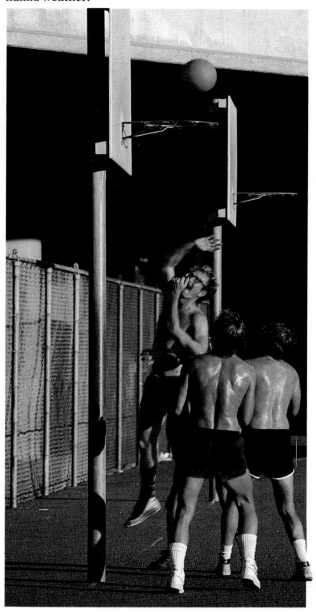

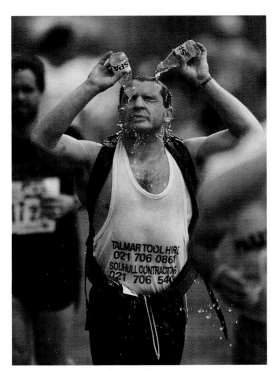

*To avoid dehydration, make sure to drink plenty of fluids. Cool water leaves the stomach quickly and helps reduce internal temperature.*

out of the body through the more than 2 million sweat glands in the skin. As this perspiration evaporates, the skin area cools.

This mechanism works well as long as the air temperature is below human skin temperature, and the relative humidity is low enough for sweat to evaporate rapidly. When the relative humidity rises above 60 percent, sweating becomes a poor cooling device; at 75 percent humidity, sweating ceases to be effective altogether. Hot, dry days can also cause problems if the body's muscles are overworked in strenuous activity. Excess sweating may deplete body salts, disrupting the body's electrolyte balance and triggering heat-induced illness.

There are a variety of heat disorders that occur when the body produces more heat than it can dissipate, especially when dehydration accompanies excessive heat production. The severity of illness can range from mild heat fatigue to potentially deadly heat exhaustion and heatstroke. Heat fatigue—characterized by headache, mental and physical sluggishness, poor appetite, fast pulse, and shallow breathing—can be treated with-

## A Jog in the Smog?

As Todd Smith learned, the great outdoors may not be so swell—air quality may be so poor that strenuous exercise, even by the very fit, may be deadly. Ozone—the primary component of smog—carbon monoxide, particulates, and sulfur and nitrogen dioxides can build up to such dangerous levels that they can contribute to a variety of ills, from wheezing and coughing to chest tightness and shortness of breath. But with care, you can still benefit from exercise in polluted areas.

Before heading out, learn the Pollutant Standards Index (PSI) level in your area from the local weather report. The PSI is a measure of air quality. Levels above 100 exceed federal safety standards, while those below 50 are considered satisfactory. On really bad days, move indoors to a gym or pool for a safer, more comfortable, and enjoyable workout.

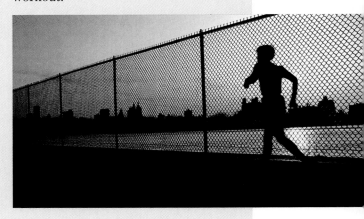

Air pollutants build up during the day and reach a peak in the late afternoon. For the best bit of fresh air, try exercising early in the morning. And avoid traffic and heavily industrialized areas. Studies have shown that runners who work out for 30 minutes near major highways may as well smoke a pack of cigarettes—they'll be inhaling the same amount of carbon monoxide.

## Storm Do's and Don'ts

If stranded outside during a storm, what do you do? Indoors, is it safe? Here are some do's and don'ts to keep you safe in storm-related situations.

**Lightning:** To tell a lightning flash's distance from you, count the seconds slowly (one-100, two-100, etc.) between the flash and its thunder. Less than a second? Head for cover; it's too close! Safe places: any shelter, inside caves, under rock outcrops, bottom of a ravine or canyon (except in a streambed). Don't take shelter under tall trees or any tree that stands alone. Keep away from metal objects, like wire fences; discard metal objects (for example, golf clubs) you may be carrying. Don't stand or walk upright on a hilltop, and avoid large open areas (if you're caught in one, lie flat on dry ground or crouch low on wet ground).

**Hurricane:** To avoid drowning, head for high ground at least several hours in advance. Leave low-lying beaches or other areas that may be swept by high tides or wind-driven waves. Stay at home during the hurricane if the house is out of danger from serious flooding and is well built. Board up windows or protect them with storm shutters or tape. Secure anything that may be blown loose. As soon as possible, get indoors. Be sure to listen to weather advisories while the storm is in progress.

**Tornado:** If a tornado warning is given, take shelter immediately. Avoid auditoriums or other large halls with poorly supported roofs. Run to the nearest tornado cellar if possible. If in open country and no shelter is nearby, move away from the tornado's path at right angles. If you are on foot with no time to escape, lie flat in the nearest ditch, ravine, or culvert with your hands protecting your head. Inside a house, lie prone in a bathtub on a lower floor, or climb under heavy furniture in the center of the house. Shut off electricity and fuel lines. To keep track of the tornado's path and degree of intensity, listen to broadcast weather advisories.

**Blizzard:** If outdoors when a blizzard begins, seek shelter immediately and stay inside. When forced to wait outside, exercise by clapping hands and moving arms and legs vigorously from time to time. If you're in a snow-stalled vehicle, stay in it. Run the motor and heater sparingly, and only with the downwind window open for ventilation. Turn on your overhead light at night to make your vehicle visible. Avoid overexertion and exposure. Exertion from shoveling heavy drifts may cause a heart attack. Don't attempt to walk your way out of blowing and drifting snow; if you become disoriented, the time spent getting back on track may lead to overexposure to the elements.

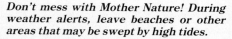

*Don't mess with Mother Nature! During weather alerts, leave beaches or other areas that may be swept by high tides.*

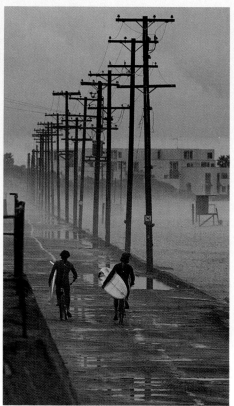

out a doctor by resting in a cool, dry place and by drinking plenty of fluids.

Heat exhaustion is more serious, with worsening symptoms of profuse sweating, dizziness, faintness, nausea, and mental confusion. The skin is pale and feels cold and clammy. Victims of heat exhaustion should lie down in a cool spot and be given cool compresses and liquids.

Perhaps the most serious heat disorder is heatstroke, in which the body's thermoregulatory system has collapsed completely. The body temperature may soar to 104° to 106° F, the skin will feel dry, and the patient may pass out. First aid must be given to the victim immediately—the person should be covered with a cool, wet sheet or plunged into an ice bath to reduce body temperature. Call for an ambulance—victims of heatstroke will probably need to be hospitalized.

Fortunately, these problems can easily be avoided as long as certain commonsense precautions are taken to make exercise in the heat safer:
• Wear loose-fitting, light-colored (sun-reflective) clothing when exercising outdoors.
• Wear adequate sunscreen protection (be sure to check out what's adequate for you) and a hat—especially between the hours of 10:00 A.M. and 2:00 P.M.
• In extreme dry heat (95° F and above, humidity below 40 percent) or moderate to extreme humid heat (85° F and above, greater than 70 percent humidity), schedule workouts early in the morning or during the evening's twilight hours.

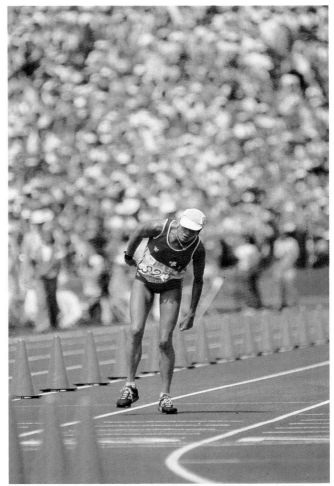

*Heat exhaustion hit Gabriele Andersen-Schiess as she struggled to finish the 1984 Olympic marathon in Los Angeles.*

> *To lessen risk, exercise in the morning or evening when the temperature is cooler.*

• If you must work out in extreme heat, take it easy. Cycle or jog 1 mile instead of 2, then go swimming. Play two sets of tennis instead of three, nine holes of golf instead of 18.
• While hot-weather winds don't usually chill the body, windy conditions add stress to any workout, decreasing physical-performance levels and stamina. For instance, in an average set of tennis on a 90° F day with 25-mile-per-hour winds blowing, an athlete expends over 800 calories of heat energy just to compensate for the wind. Jogging or cycling against the same wind also "burns up" the body's energy.
• When experiencing hot weather-conditions that your body is not used to, acclimate yourself. The body is equipped with adaptive mechanisms that can improve performance and comfort after exposure to hot weather. But these mechanisms do not work overnight, so you must *gradually* increase your workout intensity.
• Exercising in the shade is better for continuous outdoor hot-weather workouts, except in high humidity. Shade temperatures beneath trees can be 15° to 20° F cooler.
• Remember to cool down. After jogging, basketball, swimming, tennis, or cycling in the heat, walk for at least five minutes, then shower.

• Don't eat a big meal prior to a hot-weather workout. Food digestion shunts much of the blood supply away from the muscles used in activity.

• Drink plenty of water. The more intense the exercise, the more water is lost that must be replaced. Forget the water and body temperature soars, performance suffers, cardiac output decreases, and well-being deteriorates rapidly. Most people tend to drink only one-half to two-thirds the amount of water they lose in sweat, leading to progressive dehydration. You should drink at least 2 percent of your body weight to maintain body fluids during a typical workout. That's 1.5 quarts of fluids if you weigh 150 pounds, or 2 quarts if you weigh 200 pounds—enough to give yourself a safety margin.

*In cold weather, protect all exposed skin from frostbite. Try to keep dry by choosing clothes that wick moisture away from the skin.*

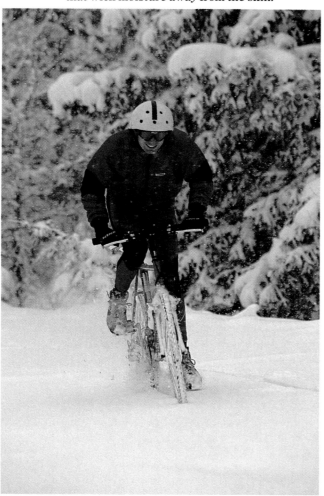

## Cold Weather

As in hot weather, exercising in cold weather conditions will make your body's heat engine work overtime to retain its temperature balance. In the cold the body has a tendency to lose heat energy rather than gain it. To counteract this problem, the body will burn more fuel to increase heat production. In addition, blood vessels and capillaries in the skin will begin narrowing (constricting), shutting off the flow of warm blood to the extremities (fingers, toes, ears, and face) in an effort to keep the body's vital organs warm.

Fingers and toes may be able to withstand a drop of 30 to 40 degrees below normal temperature, but when the internal body temperature drops below 94° F, hypothermia can develop, which can be life-threatening. One of the first signs of hypothermia is uncontrollable shivering, the involuntary contraction of muscles to generate heat. Other signs—speech may become slurred, and movements sluggish, followed by drowsiness or dizziness.

Constant activity in cold weather will certainly help fend off hypothermia. But even constant motion can cause problems if the skin becomes wet due to rain, snow, or perspiration. In order to keep the body as dry as possible in cold weather, make sure to choose clothes that absorb moisture and wick it away from the skin. When outside for long periods, bring dry clothing to change into if your first layer becomes damp.

Another cold-weather problem is frostbite. Exposed flesh can be frozen in three to five minutes in subzero temperatures or windy weather. Frozen skin can lead to frostbite and, in the most extreme cases where blood vessels are affected, to the gangrenous loss of frozen tissue, especially the fingers and toes.

The first symptom of frostbite is a pins-and-needles sensation, followed by complete numbness. The skin of the affected area appears white, cold, and hard, and then becomes red and swollen. Warm the area with hands or clothing, or, if possible, immerse the injured area in warm water (no hotter than 110° F).

To avoid these cold-weather dangers, take these precautions:

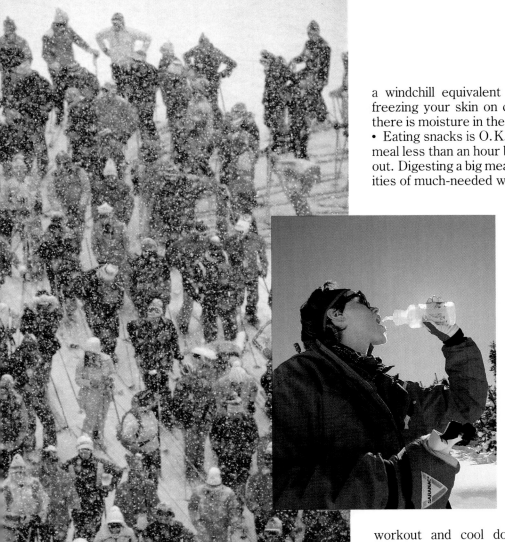

a windchill equivalent to 20° *below zero*—freezing your skin on contact—especially if there is moisture in the air.

• Eating snacks is O.K., but don't have a big meal less than an hour before a winter workout. Digesting a big meal starves the extremities of much-needed warm blood and makes

*Whatever the weather, don't leave your common sense in the locker room.*

you lethargic and lowers your level of alertness.

• Drink plenty of water — especially during one of those vigorous cold-weather workouts.

• Don't forget to warm up before a workout and cool down afterwards—the same as in hot weather.

• Acclimatize. If you're not used to exercising in cold weather, prepare for it gradually. Go outside a little bit at a time; don't immerse yourself all at once in nature's fridge.

• Keep moving. In extreme cold, no matter what exercise you've been doing, it's unwise to rest for more than a few minutes. Get out of the cold or move your muscles, stamp your feet, jog in place, or jump up and down.

No matter what the weather, it's always a good idea to stay fit. Physical fitness reduces the body's response to heat stress because it increases sweating and breathing efficiency, thereby keeping the body's core temperature stable. In cold weather, fitness helps maintain blood flow to the extremities.

Whatever the weather, don't leave common sense in the locker room. When making exercise weather out of any weather, follow the Boy Scout's credo: Be prepared. ◇

*Dehydration is a major problem during vigorous cold-weather workouts, such as cross-country skiing, above. One rule of thumb is to drink 5 to 10 ounces of water every 15 minutes.*

• Wear enough dark-colored (sun-absorbent) clothing for the conditions. You can jog comfortably in temperatures as low as 15° F if you dress warmly—wearing thermal underwear under a wind-resistant jogging suit along with a cap and mittens (gloves allow more dexterity, but they permit greater heat loss through the fingers).

• Watch the windchill factor. For instance, in a 35° F air temperature with a 25-mile-per-hour wind blowing, your flesh could begin to suffer frostbite in seven minutes. That's because the apparent air temperature—what it feels like—is 8° F. If the actual temperature is 20° F, a 35-mile-per-hour wind will produce

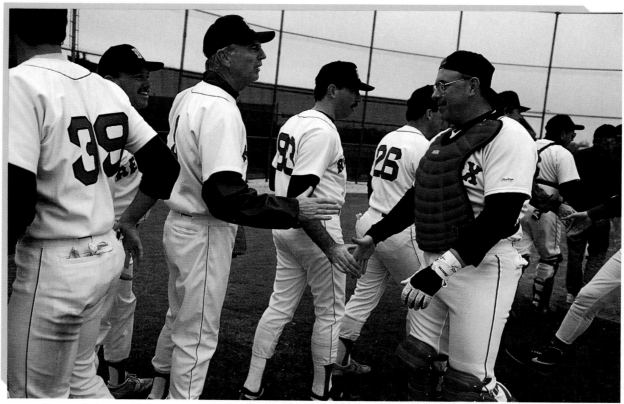

*Many of the specialty sports schools operated by major-league teams give amateur athletes the opportunity to learn from—and play side-by-side with—professional players.*

# Specialty Sports Schools

*by Christiane N. Brown*

For men and women who enjoy playing a sport—whether for competitive, social, or business reasons—perfecting form and technique is not an easy task. Many athletes find that despite their best efforts, practice does not always make perfect—often because they have been practicing with flawed techniques and without expert instruction.

Whether you are a beginner or an advanced player, if you are interested in improving your game you may want to consider attending an athletic school or clinic that specializes in your favorite sport. With the assistance of professional instructors and fully equipped training facilities, specialty sports camps can help correct (or prevent) flaws in form and technique.

More advanced athletes attend sports clinics to hone their skills and to achieve a higher level of play. Less serious-minded athletes sign up for less intensive programs to enjoy an active week of athletic activity, benefit from professional instruction, and meet new people.

As opposed to one-on-one lessons with a private instructor, specialty sports clinics are group affairs divided into training and competition sessions. Classes are broken down according to skill level so every student can be challenged without being overwhelmed by the training regimen.

Some sports schools offer the benefit of state-of-the-art training equipment. For example, The Grand Cypress Academy of Golf in Orlando, Florida, uses CompuSport, a computer video system that helps students develop their golf swing and even recommends the ideal clubs for their bags. As a matter of course, most schools videotape each student's performance to analyze his or her technique and to illustrate problems, improvements, or just to capture the player's greatest moments.

Sports-school vacation packages typically last three to seven days and include lodging and meals. Potential students should seek out a camp that suits both their budget and their personal taste. The range of available programs spans from elegant golf and tennis schools located in resort villages—complete with swimming pools, live entertainment, and gourmet meals—to baseball and basketball schools where students spend most of their time in a ballpark or stadium. For students who are not interested in complete vacation packages, some sports schools also offer commuter packages and one-day seminars and workshops.

### Training with the "Pros"
Meeting well-known sports figures is often part of the attraction of the specialty-sports-camp experience. In some cases, the sports personalities actually coach, train, and play the sport with students. For example, basketball legends Magic Johnson and Jerry West lend their names to specialty sports camps, while other superstars, including baseball Hall of Famer Jim "Catfish" Hunter and National Basketball Association (NBA) and American Basketball Association great Connie Hawkins, are well-advertised participants in other programs. However, the level of involvement of these and other famous athletes varies among the different schools and programs.

"Some camps use big-name sports figures as a marketing technique," warns Jeff Solomon, executive director of the National Camp Association. "Although the possibility of meeting a professional player can be exciting, it's more important that a qualified instructor teach students the sport."

*Weekend athletes attend sports clinics to hone their skills and to learn new techniques to improve their game.*

### Finding the Right School
Before signing up for a specialty sports clinic or school, a potential student should carefully interview its director and its instructors.

An interested attendee should ask if the school is endorsed by any professional sports associations, such as the NBA. In addition, a prospective student should find out if the course instructors have the proper credentials and qualifications. Experts recommend schools where the instructors have year-round coaching experience. For example, if you want to improve your golf game, you should look for instructors who are certified by the Professional Golf Association (PGA) or the Ladies Professional Golf Association (LGPA) and who coach golfers year-round, not just during the summer months.

Some schools have a specific coaching philosophy that all of their instructors must follow. If so, you should understand and agree with the school's philosophy of teaching before deciding to attend. For example, you may not want to attend a tennis camp that believes there is only one right way to swing a tennis racquet. You may prefer to find a tennis coach who will work with you to perfect the swing that you already have. Ask about the ratio of students to coaches, the total hours of instruction each day, and length of each training session.

Also, if you are a beginner without the "tools of the trade," look for a program that will rent or supply such expensive equipment as golf clubs or tennis racquets. At the end of the program, if you find that you enjoy the sport and wish to pursue it, ask one of the staff professionals for advice on selecting your equipment.

### Specialty Sports Camps
There is a long list of specialty sports camps —for baseball, golf, tennis, basketball, and triathlons, for example—that are offered in locations throughout the United States. The prices of these camps and the professional sports figures that attend the programs change from year to year.

## Baseball

Almost all of the major-league teams sponsor or lend their names to baseball "fantasy" camps at various times of the year. These programs re-create the major-league experience for average adult players—both male and female. "Rookies" (who average 40 in age) are taught the finer points of baseball by current and former baseball greats who serve as instructors.

"People become rejuvenated at these baseball camps," explains Mike Yaccino, marketing director of Randy Hundley's Baseball Fantasy Camps, which organizes fantasy camps for the Chicago Cubs and the St. Louis Cardinals. "Adults get to live out their childhood fantasies of playing professional baseball."

Baseball camps generally last a long weekend or a full week. They are usually conducted at the professional team's own ballpark or at the team's spring-training grounds. Rookies are coached in the fundamentals of baseball—hitting, fielding, pitching, and base running. All participants must be in good health. A listing of some popular baseball camps can be found in the opposite column.

*For many adults, attending a baseball camp helps them at least partially realize a childhood fantasy: playing in the big leagues.*

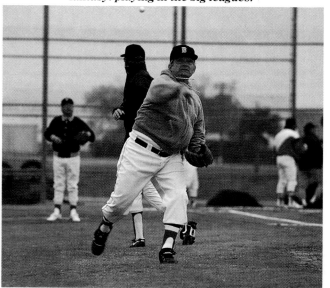

### BASEBALL

All of the camps below include hotel accommodations, most meals, playing equipment, and practice time and coaching with current or former professional players. If your favorite major-league team is not mentioned below, call its corporate headquarters and ask if they sponsor or are affiliated with a baseball camp.

| Camp Name & Address | Age | Cost*/Length of Stay |
|---|---|---|
| Dream Week, Inc. P.O. Box 115 Huntingdon Valley, PA 19006 *Camp is held at the Philadelphia Phillies spring training complex in Clearwater, FL. Includes daily practice and coaching by Phillies players, a Phillies uniform and jacket, a highlights video, and a final party.* | 30 and over | $3,595/week |
| Randy Hundley's Baseball Fantasy Camps; 675 North Court Suite 160, Palatine, IL 60067 *Conducts camps for the Chicago Cubs and the St. Louis Cardinals in their home stadiums and in Mesa, AZ. Includes a highlights video, uniform, and an awards banquet.* | 30 and over | $2,995/week; $1,600/3 days |
| Red Sox Fantasy Camp RR #3, P.O. Box 1788 Waterbury, VT 05676 *Takes place at the Red Sox spring training camp in Fort Myers, FL. Includes nightly activities, a game against former Red Sox players, a uniform, and pro player speeches.* | 30 and over | $3,500/week |
| Whitey Ford's Baseball Fantasy Camp 74 Palisade Avenue Cliffside Park, NJ 07010 *Camp is held in the spring training site of the New York Yankees in Fort Lauderdale, FL. Includes airfare, a uniform, and practice with former Yankees.* | Adult | $3,795/week |

*1994 fees

## Golf

Golf schools are in operation throughout the year with programs ranging in length from one day to one week. Details about four typical golf schools are presented on the top of the facing page.

Students of all levels can learn expert tips from highly experienced professional golfers. Many schools offer training programs that utilize video technology, practice areas with mirrors, and learning libraries with book and video references.

Although most programs cater to golfers at all levels of expertise, there are also highly specialized golf schools available. Some are geared specifically for players with low handicaps, some are for women only, others are just for left-handed players. Some programs cater to golfers who want to perfect just one aspect of their game. Golf Digest Schools, for example, offer "Short Game" schools, which

## GOLF

All of the camps listed below offer programs that include accommodations, most meals, and personal instruction from experienced professional golfers. There are over 100 golf schools and camps in the United States. Some of these schools offer camps for junior players during the summer months.

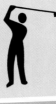

| Camp Name & Address | Age | Cost*/Time |
|---|---|---|
| The Golf Digest Instruction Schools<br>5520 Park Avenue<br>Box 395, Trumbull, CT 06611-0395<br>*The school has 18 locations around the country. Students can select programs from two to five days long and with or without accommodations. Includes full days of personalized instruction and one afternoon on the golf course with the instructors.* | 18 and over | from $1,450/<br>three days |
| Grand Cypress Academy of Golf<br>1 North Jacaranda<br>Orlando, FL 32836<br>*This program combines computer technology with personal instruction. Students receive personal instruction, take-home video analysis, and computer club fitting.* | 18 and over | from $1,425/<br>three days |
| The Golf Institute, Innisbrook Resort<br>P.O. Box 1088<br>Tarpon Springs, FL 34688-1088<br>*The institute offers three-, four-, and five-day programs with four hours of instruction daily, on-course supervised play, and video analysis for home use.* | All ages | from $1,200/<br>three days |
| The Pine Needles Learning Center<br>P.O. Box 88<br>Southern Pines, NC 28387<br>*This program utilizes high-speed video cameras to analyze golf swings and the amenities of a complete resort. Instructors include former LPGA champion Peggy Kirk Bell.* | Ages 10 to 18 | from $845/<br>week |

*1994 fees

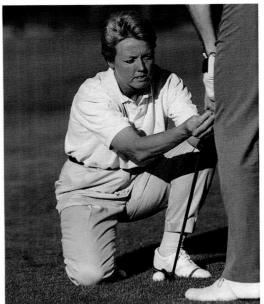

*Golf camps offer instruction according to level of expertise. For advanced golfers, the program may focus on just one aspect of the game.*

are entirely devoted to trouble shots around the green: pitching, chipping, bunker shots, and putting.

### Triathlons

Triathlons are three-sport (typically swimming, biking, and running) events that have grown very popular in recent years. Although some beginning triathletes are already skilled in one of the sports—often in running—triathlon clinics or camps help athletes train for all three segments of the race.

"Triathlon camps can save beginners years worth of training by teaching them how to

*Triathlon camps concentrate on teaching athletes how to physically train and psychologically prepare for the grueling three-sport races.*

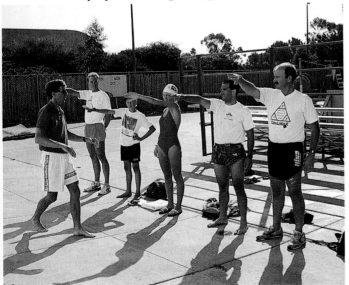

## TRIATHLON

The two programs listed below include lodging, meals, physical training, nutrition education, and technique instruction from experienced triathletes.

| Camp Name & Address | Age | Cost*/Time |
|---|---|---|
| National Triathlon Training Camp<br>1015 Gayley Avenue, Suite 217<br>Los Angeles, CA 90024<br>*Offers triathletes an intensive weekend of training and an education in race strategy, training techniques, and nutrition. Groups are divided by skill level.* | 14 and over | $275/four days,<br>$185/three days |
| Women's Quest<br>25 Arapahoe Avenue<br>Suite E4-181, Boulder, CO 80302<br>*A program for women only. Emphasis is placed on all-around health and fitness. Campers receive physical training, as well as instruction on mental preparation, yoga, and nutrition. Sessions are geared to a particular skill level.* | Adult | $750/five days |

*1994 fees

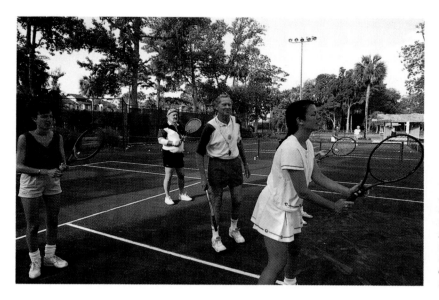

*Tennis schools work with players of all ages and abilities to analyze and improve their games. Many novice players find that their mastery of the game improves dramatically after attending tennis camp.*

## TENNIS

All of the programs below include hotel accommodations, most meals, court time, and instruction from tennis professionals. Most clinics divide guests into groups according to ability. Many tennis programs offer camps for junior players during the summer months.

| Camp Name & Address | Age | Cost*/Time |
|---|---|---|
| Van der Meer Tennis Center<br>P.O. Box 5902<br>Hilton Head Island, SC 29938<br>*Various clinics are geared toward players of all abilities. Includes intensive instruction, video analysis, and strategy sessions.* | All ages | from $455/<br>five days |
| John Newcomb Tennis Ranch<br>P.O. Box 310469<br>New Braunfels, TX 78131-0469<br>*Includes video critique, free court time, and a pro-to-guest ratio of one to four.* | All ages | $850/week,<br>$305/weekend |
| Stan Smith Tennis Academy<br>11 Lighthouse Lane<br>Sea Pines Racquet Club<br>Hilton Head Island, SC 29938<br>*This camp is geared for intermediate and advanced players. The program includes stroke and strategy instruction, drills, and video analysis.* | 18 and over | $245/four days<br>(excluding<br>accommodations) |
| Harry Hopman/Saddlebrook<br>International Tennis<br>5700 Saddlebrook Way<br>Wesley Chapel, FL 33543<br>*The five-day program includes a minimum of five hours per day in small clinics. Also included is match play with instructors, video analysis, and unlimited court practice time.* | All ages | from $800/<br>five days |

*1994 fees

about preparing for a race." Information about two popular triathlon camps is presented on the bottom of page 121.

## Tennis

Tennis clinics typically last anywhere from two days to one week. Some offer resort vacation packages, which provide a host of recreational activities, along with tennis instruction. Other tennis programs are devoted entirely to the sport, and expect participants to work intensely to improve or even overhaul their tennis game.

Most clinics are divided into groups graded by ability. There are drills for every aspect of the game, including match play for adults, audiovisual aids, fitness and agility exercises, and stroke and strategy instruction. Some tennis clinics are detailed in the box at left.

## Basketball

Many teams in the NBA—including the Washington Bullets, Los Angeles Lakers, and Phoenix Suns—sponsor or are affiliated with adult basketball camps. These camps offer ordinary basketball fans a chance to train with past and present professional basketball players, coaches, and trainers.

Players who want to attend these camps must be in good health, and some programs ask that attendees meet certain age requirements (usually age 30 and over). Three well-known camps are described on page 123.

train properly in the first place," says Colleen Cannon, who runs Women's Quest triathlon camps. "Campers receive expert advice from professional triathletes who know everything

## BASKETBALL

All of the camps listed below include hotel accommodations, most meals, and instruction from current and former professional players and coaches. These camps ask that all players be in good health before attending. If your favorite pro team is not mentioned below, call its corporate headquarters and ask if they are affiliated with a basketball camp.

| Camp Name & Address | Age | Cost*/Time |
| --- | --- | --- |
| Wes Unseld's Washington Bullets Adult Basketball Camp 1 Harry S. Truman Drive Landover, MD 20785 *Daily workout sessions take place at the Washington Bullets' training center in Sheperdstown, WV. Camp members train with Bullets coaches, running big-league drills. Includes Bullets workout gear, an awards dinner, and visits from Bullets players.* | Adult | $1,350/four days |
| Magic Johnson/Jerry West Executive Camp 10100 Santa Monica Boulevard Suite 316, Los Angeles, CA 90067 *The camp offers instruction and play with Magic Johnson, Jerry West, and the Laker coaching staff. The program includes a Laker uniform, a banquet, and a video. The camp is held in Maui, HI.* | 30 and over | $5,900/four days |
| Cotton Fitzsimmons/Kurt Rambis Fast Break Fantasy Camp P.O. Box 1369, Phoenix, AZ 85001 *Two practices are held each day, featuring instruction from Phoenix Suns coaches, Kurt Rambis, and Hall of Famer Connie Hawkins. The camp is held in Lake Tahoe, NV.* | 30 and over | from $2,600/ five days |

*1994 fees

*Professional athletes can be a major draw for a sports camp. Below, superstar Magic Johnson dribbles and shoots hoops with youngsters at a basketball camp.*

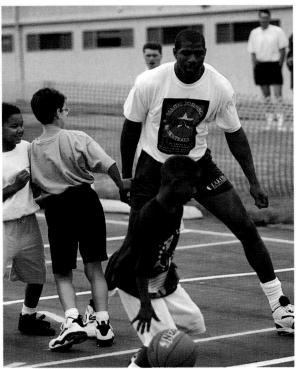

## Camps for Kids

A camp experience can have a significant impact on a child, so parents should always choose a camp carefully. Most experts agree that young children are generally better off at traditional camps that offer a variety of activities such as archery, arts and crafts, fishing, hiking, horseback riding, and swimming. Young children may find themselves overwhelmed by the intensity and competitiveness they are likely to experience at specialty sports camps. And if they have a negative experience at such a camp, it may well turn them off to a particular sport forever.

However, a specialty sports camp might be the perfect choice for an older child or teenager who is interested in learning the game or improving his or her performance in the particular sport. The decision depends on the maturity of the child. At specialty sports camps, staff and facilities are geared to provide a concentrated experience in a single sport, such as tennis, soccer, basketball, or baseball.

Before you make a commitment, talk to your child about the type of camp he or she would like to attend. Children are much more likely to enjoy the experiences if they have a hand in the selection process.

Parents should meet with camp directors to get specific information about facilities and programs. Make sure to ask about food service, sleeping and bathroom arrangements, medical service, safety provisions, insurance costs, and whether the camp is accredited and, if so, by what organizations. Also ask the camp about staff credentials and for references in your area.

Before choosing any camp program (whether it be a general camp, sports specialty camp, or another specialty camp), it is best to get expert advice from an impartial advisory group, such as the *American Camp Association* (ACA), which will send you a free directory of the camps in an area and give general camp referrals. The ACA can be reached at 5000 State Road 67 North, Martinsville, IN 46151.

As might be expected, camp prices can vary considerably. Four weeks at a private sleep-away camp can cost between $1,700 and $2,800; eight weeks will typically range

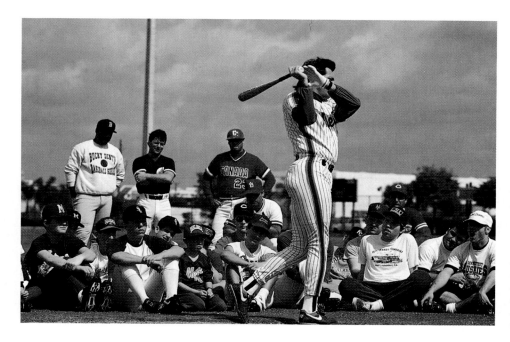

*Many parents prefer to send their children to specialty sports camps rather than to the more-traditional summer camps. Even those sports camps that feature appearances by professional athletes are reasonably affordable.*

from about $2,800 to $5,000. The following is a sampling of some specialty sports camps for children.

**Swarthmore Tennis Camp,** 444 East 82nd Street, Suite 31D, New York, NY 10028. Located in Swarthmore, Pennsylvania, this camp is open to students of all abilities, ages 9 to 18. The program at Swarthmore includes five hours of team play, private lessons, and group instruction each day. The 1994 cost of a one-week program is $560, which includes instruction, food, and housing. The cost of each additional week is less.

**Play Ball Baseball Academy,** P.O. Box 4855, Fort Lauderdale, FL 33338. Camps are located in Fort Lauderdale, Florida; Cape Cod, Massachusetts; and West Virginia. Campers aged 8 to 23 can spend as many weeks as they wish improving their batting average, base-stealing strategies, and other baseball skills. All levels of players are welcome. The 1994 cost of a one-week program is $460, which includes instruction, food, and housing. Additional weeks are discounted.

**The Big League Sports Camps,** 2546 Croppsey Avenue, Brooklyn, NY 11214. Located at Montclair State College in New Jersey,

this organization provides three different sport programs for kids: Big League Baseball, Hall of Fame Soccer, and Hall of Fame Basketball. All programs are geared for children at all levels of ability, ages 8 through 19. Each child's skill level is evaluated early in the program; then he or she is placed into an appropriate competitive group. All Big League Sports Camp participants receive roughly 7.5 hours of instruction, drills, practice, and games each day.

There is a minimum stay of one week, at a 1994 cost of $450, although campers are permitted to stay the entire nine weeks of the camp. The cost includes three daily meals, expert instruction, and housing.

**Aim High Basketball Camp,** P.O. Box 183, Kingston, RI 02881. This camp is located on beautiful ocean-front property at St. George's School in Newport, Rhode Island. The camp has a developmental program for kids aged 8 to 17. Campers are divided by age and ability and coached in basic fundamentals of basketball. Each day campers can learn from a different guest speaker who is either a professional basketball player or coach. The program runs one week in August and costs $350 for instruction, food, and housing. ◇

# HOT TUBS AND SPAS:

## Healthy or Hazardous?

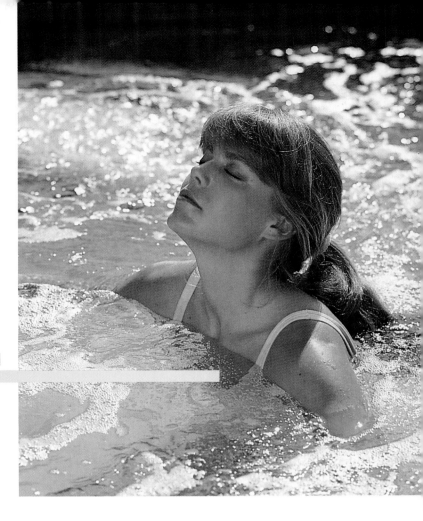

*by Susan Nielsen*

Ahhh! In today's hurried and harried world, there's nothing like slipping into a hot tub or spa to melt away the day's tensions and to pamper sore muscles. The warm, bubbling jet streams of water not only feel good—they are good for you.

For centuries, people have enjoyed soaking and bathing in natural hot springs. The ancient Romans went so far as to build public baths to which thousands of people flocked for the pleasure of luxuriating in warm water. Today people are drawn to the same physical and mental benefits of soaking in hot water as were the people of ancient cultures.

Then, as now, hot water's primary health benefit is its ability to cause the body's blood vessels to dilate, a process called vasodilation. When blood vessels are dilated, circulation to the entire body improves. At the same time, the pulse rate slows because, as the body floats in water, the heart no longer has to contend with gravity. The heart also enlarges slightly and works 10 to 20 percent more efficiently.

According to a study conducted by Mary R. Duncan, M.D., for the National Spa and Pool Institute (NSPI): "The first response to immersion [in a hot tub] . . . is a general and muscular relaxation. The hot water is beneficial to the functioning of weak or spastic muscles, and is usually sedative for those with arthritis, muscle pains, and neuralgia."

From arthritis sufferers seeking temporary relief to professional athletes nursing sports injuries, a hot soak can ease painful joints and muscles. The buoyancy of the water supports the joints and muscles, and lessens the stress on them, resulting in freer movement. For those without any physical pain, a hot soak can simply ease the mind. However, some precautions should be considered when using a hot tub or spa.

### Before You Soak

Before entering the tub, inspect the water. If it is cloudy, foaming, or has a strong chlorine smell, the water needs maintenance and treatment. Soaking in such water increases

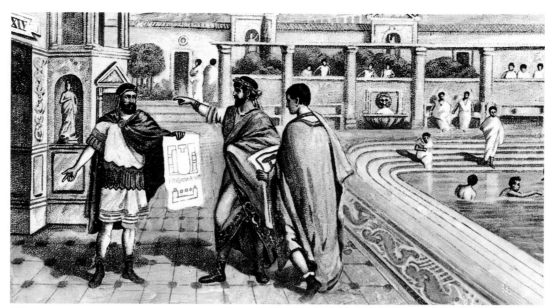

*Where possible, the ancient Romans located their public baths over natural hot-water springs. Ancient bathers often ended their visit to the baths with a dip in the cold-water frigidarium.*

your chances of getting a skin rash or respiratory infection caused by a strain of bacteria called pseudomonas. Similarly, people with skin, ear, genital, or other body infections, or open sores or wounds, should not use a hot tub, because of the risk of spreading infection. It is essential to chemically treat a hot tub as directed by the manufacturer.

Showering before using a hot tub removes creams, lotions, and deodorants from the skin. These products can reduce the effectiveness of the hot tub's disinfectant treatment and decrease the filter's efficiency. To wash away skin bacteria that may have been picked up in the tub, showering after a soak is a good idea.

Another point to consider before slipping in for a soak: Medication and hot water don't always mix. A hot tub can intensify the effects of some medications, leading to dizziness, light-headedness, and other severe reactions. If you are taking any prescription or over-the-counter medication, consult your doctor about potential side effects.

### During Your Soak

Certain body changes take place as you sit in a hot tub. "The circulatory system must dissipate excess heat so the internal organs do not get overheated," says Jonathan L. Halperin, M.D., director of Clinical Services in the Division of Cardiology at Mount Sinai Medical Center in New York City. "The hotter the water, the harder it is for the body

to regulate its temperature." This reaction, coupled with the force of gravity, he says, causes blood to be pooled in the parts of the body under the water and in the skin as the body attempts to rid itself of the excess heat. At the same time, gravity is pulling blood downward. That is why, if you stand too quickly after soaking, blood pressure may drop, reducing blood flow to your brain. The result: you may feel dizzy, light-headed, and may even faint. This is known as *orthostatic hypotension.*

Always check the water thermometer before entering the tub. The water should feel soothing to the skin, not hot; ideally, it should not exceed 104° F (40° C). At this temperature, you can safely soak for no more than 15 minutes at any one time. In lower temperatures, however—closer to the body's own of 98.6° F—you can generally soak for longer periods. Try various temperatures to determine which is the most comfortable for you. But be aware of the soaking time. During a prolonged soak, your body can't dissipate the heat, and *hyperthermia,* an unsafe level of body temperature, may result.

As you relax, the temptation may exist to complement your mellow state with alcoholic beverages . . . but think again. Alcohol combined with the vasodilating effects of hot water acts to expand blood vessels and increase body temperature—a deadly mixture. Your body temperature may accelerate too quickly to dangerous levels. Worse yet, when under the influence, you may not realize how hot you are getting. Meanwhile, the alcohol may cause nausea, dizziness, or light-headedness. This lethal combination may lead to loss of consciousness, heart attack, injury, or even death from drowning (caused by passing out or falling in the tub).

As the body attempts to rid itself of the excess heat, you perspire, losing valuable water and salts. Alcohol, a diuretic, amplifies this effect. As a result, you become quite dehydrated. If the water and salt are not replenished, hyperthermia may occur.

### Users Beware

Certain people may be at particular risk for some of the dangers associated with hot tubs. For instance, many diabetics have an impairment of the nervous system that reduces skin sensation. Thus, a diabetic may not realize how hot the water or tub surfaces are, and get burned. Moreover, the diabetic's autonomic, or involuntary, nervous system sometimes malfunctions. When the reflexes are not working properly, blood pressure may fall, and light-headedness may result.

Pregnant women should use a hot tub only on a doctor's advice. During pregnancy, there are a number of changes in the cardiovascular system as well as a redistribution of body mass. For example, the uterus presses on veins that normally drain blood flow from the legs. This makes it more difficult for blood flow to return to the heart for pumping to other parts of the body. As a result, light-headedness or dizziness may occur when standing to exit the tub. Furthermore, the uterus does not have any way to dissipate the heat from a hot tub. A small mass, such as the fetus, heats up faster than a large one, such as the adult female carrying the fetus. And a mother has no way of monitoring the temperature of the fetus.

Similarly, children also "heat up" faster than adults. "Parents often make the mistake of projecting their thermal comfort level on their children," says Thomas Adams, Ph.D., professor and associate chair of undergraduate studies in the Department of Physiology at Michigan State University in East Lansing. "A child's smaller body will heat up much quicker than an adult's in a hot tub. That is

## Hot-Tub Tips

Here are steps you can take to keep your cool in a hot tub:
• To help the body dissipate the excess heat, keep part of your body above the water.
• Limit hot-tub soaks to short intervals so the body can rid itself of excess heat.
• Shower between soaks.
• Never use a hot tub when alone.
• Do not hesitate to leave the tub if you get too hot or feel nauseous or dizzy, even if others stay in. Everyone reacts differently to heat.
• Wait a bit after eating before using a hot tub. The body's blood flow will be concentrating on aiding digestion.
• Slowly step out of the tub so you don't get dizzy or light-headed. This way your body has a chance to redirect the blood flow from your skin to your brain.
• If you are unsure about whether you should use a hot tub, contact your physician for advice.

why children should not remain in a hot tub for any extended period of time, and they should always be under adult supervision when using a hot tub."

People with certain cardiovascular ailments should also be careful when using a hot tub. As the body attempts to cool down, the blood vessels in the skin dilate, which in turn causes blood pressure to drop. For those with high blood pressure, a sudden drop in pressure can cause dizziness and light-headedness—especially if the high blood pressure is being treated with medication. Similarly, for those with low blood pressure, the pressure can drop even further with the same effects.

For those with heart palpitations or mitral-valve prolapse, for example, the hot water may aggravate their symptoms, possibly producing an irregular heartbeat. People with any type of cardiovascular disease or those taking medication should consult a physician before using a hot tub.                    ◇

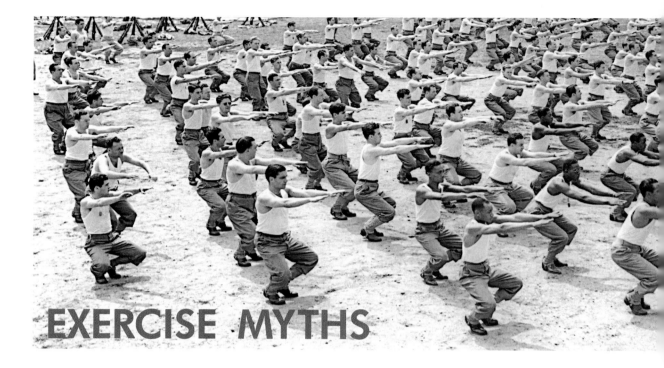

# EXERCISE MYTHS

*by Ralph LaForge*

Over the years, many myths about exercise have been dispelled as physiology research has matured. Every year, exercise behaviors still used by many people are found to be nonbeneficial or even downright harmful. Here's a list of eight of the worst offenders.

### Myths from the Good Old Days . . .

1. **Sit-ups.** Traditionally done straight-leg sit-ups win the prize for being one of the greatest exercise myths to this day. One of the most commonly prescribed exercises for generations of young and middle-aged people, the sit-up can stress the lower back. As done with straight legs, pulling oneself up to a sitting position with hands locked behind the neck and knees straight, it can also strain the neck. Today's bent-leg sit-up, or "abdominal crunch," is easier on backs and necks, yet tones the tummy effectively. Here's how: Knees bent and the hands on either side of the head near the ear, use your abdominal muscles to pull up your head and upper chest.

2. **Leg lifts.** "Lie down flat on your back, lift your legs 6 to 8 inches off the ground—now hold it!" Another legacy of the good old days, this torturous exercise was done to tighten the gut and abdominal muscles. A strained lower back could also result if you weren't strong enough to keep the small of your back on the floor. Today we know better. Don't hold both outstretched legs up in the air for any period of time at all. Instead, lie on your back, flex one knee, extend the leg up and hold it. Then bring it down and lift the other leg, bicycle style.

### . . . And from the '90s

3. **Exercise burns cholesterol.** Contrary to popular belief, cholesterol is not a fuel for exercise. You *can* burn fat and triglycerides. Cholesterol is a fat-soluble sterol in your blood, bile, nerve sheaths, and various organs. As a rule, to significantly reduce cholesterol, you must expend 1,500 calories or more weekly, the equivalent of running 15 miles at 100 calories per mile. Cholesterol levels are a matrix of many factors: genetics,

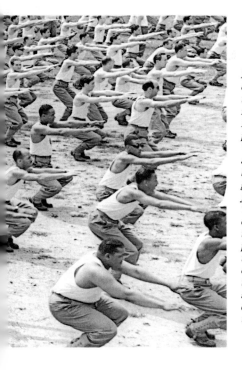

*Many myths about exercise persist; some of them can have downright harmful results. Deep knee bends, as performed by these World War II soldiers at left, have since been found to endanger the ligaments and joints of the knees. Today, exercise physiologists recommend that knee bends be performed by keeping the feet flat and lowering the body to a sitting position, making sure that the knees do not project beyond the toes.*

diet, and, to some extent, fitness. It is not unusual for reasonably fit people to have borderline or—in more than a few cases—high total cholesterol levels.

**4. Exercise converts fat into muscle.** Wrong! Research shows that muscle is protein; flabby muscle cannot change into fat, nor can exercise convert fat into muscle. Certainly, if you do not exercise, chances are you will gain weight and find yourself growing flabby. Training can tone up a flabby muscle, and such toning will help produce the desired slimming effect.

**5. Exercise can help you spot-reduce.** Wrong again. The body doesn't operate on the convenience store approach. It does not draw all of its fuel from fat stored closest to the muscle being exercised. Take abdominal fat. Doing crunches will not necessarily pull energy from the fat roll around the hip, waist, and abdomen. Instead, fuel is pulled from all metabolically available fat stores. Crunches will tone up flabby abdominal muscles, thereby whittling inches. But you must do prolonged endurance exercise—30 to 40 minutes or more—to burn fat from any available stores.

**6. Walking and running both burn about 100 calories per mile.** New evidence shows running a mile takes about 35 percent to 40 percent more energy. In general, walking burns a net of 65 to 75 calories per mile. Only by stepping up the pace to 4.5 to 5 miles per hour can you approach jogging's 100 calories per mile.

**7. High-intensity aerobic exercise is needed to affect depression.** New research shows that to reduce the symptoms of anxiety and depression, low-level exercise can make a big difference. The same is true for stress management and tension reduction. Many new research reports indicate that just about any exercise, done on a regular basis at as little as 35 percent of maximum capacity, can help these symptoms. Significant reduction of anxiety and depressive symptoms has resulted from such diverse activities as T'ai Chi, yoga, and circuit weight training, among others.

**8. You must exercise 2,000 calories (about 5 to 7 hours) per week to lower your risk of cardiovascular disease.** According to new studies from Dallas, Texas, and elsewhere, the biggest drop in risk occurs when couch potatoes go from zero activity to a mere 500 to 800 calories a week—the equivalent of jogging 5 to 8 miles.

Furthermore, the risk continues to drop as you expend more calories. The peak is a weekly level of 1,500 to 2,000 exercise calories. After that, cardiovascular health benefits seem to top out—remember, we're talking about a *specific* health benefit to your cardiovascular system, not overall fitness.

Nancy Owens, Ph.D., of the University of Pittsburgh reported similar results based on the Healthy Women's Study. When more than 500 middle-aged women went from doing zero exercise to the equivalent of a 20-minute walk three times a week, their cardiovascular risk dropped significantly.

The control group, which did not exercise at all, lost more beneficial HDL cholesterol and gained more weight than those who added 300 calories of weekly exercise. The nonexercisers also had higher perceived stress levels. ◇

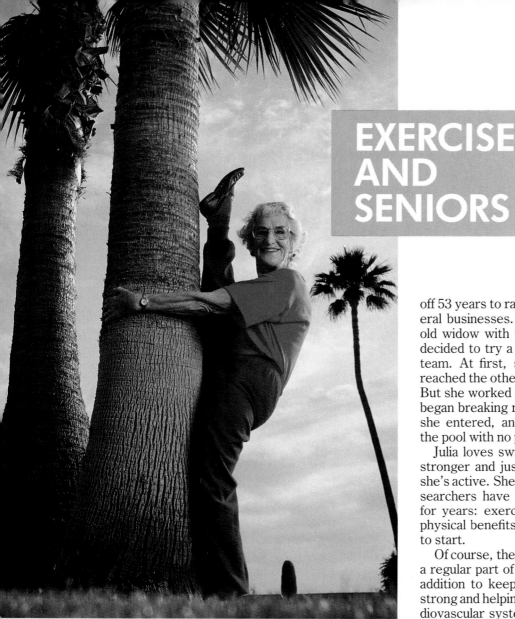

## EXERCISE AND SENIORS

*Exercise is beneficial at any age. But for senior citizens, staying in shape is particularly essential for remaining healthy, strong, and limber.*

*by Linda J. Brown*

Julia Dolce never expected to make it into the pages of *Sports Illustrated*—especially at 84 years old. But she did just that last November, thanks to her considerable prowess as a late-blooming Masters swimmer. A grandmother of seven and great-grandmother of four, Julia holds national and world records in various distance freestyle races. Although she swam competitively while growing up in New York City, she had taken off 53 years to raise a family and run several businesses. In 1981, as a 72-year-old widow with time on her hands, she decided to try a local Y's Masters swim team. At first, she says, "I just about reached the other end of a 25-yard pool." But she worked at it, regained her form, began breaking records in the first meet she entered, and continues to burn up the pool with no plans to stop.

Julia loves swimming and finds she is stronger and just feels better now that she's active. She has discovered what researchers have been telling Americans for years: exercise can provide myriad physical benefits, and it's never too late to start.

Of course, the earlier you make fitness a regular part of your life, the better. In addition to keeping muscles and bones strong and helping maintain a healthy cardiovascular system, exercise may delay the onset of non-insulin-dependent diabetes, and may provide protection against some forms of cancer. On top of that, many exercisers find that they have less stress and that they enjoy other psychological benefits from getting physical. A recent report from the National Institute of Aging states, "If exercise could be packed into a pill, it would be the single most widely prescribed and beneficial medicine in the nation."

### Quality and Quantity

All these benefits can certainly improve not only the quality of life, but maybe the life span as well. In comprehensive research done by Ralph S. Paffenbarger, Jr., M.D., Dr.P.H., and his colleagues at Stanford University in

Palo Alto, California, a group of nearly 17,000 Harvard alumni followed for more than 25 years clearly illustrated an exercise-longevity link. The study found that the more a man exercises, the better his chances to outlive his peers. In fact, exercise that burns as little as 500 calories per week improves life expectancy.

While the Stanford study only looked at self-reported exercise habits for well-educated white men, a study by the Institute for Aerobics Research in Dallas, Texas, put subjects of both sexes to the test. More than 10,000 men and 3,000 women were given treadmill exercise tests to measure fitness. Based on the results, subjects were categorized into five fitness levels and followed for the next eight years. Those with high and even moderate levels of physical fitness had much lower death rates than those near the bottom of the fitness scale. The fitter folks also had less incidence of cardiovascular disease and cancer.

The gains from exercise stack up high, but it does require some effort and commitment to join the ranks of regular exercisers. It is particularly important for people to take the initiative and keep moving in their golden years. With age, our bodies change. Aerobic capacity (the ability of the cardiovascular system to deliver oxygen to working muscles) declines slightly every year after age 30. At the same time, the ability of heart muscle to contract slowly declines, as does the general strength of muscles. The percentage of body fat, as opposed to lean muscle tissue, tends to increase with age. The good news is that we have some control over these declines through our diet and lifestyle habits, with exercise heading the list. And whether you're in your 40s or your 80s, it's never too late to get moving and reap significant gains.

## Healthy Hearts

The tie between exercise and healthy hearts is well established. In July 1992 the American Heart Association (AHA) added punch to that message by placing physical inactivity on its list of risk factors for coronary heart disease. According to the AHA, "regular aerobic physical activity plays a significant role in preventing heart and blood-vessel disease."

Even sedentary older adults can improve their cardiovascular function once they start exercising, as researchers at Washington University School of Medicine in St. Louis, Missouri, discovered. They enlisted 110 sedentary but healthy men and women aged 60 to 71 to engage in a regular endurance exercise program and measured how well their hearts adapted. After one year of walking or jogging for 45 to 50 minutes, four times a week, both men and women im-

*People who exercise frequently find that their level of stress becomes greatly reduced.*

*Always consult a physician before embarking on an exercise program. People who have not engaged in strenuous exercise for years should be extremely careful about suddenly undertaking an intense workout. It's wiser to take it very slowly at first.*

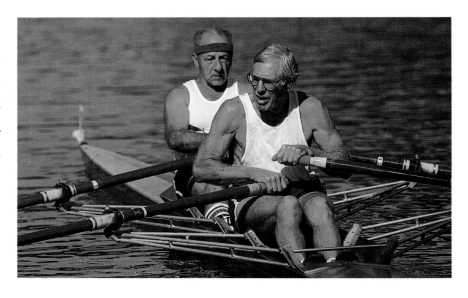

proved their cardiovascular function by 20 to 25 percent, right on par with improvements noted in similar studies of much younger people. Also, all subjects made gains regardless of their initial fitness levels (determined by a treadmill test). "We had some true couch potatoes in the study and we had some who were very physically active, but our results indicate that in this age group, virtually everyone could benefit from endurance exercise training," concluded Wendy Kohrt, Ph.D., research assistant professor of medicine and principal investigator of the study.

Before embarking on any exercise program, you must get your doctor's approval. The next step is to choose an activity that involves motion, uses large muscle groups, and is repetitive and rhythmic. Walking, jogging, hiking, cycling, cross-country skiing, dancing, swimming, stair climbing, and skating all fit that description. To get the full benefits, the American College of Sports Medicine recommends that you work out for 20 to 60 minutes, three to five times a week, at 60 to 90 percent of your maximum heart rate. You may need to work up slowly to that standard, but anything you do is better than nothing. Everett Smith, Ph.D., director of the biogerontology labs at the University of Wisconsin's department of preventive medicine, suggests that even walking in place at home for three to four minutes, resting, and repeating that exercise two to three times a day would be a good start for some.

*Weight-bearing exercises can help adults to maintain healthy bone mass.*

### Pump It Up
Bodybuilder muscles aside, we all need a certain level of muscle strength to function comfortably and safely. But as a person ages, muscle fibers slowly shrink and are replaced by fat or connective tissue. This occurs quite gradually, but with normal aging and a fairly sedentary existence, most people will lose 20 to 40 percent of their muscle mass by age 80, according to the Human Nutrition Research Center on Aging at Tufts University in Boston, Massachusetts. This strength loss plays a big part in the frailty of many seniors, which in turn contributes to the serious problem of falls among the elderly. Strengthening programs can have a profound effect, even among those in their 80s and 90s. Dramatic results were obtained in a study done with 10 subjects, aged 86 to 96, eight of whom had a history of falls and seven of whom used canes or walkers. Simple weight-lifting exercises for thighs, done three times a week for eight weeks, yielded an average strength gain of almost 200 percent. Midthigh muscle area increased nine percent, and gait speed improved 48 percent. After the study, two subjects ditched their canes and three could rise from a chair without using their arms. Study leader Maria Fiatarone, M.D., of the Human Nutrition Research Center on Aging at Tufts University said the results "challenge the expectation of decline in muscle strength associated with aging."

With an eight-week combination of strength training and aerobic exercise, 116 people with an average age of 65 gained 2.5 pounds of new muscle in a study at the South Shore YMCA in Quincy, Massachusetts. The subjects trained two or three days per week for an hour session divided into 25 minutes of strength training and 25 minutes of walking or stationary cycling. Wayne Westcott, Ph.D., the national YMCA strength-training consultant who led the study, said people were excited by their progress. "Once they do enough to start seeing some benefits they realize this is a positive addition to their lives and they look forward to exercise."

### Building Bones
Bones decrease in mass as we get older. For women, the rate of bone loss accelerates rapidly after menopause, especially in those with osteoporosis. The National Osteoporosis Foundation says that a whopping one out of two women over the age of 50 will have a fracture caused by osteoporosis. Men aren't exempt, either: one in five men will develop osteoporosis. Weight-bearing exercises such as weight lifting, jogging, aerobics, racquet sports, and dancing can help maximize bone mass in young adults, maintain bone mass in adults, and reduce bone loss in postmenopausal women.

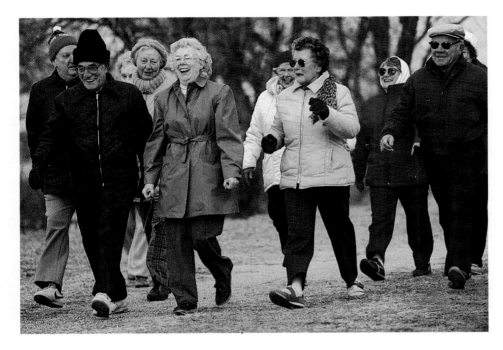

*An invigorating walk several times a week represents a good first step in a regular exercise program— and it's fun, too. During periods of inclement weather, many people prefer to do their walking in a shopping mall or some other indoor facility.*

A four-year study that had women (average age: 50) combining light weight lifting (three to five pounds) with endurance dance cut bone loss in the arms by better than 50 percent. The study leader, Dr. Smith of the University of Wisconsin, has also just finished a study that shows weight-bearing exercise plus calcium intake can almost completely stop bone loss in middle-aged women.

A study comparing low- and high-impact exercise done for 20 minutes, three days a week, for a year found that both types of workouts helped maintain spinal bone among the previously sedentary, postmenopausal female subjects. The study, conducted at the University of Missouri, bodes well for those who only want a moderate fitness program. "It didn't take a lot of exercise to maintain the bone," said study leader Katie Grove, Ph.D., now an assistant professor at Indiana University in Bloomington.

### Exercise/Arthritis Connection

Arthritis in its many forms affects 37 million Americans. Of this group, 15.8 million have osteoarthritis, a degenerative joint disease. Doctors long told arthritis sufferers to avoid vigorous activity. But by the mid-1980s researchers had begun to discover that exercise could help arthritis patients.

Marian Minor, Ph.D., assistant professor of physical therapy at the University of Missouri-Columbia School of Medicine, was one of those early researchers. In her studies she has found great success with a three-day-per-week program that combines 30 to 40 minutes of aerobic endurance with flexibility and strengthening exercises. Exercise seems to lessen the effects of arthritis. "People don't have as much pain, the swelling goes down, they show less depression and anxiety, and they become more active in other aspects of their lives," said Minor. Incorporating several types of exercise is also helpful. "It's important for people with arthritis— partly because the disease changes—to learn to do different kinds of exercise. Walking's fine, but when your hip is sore, it may be better to swim or choose another exercise for awhile."

Whatever you do, you should check with your doctor first and start slowly. You can call the Arthritis Foundation's information line at 800-283-7800 to get an exercise brochure; the Foundation also offers exercise videos. The University of Missouri has a brand-new exercise video entitled "Good Moves for Every Body" for $30. For details, call 314-882-1718.

So while we all grow older each day, we don't need to accept the fact that aging means getting fatter, weaker, and slower. "Fifty percent of what we commonly call aging as far as muscle strength and fitness is disuse atrophy," said Dr. Smith. The choice is yours —use it or lose it. ◇

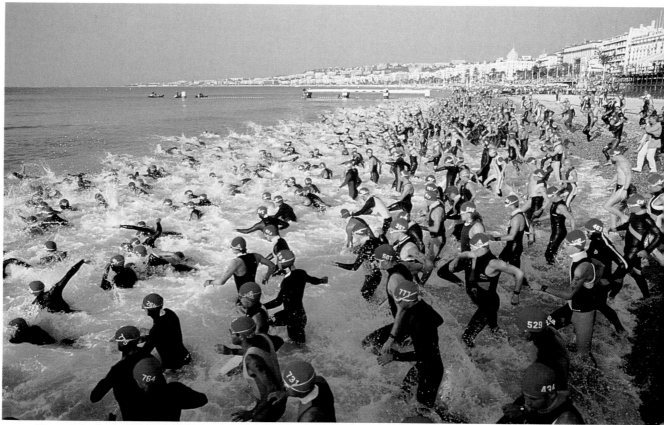

*The original triathlons featured a 2.4-mile swim, a 112-mile bike race, and a 26.2-mile run. Today's distances vary, but all triathlons still include a sequence of swimming, biking, and running.*

# Trying Out Triathlons

*by Linda J. Brown*

Some people just can't resist a challenge. Not content to simply run a race or sweat it out on a bike or take to the water, they have to tackle all three in succession, all in the same day.

Enter the triathlon, a sport designed to appease these not-so-few zealots, an estimated 20,000 in this country alone. That's an amazing number, considering this American-born supersport really came into its own only a little more than a decade ago.

It all started in 1974, when the San Diego Track Club began holding low-key swim-bike-run races as a way to break up their training routines. One participant, a U.S.

Navy officer named John Collins, took the idea to Hawaii, and several years later he merged three long races (the Waikiki Rough Water Swim, the Around-Oahu Bike Ride, and the Honolulu Marathon) to form a triathlon. Collins figured whoever could do all three events in one day "could surely call himself an Iron Man," author Mike Plant writes in his book *Triathlon—Going the Distance*. Only 12 men finished the first Ironman's 2.4-mile swim, 112-mile bike, and 26.2-mile run in 1978. The next year the number rose slightly to 13 men and one woman. Then, according to Plant, the sport took off: by 1980, the number of competitors had increased tenfold.

"It was the Ironman that burned triathlon into the hearts and minds of the general public," Plant writes, especially the unforgettable 1982 race, where the second-place women's finisher, Julie Moss, crawled across the finish line. That year also marked the formation of the United States Triathlon Association, the sport's national governing organization (now called Triathlon Federation/USA, or Tri-Fed), the first race of the United States Triathlon Series, and the premier issue of *Triathlon Magazine.*

Now, with an estimated 1,700 events each year, and more than a quarter of a million

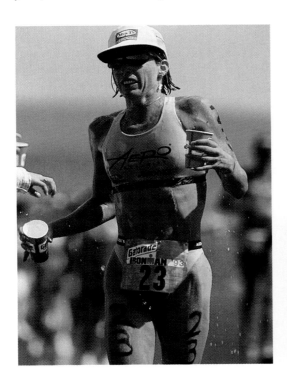

participants, the sport stands firmly entrenched. Distances covered in triathlons vary tremendously, from short sprint races to the popular international distance of a 1.5-kilometer swim, 40-kilometer bike, and 10-kilometer run, all the way up to the ultradistance Ironman and longer. For real hard-core triathlete junkies, there's another triathlon in Hawaii called the Ultraman Triathlon, with a 6.2-mile swim, 260-mile bike, and 52.4-mile run.

While triathlon generally means swim-bike-run, that's not always the case. You can find cross-country skiing, snowshoeing, canoeing, speed skating, in-line skating, and horseback riding mixed in occasionally. The Taylor Quadrathlon in Taos, New Mexico, for instance, consists of a bike, run, cross-country ski, snowshoe, run, and bike, and covers about 50 miles in total. To boost the spectator appeal of triathlons, some race organizers are even taking them indoors. Competitors swim in a pool, ride a bike trainer (for distance in a certain time or for the time it takes to go a specific mileage), and then run on a track.

Since the early Ironman days, triathlons have opened themselves up to a much larger slice of the population, not just elite athletes. "We're trying to make triathlons 'user-friendly' to as many groups as possible," says Tim Yount, deputy director of Tri-Fed/USA. The inclusion of shorter-distance races has made triathlons accessible to athletic homemakers, businesspeople, kids, and senior citizens. Race results typically are divided into five-year age groups, so participants can see how they fare among their contemporaries.

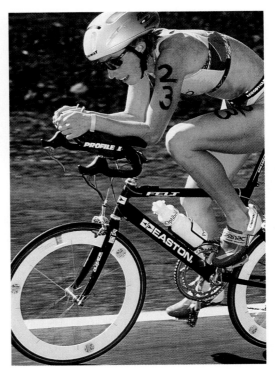

### Child's Play

Seven- to 14-year-old boys and girls can enter youth races, with the youngest among them typically swimming 100 meters, cycling 5 kilometers, and running 1 kilometer. The number of races for junior jocks has risen rapidly. Yount says that almost every major triathlon also holds a youth event; he predicts there will be close to 100 youth races in 1994. The Rainbo Bread Ironkids Series alone hosted 17 races in 1993 in different cities nationwide. "If you asked me about youth races four years ago, I would have said they rarely exist," Yount adds.

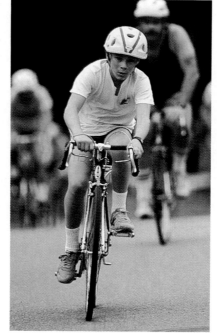

*In a youth triathlon, the distances are for the most part considerably shorter than they are in an adult race.*

The reason for the jump is simple. "A lot of different race directors understand that this is the future of the sport, to get these kids associated with triathlons at a very young age," says Yount.

Race sponsors also draw more women to the sport (now around 23 percent) by holding races for women only.

Another group found in very small numbers, but which often packs a huge, inspira-tional punch, is disabled triathletes. Jim Mac Laren, who lost his left leg just below the knee in 1985, is perhaps the best known. He has competed in numerous triathlons, including several Ironmans during which he cut close to two hours off the Ironman amputee record. Another incredible pair of athletes successfully completed their first triathlon in October 1993 in Islamorada, Florida. Mike Chastain is blind, and his partner, David Lindsey, lost both legs in a boating accident. David and Mike rode a tandem bike and worked together in the swim and run to finish the Bud Lite Sprint and Triathlon in 2:05:00 amid the cheers of 1,500 spectators and athletes.

At the forefront of the special segments of triathletes are the professionals, those sleek, tan, muscular men and women who carve a living out of pursuing triathlon prize money. Five-time Ironman winner Mark Allen and six-time Ironman champ Paula Newby-Fraser currently lead the pro field, an honor they earned by each capturing the 1993 Ironman.

### Geared to Go

From the pros on down to the most neophyte triathletes, everyone needs certain equipment to get into the game. Pared down to the basics, a swimsuit, cap, and goggles; a bike (road bike, mountain bike, or "hybrid," usually offering 18 or 21 speeds); bike helmet; and a pair of running shoes are all you need.

On the high end, if money's no concern, you can equip yourself to the hilt. Bicycles are the biggest-ticket items. Yount notes that you can spend $10,000 to own the ultimate bike, which would include lightweight tita-

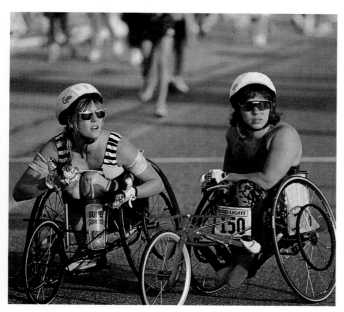

*Disabled triathletes add an inspirational aspect to the sport. Such participants sometimes work in tandem to compensate for each other's disability.*

nium parts, a disc wheel on the back that looks like a solid circle, and a carbon-fiber front wheel or a tri-spoke wheel (both very aerodynamic, fast, and costing about $400 to $500). You'd have tri-bars (more comfortable and aerodynamic), pedals that clip onto your shoes, biking gloves, vented helmet, padded biking shorts, water bottles, sunglasses, and biking shirt. Running is a bargain compared to biking, but shoes can set you back in excess of $100 (high-mileage runners go through at least one pair every six months). Many triathletes also opt for wetsuits in races where they are permitted. So once you start getting fancy, this sport doesn't come cheap.

## Time to Train

All the high-tech equipment in the world won't help without the training base to back it up. For most people, that means juggling job and family to chisel out a training schedule that is adequate for whatever goals you've set for yourself. If you are motivated and make wise use of your time, settling into a training routine is not impossible.

Of course, deciding to take on a triathlon is the first step. If you are in reasonably good shape and can do all three sports fairly well, a sprint triathlon should be within your grasp. Sprint triathlons usually consist of a 1-kilometer (0.62-mile) swim, a 25-kilometer (15.3-mile) bike ride, and a 5-kilometer (3.1-mile) run. Pick a race that's about four months away. That allows a sufficient period of steady, consistent workouts to get yourself ready. The training schedule opposite can serve as a good guide. You may need to adjust it a bit or work up to those distances for your weaker sports, but with this plan, you should build the base you need to become a full-fledged triathlete.

Just so you don't get cocky, here's the mileage a pro might chalk up in one week: at least 10,000 yards (9,144 meters) of swimming, 175 to 300 miles (280 to 480 kilometers) of biking, and 35 to 75 miles (56 to 120 kilometers) of running. How much they log varies with the distance race they are training for and their injury history. "If they're injury-prone, you'll find them doing more quality workouts," says Yount. Top triathlete pro Melissa Mantak sometimes goes by time

rather than distance in her workouts, especially if she's traveled to a place where she doesn't have the routes measured off.

## Hanging Tough

Once you've got your body in shape, you need to toughen your mind, too. Despite faithfully sticking to your training program,

## Beginner Triathlon Training Schedule

Four months from novicehood to a short-distance triathlon. During the first month, forget the schedule and just play around a bit in all three sports. Get used to the bike, explore your running routes, get strong in the pool. During the second month, settle into your training schedule and make adjustments where necessary. Eventually you'll work into a training rhythm.

During the last two months, build the quality of your training, not your mileage. Feeling tired after a hard workout is good; feeling exhausted at the end of the week is not.

| DAY | SWIM | BIKE | RUN |
|---|---|---|---|
| Monday | 1,500–2,000 yds. (continuous, steady pace) | 0 | 3–4 miles (first mile easy, miles two and three hard, fourth mile easy) |
| Tuesday | 0 | 0 | 0 |
| Wednesday | 1,500–2,000 yds. (time trials) | 10–15 miles (steady pace) | 3–4 miles (steady pace) |
| Thursday | 0 | 0 | 0 |
| Friday | 1,500–2,000 yds. (varied pace) | 10–15 miles | 0 |
| Saturday | 0 | 10 miles (very easy pace—after run) | 6–8 miles (easy pace) |
| Sunday | 0 | 25–30 miles (steady pace) | 0 |

**Source:** *Women's Sports and Fitness*

# Tips From the Pros for Smooth Transitions

Switching from the swim to the bike and then from the bike to the run requires you to drop off gear from one segment and put on what you need for the next. The clock keeps running during these times, so those with speedy transitions can gain "free" time over those who fumble around. Here are some tips for snappy transitions:

• *Know race layout* before the gun goes off. Your race number corresponds to an assigned spot in the transition area, where your bike and clothes will be stowed. Know where that spot is, as well as where you enter the transition area after the swim, which way you leave and come in on your bike, and which way you run out. This will prevent you from wasting time searching for your stuff.

• *Plan* how to logically lay out your equipment. "Your running shoes shouldn't be the first thing you get to

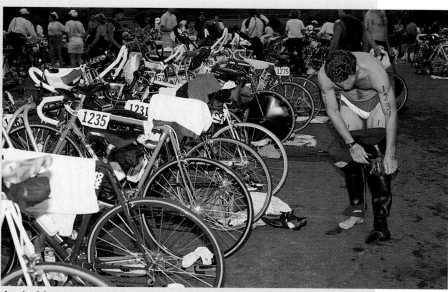

*A triathlete must make rapid transitions from one sport to another. The transition from swimming to biking is particularly difficult.*

when you get to the bike; it should be your cycling shoes," says Campbell. Set things up to minimize the number of movements. "I pick up my glasses, and they go right on my head," says Smyers. "I don't have to turn them around or open them up."

• *Practice makes perfect,* and it's the most important thing you can do. "Set it up in your living room so you can jump out of the shower and try to get into your bike clothes, or toss your bike into your garage, throw on your shoes, and run out," suggests Mantak. You want your actions to be almost rote by race time.

• *Run from the swim* to the transition area.

"People forget sometimes that you've got to run up from the swim to the bike. It's part of the race," says Smyers. She thinks of this portion as a 100-meter dash, and says you can gain 30 seconds to a minute on competitors, time that may be hard to come by on the bike or run.

• *Do it the same every race.* Once you develop an efficient way of transitioning, stick with it every race. Use lace locks or elastic laces on your running shoes. Lace locks eliminate bow-tying, and elastic laces let you slip on your sneakers like slippers. "You're not the most dexterous person when you're done hammering out 25 miles on the bike and you're fiddling around with laces when your hands are shaking," says Campbell.

• *Think ahead* the last few meters of the swim and bike. Visualize what you have to do to achieve the fastest transition time possible so you're completely ready when the time comes.

you may be surprised at how tired you may feel during your first race or at the burn in your leg muscles. You may ask, "What am I doing here?" That's when a positive mental attitude has to kick in to take up the slack.

The pros know this only too well—say when they're riding through the sunbaked lava desert on mile 100 of the Ironman's 112-mile bike with a full marathon yet to come. Mantak engages in what Sean McCann, Ph.D., a sports psychologist with the U.S. Olympic Committee, calls positive self-talk. Mantak repeats to herself affirmations like, "I feel good, I feel strong, I believe in myself," when she's preparing mentally for an event and throughout the race.

Many people also use distraction techniques to take their mind off fatigue or pain. They might think about the cold beer or ice-cream sundae they're going to indulge in after the race, or about keeping a certain distance between themselves and the athlete in front of them, or about their next vacation.

McCann has studied elite athletes and found that, surprisingly, they often focus on exactly how their bodies are feeling rather than distracting themselves. He believes that because these athletes know their bodies so well, they can gauge exactly how far they can go before they take themselves over their anaerobic threshold. So for them, intense fatigue and a high heart rate may mean, "this is how I feel when I'm going fast"—not, "I feel terrible." Top pro Karen Smyers agrees, saying, "You're usually right on that anaerobic threshold on the shorter races, so you try to push as hard as you can without going over the edge."

### Healthy Eats

Common sense dictates that what you put into your body affects its performance, and that holds true for triathletes, who burn large numbers of calories while training. Clark Campbell, coach of the junior national Tri-Fed team, head swim coach at West Virginia Wesleyan College, and a recently retired pro triathlete, believes that both what and when triathletes eat is important. Campbell feels the optimum mix of calories eaten daily should be 65 percent complex carbohydrates, 20 percent fat, and 15 percent pro-

tein. Compare that to the typical American diet, where 45 percent of the calories come from carbohydrates, 35 to 40 percent from fat, and the remainder from protein. That means a triathlete should down lots of fruits and vegetables, whole-grain breads and cereals, low-fat or skim-milk products, lean meats, and no junk food. Smyers tries to eat 70 percent of her calories from carbohydrates, and says she "craves bread, rice, pasta, and fruit." The less the food is packaged, wrapped, cooked, and processed, the better, Campbell also believes. "It's not rocket science; it's a lot of what your mom taught you, but just fine-tuned," he adds. Mantak thinks the bottom line is: "Whether you're an athlete or an executive, the better quality of food you eat, the better you feel, and the better your body will perform for you."

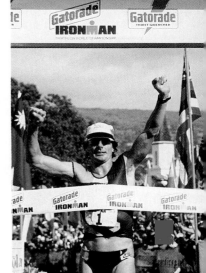

*After hour upon hour of exertion in the blazing Sun, a triathlete crossing the finish line experiences a sense of accomplishment that's all but impossible to match.*

Eating a little something 15 minutes after training or racing and a couple hours before competing will supply needed energy and cut recovery time, advises Campbell. People should experiment to find what sort of food combinations work best for them, whether it's a banana or two, an energy bar, fruit juice, or a sports drink. Don't try a new food or drink for the first time on race day—you may find it disagrees with you.

Above all, enjoy your first triathlon and the training that leads up to it. Most likely, you'll meet new people and feel healthier and fitter than you have in a long time. ◇

# Housecalls

by Jennifer Kennedy, M.S.

Q *Are football helmets safe? If so, why does it seem that every so often a football player breaks his neck? What about bicycle helmets?*

A Football helmets are generally safe, but keep in mind that they are meant primarily to protect the head and face, not the neck. To the degree that a helmet cushions a blow to the head, and thus lessens the force transmitted to the neck, it can help guard the neck. When a neck is bent in any direction, the helmet will often meet the shoulder pads and help to keep the neck from overextending. Some football players also wear large, padded collars for the same purpose.

However, these aspects of neck protection are only moderate. Helmet manufacturers are researching ways to protect the spine and spinal cord in the neck area, but for now the best way to do so on the field is through proper technique and conditioning. Correct tackling never uses the helmet as a weapon, thus avoiding throwing the head and helmet forward as the main point of contact, otherwise known as "spearing." Before contact, good tacklers "bull" their shoulders around their neck first and use the shoulders to take most of the force of the hit. Strengthening the muscles of the neck is very important, too. Football players and other athletes use a variety of equipment and exercises to do this.

Most bicycle helmets are safe. Compared to football helmets, bike helmets are even more specifically meant to protect against brain injury rather than neck injury. Major traumatic brain injury (TBI) is a more typical type of serious injury in bicycling than in football.

In determining whether any helmet is doing the job it is meant to, here are a few points to consider:
• Does the helmet meet safety-regulation standards? The most common certifications for bicycle helmets are the American National Standards Institute (ASNI), the Snell Memorial Foundation (Snell), and the American Society for Testing and Materials (ASTM). Some helmets have all three certifications. On football helmets, look for the NOC-SAE certification (National Operating Committee, Standards for Athletic Equipment).
• Is the helmet the correct size? If too large or too small, it won't offer proper protection.
• When was the helmet bought, how was it used, how often has it been checked to make sure that no parts are broken or missing, and how has it been maintained or reconditioned if necessary?

---

Q *My son would rather sit inside and read a book than play baseball with his friends. Should he be encouraged to develop a stronger interest in sports? He otherwise seems well adjusted, and he is an excellent student.*

A Emphasis on sports is very much an individual choice among parents and children. If you want to stimulate his interest in physical activities, try family fitness outings, such as biking or hiking, or other fun events involving physical activity with siblings or friends. This may lead him to take interest in a more organized sport, and it starts him out in a noncompetitive environment. Competition in children's sports has become increasingly intense, and many kids are understandably intimidated by it.

*Football helmets are designed primarily to protect the head, not the neck. In football, using the helmet as a weapon when tackling is not only dangerous, it's illegal.*

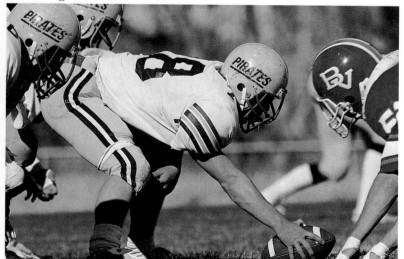

Certainly aspects of the "couch potato" syndrome can be present in a child, even if he doesn't watch a lot of TV. But keep in mind that if your child is physically active at recess, rides his bike, and plays with other children in the neighborhood, he is getting good exercise. Your child does not have to be in a formal sports league to be athletic.

Q *I find that if I drink a couple of cups of coffee before exercising, I have more energy and seem to perform better. Is that effect the result of caffeine?*

A It may be. Caffeine is a stimulant that increases alertness and energy, and decreases reaction time. But it also increases metabolism and stimulates the flow of urine and stomach acid.

Studies have shown that endurance athletes may benefit from imbibing a moderate amount of caffeine before competition. But results on this question are still inconclusive, and the effect depends in part on the individual and his or her tolerance to caffeine. If you plan on trying caffeine, don't do it for the first time in competition; try it in training first.

The question of whether caffeine can contribute to irregular heart rhythms has caused controversy, but studies in recent years appear to have cleared it of this side effect, at least under normal conditions in both healthy individuals and in those with heart disease. Its effects under exercise conditions, though, have not been looked at as closely.

Q *What's the best way to break in new running shoes? It seems as though every time I get a new pair of running shoes, I develop blisters on the back of my heel that take a week or so to heal.*

A Any new pair of shoes can give you a rub here or there, until your foot and shoe get used to each other; however, normally you should not experience blisters from running shoes. They are a soft, orthopedically designed shoe that should feel good right from the start. You should not have to break them in. You should be able to put them on right away and go for a run.

If you do experience blisters:
• Try wearing the shoes around the house for a day or so before running in them.
• Make sure you have the right fit. If the shoe is too big or too small, you will create pressure stresses or sliding (shear) stresses on the skin.
• Don't go for your longest, hardest workout on the first day with new shoes.
• Wear thicker socks.

If nothing else works, you may want to see an orthopedist, podiatrist, or sports-medicine specialist who can evaluate your gait. Certain people are "heel impactors" who may benefit from a heel orthotic, a shoe lining designed to support the foot.

Q *Why do so many amateur and professional athletes wear spandex shorts? Is it just a fad, or do such shorts somehow improve athletic performance?*

A Synthetic fibers such as Lycra, when woven with cotton (to make spandex) or with nylon, have resulted in a new generation of light, warm, flexible garments. The shorts, sweats, and other garments made of these materials fit closely, but are thin and pliable; as a result, they provide a good range of motion, keep muscles warm to prevent injury, and dry quickly. They tend to have a smooth texture that can protect from chafing. They may also improve aerodynamics for certain athletes such as bikers or runners.

Do these characteristics result in improved performance? This has not been determined, and would be a difficult question to answer conclusively. Perhaps only the individual athlete knows.

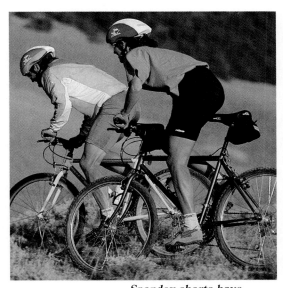

*Spandex shorts have become all the rage for runners, bikers, and other athletes. Such shorts offer more in the way of comfort than they do in improved performance.*

*Do you have a fitness question?*
Send it to Editor, Health and Medicine Annual, P.O. Box 90, Hawleyville, CT 06440-9990.

# Psychology

Understanding how and why humans behave as they do continues to be one of the most challenging areas of medicine. Yet scientists are steadily broadening our knowledge of the complexity of human behavior, particularly its links to genetics and its close association with the body's biochemistry.

For instance, during 1993 Peter Hauser, M.D., and coworkers at the National Institute of Diabetes and Digestive and Kidney Diseases reported that an inherited defect in the body's thyroid hormone system appears to be responsible for attention-deficit disorder in some children. A study by Theodore Weltzin, M.D., of the University of Pittsburgh School of Medicine suggests that low levels of serotonin in the brain trigger binge eating by women with bulimia. And while studying the gigantic brain cells of sea snails, neuroscientists Thomas Carew and Nigel Emptage at Yale University found evidence to support what many people probably suspect every time they misplace their car keys: short- and long-term memories are fundamentally different. Short-term memories appear to form rapidly at the synapses, where connections are made with neighboring brain cells. In contrast, long-term memories require protein synthesis in the cell nucleus, followed by transport of the proteins to the synapses—a process that can take several hours or longer.

New findings also demonstrate that placebos—inactive, harmless substances prescribed as if they were effective drugs—can be more powerful healers than has previously been recognized. Apparently, for many patients, the belief that a therapy will work is sufficient to result in actual improvement. The study, led by Alan H. Roberts, M.D., of Scripps Clinic and Research Foundation, reviewed the cases of 6,931 patients who had received treatments considered effective during the 1960s and 1970s, but later shown to be useless. Of the patients, 40 percent were reported to have had excellent results, and 30 percent to have had good results; only 30 percent had poor results from the treatments.

Misunderstood, often feared, and still stigmatizing, mental disorders affect 22

**See also:**
Individual articles in the second half of this book, arranged in alphabetical order, for additional information.

percent of the U.S. population in any given year, says the National Institute of Mental Health (NIMH). One of the most widespread of these illnesses is depression. According to a study led by Paul Greenberg, a health economist at the Analysis Group, about 11 million Americans a year suffer from depression, at an annual cost to the nation of $43.7 billion, including direct costs for treatment and indirect costs for lost productivity. Yet, for most of these people, the disorder goes undiagnosed and untreated.

A problem that received widespread attention during 1993 was post-traumatic stress disorder, which develops as people try to cope with terrifying events. Victims of the bombing of the World Trade Center in New York City, widespread flooding in the U.S. Midwest, and wildfires and earthquakes in Southern California experienced emotional turmoil and serious symptoms of stress in the weeks and months following their ordeals. Counseling by social workers, participation in group therapy, and other interventions are used to help people deal with depression, anxiety, irritability, and other symptoms caused by such catastrophes.

One of the nation's most serious health problems is a learned behavior: violence. Particularly disturbing is the disproportionate number of young people involved in killings and other violent crimes. In Cleveland, Ohio, for example, half the homicides committed in 1993 were by people younger than 25. In Washington, D.C., the number of homicides increased only 3 percent from 1992 to 1993, while the number committed by people 17 and younger increased 17 percent.

Physicians, especially those who treat the victims of violence, are increasingly adding their voices to national debates on issues such as gun control and TV violence. Together with public-health officials, they are initiating programs to teach children alternatives to violence.

At the other extreme from TV violence is public television's "Barney & Friends," a preschool program featuring an overstuffed purple dinosaur. Many adults have ridiculed the show, but according to Yale psychologists Jerome and Dorothy Singer, the program provides the unconditional love that children crave, and is "nearly a model of what a preschool program should be." The Singers praised the show for its simplicity and slow pace, its use of a single theme per episode, and its familiar songs and simple verses.

*Scientists are finding more links between human behavior and genetic factors.*

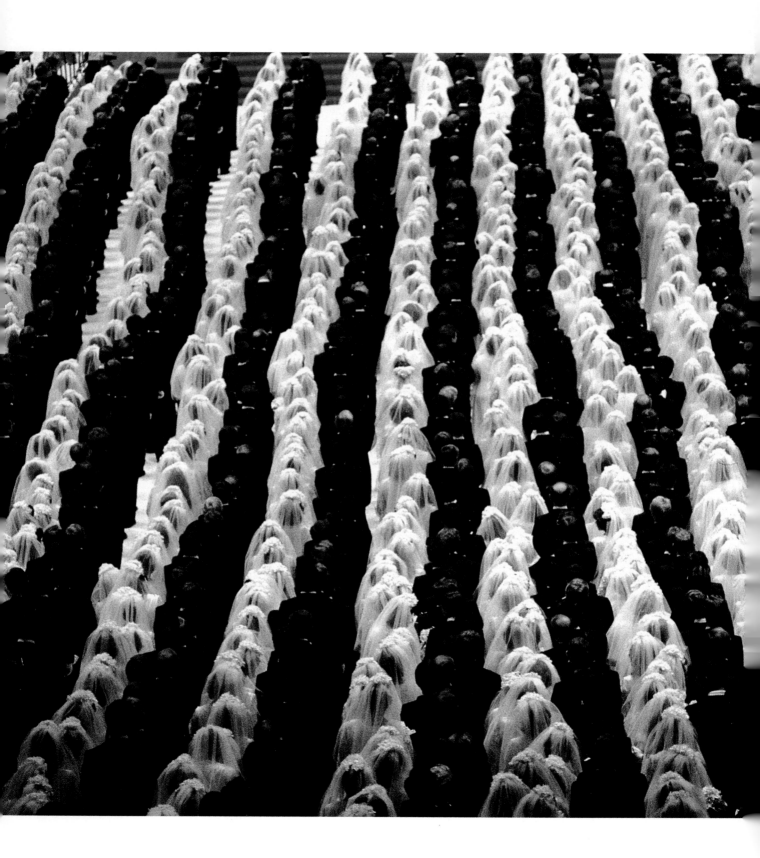

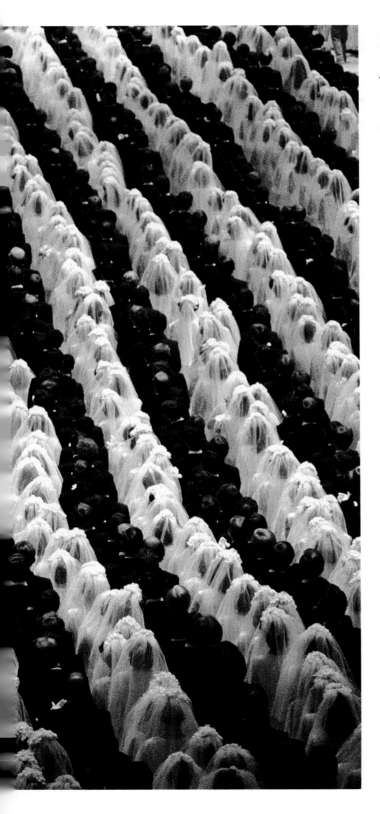

# CULTS
## The Ultimate
# MIND TRAP

*by Marcy O'Koon*

Last year, night after night, the nation watched on the evening news as a dramatic standoff unfolded between federal agents and the Branch Davidians, a religious group whose members had holed up in their well-armed compound in Waco, Texas. The defiant behavior of the group's leader, David Koresh, ultimately led 76 people to their deaths. The Waco tragedy recalled the mass suicide in Guyana 15 years ago, when 900 members of the People's Temple killed themselves by drinking poison at the behest of their leader, Jim Jones.

Less well known, but just as mystifying, was the case of 19-year-old Steve Hassan, who became a "Moonie," a follower of Sun Myung Moon, a Korean who claims to be the messiah. In a matter of weeks in 1974, Hassan dropped out of college, threw away all of the 400 poems he had written (even though he wanted to be a writer), donated his savings to the Unification Church (even though he was Jewish), cut his hair unfashionably short, and traded his jeans and T-shirts for a suit and tie. For 40 days, he refused to speak to his family members or friends. His family and friends were baffled.

Whether the tragedy is public or private, large-scale or small-scale, the overriding question remains: *WHY?* Why do intelligent, healthy people turn from their family and friends and place control of their lives in the hands of cult leaders?

*Cults exert much control over their members. In 1982, for instance, the Unification Church arranged the marriages of 4,200 of its members and then conducted a mass wedding at Madison Square Garden.*

## What Is a Cult?

The term "cult" is typically used to label organizations that physically, financially, or psychologically exploit, abuse, manipulate, or deceive their members, or isolate them from their family and friends. Such groups have one or several leaders who claim divinity, power, or privilege, and who require unquestioning obedience.

An estimated 5 million people belong to cults, and several thousand new recruits join every year, according to the Cult Awareness Network (CAN), a nonprofit educational association. Depending on who does the counting, there are anywhere from 700 to 6,000 cults in America.

Cult ideologies are typically religions, often a new branch of a traditional church or a Bible-based religion, or a bizarre form of worship such as Satanism. But there are also secular cults—the fastest-growing category of cult—which are based on such varied themes as psychotherapy, self-improvement, career advancement, UFO obsession, New Age awareness, or political change.

Whatever its creed, its means of abuse, or its facade of respectability, a group that abuses or exploits its members in any way can be considered a cult. Some cult groups behave, appear, or live in a way that sets them apart from the rest of society. The International Society of Krishna Consciousness members, for example, shave their heads, dance on street corners, wear long robes, and live communally. Today some cult leaders seek to avoid negative attention by having their members continue to live seemingly normal lives, hold down responsible jobs, and live independently. It is, however, the way the members are treated—not a lifestyle characteristic—that determines which groups are labeled cults.

In addition to the mistreatment of their members, cults have been known to engage in numerous illegal activities, such as child abuse and neglect; drug dealing; tax evasion; fraud in recruiting, business, and fund-raising activities; harassment of critics and former members; stockpiling and smuggling of weapons and ammunition; physical and sexual abuse of members; prostitution; kidnapping; and murder.

## The Setup

Steve Hassan's state of mind just before joining the Moonies is typical of someone ripe for cult recruitment. His senior year at college marked a time of difficulties. He struggled to find a career in which he could be a writer and still earn a good living, and was depressed over a recent romantic breakup. During this time, Steve was also searching for answers to some of life's biggest questions: If there is a God, why are so many people suffering? What can I do to make a difference in the world?

Recruiters intentionally seek out people who are emotionally vulnerable, perhaps due to a major transition, such as beginning college, graduating, divorcing or separating, grieving for a loved one, moving away from family and friends, or simply searching for meaning and purpose in life.

Contrary to the common assumption, people who join cults are by and large mentally healthy. "They are simply in one of the transition stages that we all face at one time or

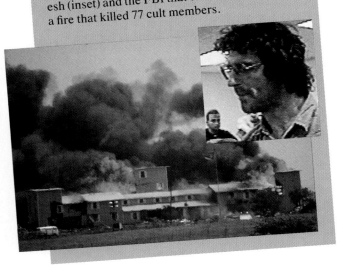

### Branch Davidians Perish in Fiery Finale

On February 28, 1993, four federal agents died in a raid on the Branch Davidian compound near Waco, Texas. The raid touched off a nearly two-month standoff between cult leader David Koresh (inset) and the FBI that ended dramatically in a fire that killed 77 cult members.

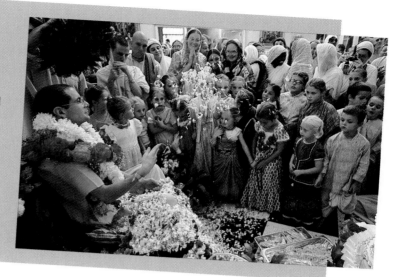

## Hare Krishnas Hover at Major Airports and Local Supermarkets

The distinctive clothing and shaved heads of members of the International Society of Krishna Consciousness have made Hare Krishnas perhaps the most easily recognizable cult members in the United States. Since its heyday in the 1970s, the movement has lost much of its cohesiveness, due partly to persistent rumors (and charges) of illegal activity.

another. They tend to be bright, curious, idealistic, and altruistic," says Carol Gimbalvo, a cult-information specialist who was once involved in a self-improvement cult called est/ the Hunger Project.

Cult members are trained to spot "ripe" or vulnerable people. One former Branch Davidian (who is alive today because she happened to be out of town during the raid in Waco) says that a man she had met socially got her involved in the group. He knew she was disenchanted with her traditional religion and was searching for a spiritual base, so he invited her to the Branch Davidian compound for a visit.

Cult insiders zero in on the needs of potential recruits. Recruiters for the Unification Church attract members by practicing "love bombing," a technique that makes people feel well-liked and appreciated. They disarm potential members with kindness, says Hassan, who has written about his experience with the Moonies in *Combatting Cult Mind Control* (Park Street Press, 1988). "I was told over and over what a nice person I was, what a good person I was, how smart I was, how dynamic I was, and so forth," he recalls from his experience.

While college campuses are still prime recruiting spots, cults increasingly prey on middle-aged and older women, especially those whose children are grown and those who are recently widowed or divorced. Such women are not only particularly vulnerable, but they are often well-off financially. Once

these women have joined an organization, they are asked to help support the cult with their own money.

In 1991, 81-year-old Helen Overington of Baltimore, Maryland, was convinced by recruiters from the Lyndon LaRouche organization, a political cult, that LaRouche's political plan could save the world . . . with her financial help, of course. Within a year, Overington was bankrupt: She had given the group $741,268 in cash, checks, and stock certificates.

Almost all cults lure people into their grip with deception. Using false fronts, aliases, or blatant misinformation, cults often deceive the public and potential recruits as to their true identity. Cult specialist Gimbalvo says she has a 31-page list of front groups, for both recruiting and business purposes, run by the Unification Church alone. CAN also receives many complaints about the Boston Church of Christ, and has compiled a six-page-long list of front names used by that organization.

The people who approached Steve Hassan in his college's student union said they were involved in a small community of "young people from all over the world." He accepted their invitation to join them for a casual get-together. At the meeting, he asked if they were part of a religious group. They laughed and said, "Oh no, not at all," and claimed instead to be part of the One World Crusade, a group dedicated to combating major social problems—something Steve cared about deeply, too.

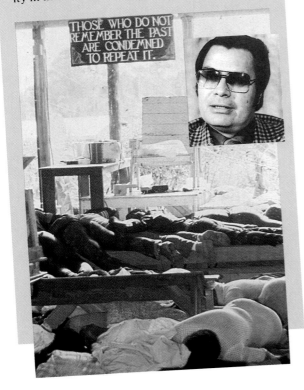

## Reverend Jim Jones and 900 Followers Commit Suicide

In what is likely the most tragic example of cult mind control, the Reverend Jim Jones (inset), founder of the People's Temple, led—or coerced—914 followers to commit suicide by drinking poisoned fruit drink at the cult's encampment in the jungles of Guyana in South America. The 1978 event shocked the world and, at least temporarily, caused a substantial drop-off in cult activity in the United States and elsewhere.

Steve then accepted their repeated invitations to a weekend retreat. Not until he arrived did someone mention that this was a "joint retreat with the Unification Church." And it was not until he was ready to leave Sunday night that he learned that the two-day retreat was really a three-day retreat. No one could drive him back to the city until the next evening.

As a member, Hassan found out that the Moonies call such duplicity "heavenly deception." The Krishnas call it "transcendental trickery." Cults rationalize this dishonesty with the belief that people otherwise could not be induced to join.

### The Trap

The most notorious technique used by cults is mind control, perpetrated without a person's knowledge by people acting as friends. Brainwashing, in contrast, is carried out by a known enemy on someone who is resistant —by a jailer on a prisoner of war, for example —and usually involves physical torture. Though the methods differ, the end results are the same. Through a wily abuse of the human psyche, cults transform people's minds into putty and re-form them in accordance with cult doctrines.

After fewer than five encounters with the Unification Church, Steve firmly believed that his thoughts were being influenced by Satan, an idea planted by the insiders. "One week earlier, I had had no belief in Satan," he says. He was also emotionally high after being convinced that God had chosen him to bring about what Reverend Moon called the Garden of Eden, a world of "just love, truth, beauty, and goodness."

Cults apply a strategic combination of hypnotic techniques and group pressures to radically change a person's beliefs and personality. Hypnotic techniques create an altered state of consciousness in which even well-adjusted and strong-minded individuals become easily persuaded. "It's like being covertly drugged," explains Cynthia Kisser, executive director for CAN. "You don't have a choice of whether or not you respond. Your body physiologically will respond, without your volition or awareness."

Lengthy, repetitive indoctrination lectures; excessive, fast-paced prayers or chanting; and meditation induce a trance that opens people's minds to suggestion, and halts their ability to think critically. Once indoctrinated, members are taught to spontaneously begin meditating or praying in response to their own "unacceptable" thoughts, that is, thoughts that question the group's purpose or leaders.

The Church Universal and Triumphant, run by Elizabeth "Guru Ma" Prophet, in Paradise Valley, Montana, directs its members to "decree"—repeat a rhythmic, fast-paced form of prayer over and over for hours.

Sleep and nutritional deprivation can create altered states of consciousness, too. Cult leaders often concoct a sense of urgency for projects, requiring members to work all night. As a Unification Church member, Hassan says that during his first year, "I was in a high-speed daze of exhaustion, zeal, and emotional overload. I generally slept between three and four hours a night." One-day or multi-day fasts are common as well. Hassan first learned how to go for three days with only water, but later was able to fast for seven days at a stretch.

Cult recruiters also know how to exploit the social nature of humans to make a person vulnerable. "Whenever human beings are in a group," says Hassan, "we have a tendency to shift our behaviors to blend in." Surrounded three to one, potential recruits naturally experience peer pressure and a desire to accommodate. People in such situations are hesitant to persistently ask questions, to decline further invitations, to reject the group's purpose, or to resist the group's efforts to control the situation.

Life in a cult is strictly controlled by the cult's leadership. Cults dictate members' behavior: what they will do every minute of the day, including what they will wear; what they will eat (and how much and when); what jobs they will be assigned; and where they will sleep and for how long.

Cults exert enormous emotional influence, primarily through guilt and fear. Forced confessions and regular doses of misplaced blame cause members to believe themselves responsible for all kinds of personal problems and world tragedies. For example, followers of Elizabeth Prophet "decree" to ward off disasters, such as earthquakes and nuclear war. If the predicted disaster does not happen, they have decreed successfully. If it does occur, they did not decree long enough or sincerely enough, and they are at fault. Such guilt inducement cements the members' need for salvation as offered by the cult leader. It also causes the members to repeatedly put themselves into hypnotic states by chanting, which maintains their inability to think for themselves.

Cults also isolate their members so that alternative opinions and facts are difficult to access. Typically, members are inculcated with the idea that the outside world harbors evil and seeks to destroy their group. This instilled fear creates phobias and convinces members to stay away from friends, family, or society at large. When they visit with people from the outside, cult members use their training to deflect any criticism by adopting a placid demeanor, glassy stare, and a mentally created deafness to unacceptable words or questions.

By controlling members' thoughts, behavior, and emotions, cult leaders manipulate the members until they are "willing" to stay. Although cult spokespeople state that their members are free to leave at any time, and members truly believe they remain of their own free will, the members actually have been stripped of their ability to choose.

### Paradise Valley— A Heavenly Hoax?

"Guru Ma" Elizabeth Prophet and her followers in the Church Universal and Triumphant await the end of the world in a huge, fallout-shelter-equipped compound in Paradise Valley, Montana. Prophet and her followers have been accused of amassing an enormous amount of arms in a mountainside arsenal.

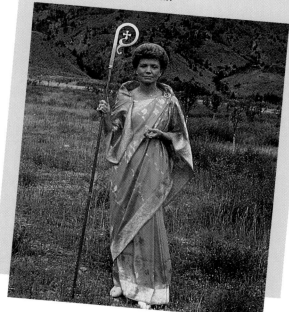

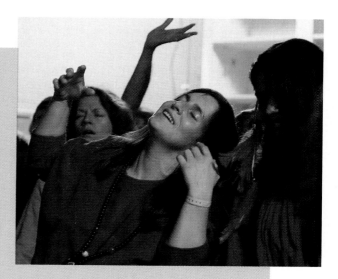

## Is This Group a Cult?

If you are being pursued by members of an organization that you are not sure about, ask the following questions, remembering that destructive cults may deceive you about these issues until you are fully involved.
• What commitments of time, money, and other resources will they expect from me?
• Would I be assigned recruiting or financial quotas?
• Would they discourage me from associating with family and friends?
• What will I gain from being a member of this group? How does that fit with my own goals and ideas?
In addition, find out if the group or organization does the following:
• Encourages you to advance professionally or to continue your studies, to succeed academically, and to graduate; or does the group say that its activities are more important than school or career?
• Answers the questions that you ask; or are you repeatedly told that the answers will come later?

• Discourages discussion of its beliefs, either with other members or with your family or friends.
• Wants its members to give up traditions and beliefs.
• Requires absolute obedience and devotion to its leader or to people in the group's hierarchy.
• Allows members to have quiet times alone, or time with other friends outside the group.
• Predicts tragedy will befall anyone who leaves the group.

The prevalence of these mind-control techniques and their effectiveness is disputed, particularly by those involved in groups accused of cult activity. The group known as The Family (formerly Children of God) issued a statement in 1993 "categorically deny[ing] all accusations, allegations, and insinuations which suggest that our members are not free-willed and mentally responsible individuals. We reject, as does much of the scientific community, the attempts by anti-cult advocates to foist fanciful and mythical 'robot' brainwashing theories."

Some cult experts acknowledge the positive aspects some members derive from these groups. For instance, The Family has won praise from law-enforcement officials for its work with youth gangs in Los Angeles and with victims of 1992's Hurricane Andrew in Florida. Some current members have claimed that their participation has changed their lives for the better, citing their new-found ability to kick drug addiction or become more focused and productive people.

"No experience is totally bad in the mainstream cults," says CAN's Kisser in an interview with the *Congressional Quarterly Researcher.* "No one would join if it was so oppressive on the surface; it's oppressive below the surface. Something has to be offered—a better relationship with God or a spouse, or a better job. One former cult member said, 'I'm no longer afraid of speaking in front of large crowds.' " But, Kisser adds, "The sense of companionship, of being in a special elite, and the affection . . . are conditional and can be withdrawn. It's a trade-off. Some cult members learn carpentry skills, but there was another career given up, and then there's the severed family ties."

## The Escape

A 1991 CAN survey of 500 former cult members found that 59 percent left of their own accord. Others required intervention by cult deprogrammers (21 percent) or exit counselors (16 percent) hired by their families. (Four percent were kicked out of the cult for physical or mental-health problems, low productivity, or other reasons.)

Deprogramming involves abducting a person from a cult or holding a member prisoner when he or she goes home to visit. Over days or weeks—however long it takes—deprogrammers use information to help the person snap out of the cultic mind-set. Because members have been taught to fear "Satan's deprogrammers," they sometimes grow violent and chant or meditate to ward off the "evil" thoughts that the deprogrammers, typically former cult members, are trying to communicate. Because the cults will often press kidnapping charges following an abduction, deprogramming is seldom used today.

Steve Hassan's departure from the Unification Church began after he completed an all-night fund-raiser in front of a convenience store. On the way home, he fell asleep at the wheel, crashed, and broke his leg. While he was recuperating at his sister's house, his father brought in a team of cult deprogrammers. Hassan initially believed these people were the soldiers of Satan, so he plotted to kill his father and threatened to kill himself. But after five days with the team, Hassan began to see the Moonies in a different light, and he eventually came to realize that they had taken over his mind. "In comparison with the pain of the accident," says Hassan, "I felt much worse. I cried for a long time." It had been just over two years since he was first approached at the student union.

Once free of the Moonies, Hassan completed his education in counseling psychology and began helping others leave cults. He uses a technique called exit counseling, practiced today by more than a dozen former cult members. A gentler approach, exit counseling requires a mutual trust among the exit counselor, the cult member, and the family. The family and the counselor provide the cult member with alternative information over a period of time and conduct nonthreatening meetings. The cult member can get up and walk out if he or she wishes.

Now, 18 years later and with more than 300 exits to his credit, Hassan says, "I never imagined that I'd be doing cult education and exit counseling after this many years. But the problem keeps getting worse, and there are very few people who know how to help someone trapped in a cult." ◇

The Cult Awareness Network receives many complaints about the following organizations (some aliases are included in parentheses):

Alamo Christian Fellowship
Ananda Marga
Bible Speaks (Greater Grace World Outreach)
Boston Church of Christ (Multiplying Ministries)
Children of God (Family of Love)
Church Universal and Triumphant (CUT)
Faith Assembly
Fellowship of Friends
The Forum (est/The Hunger Project)
International Society for Krishna Consciousness (ISKON, Hare Krishnas)
Jehovah's Witnesses
Lyndon LaRouche organizations
Lifespring
Maranatha Ministries
MOVE
Nichiren Shoshu of America (NSA, Soka Gakkai)
People's Temple (Jonestown)
Rajneesh Movement Ramtha (J.Z. Knight)
Scientology (Dianetics, Narconon)
Sullivan Institute
Synanon
Transcendental Meditation
Unification Church (CAUSA, CARP)
University Bible Fellowship
The Way International (PFAL, TWIG)

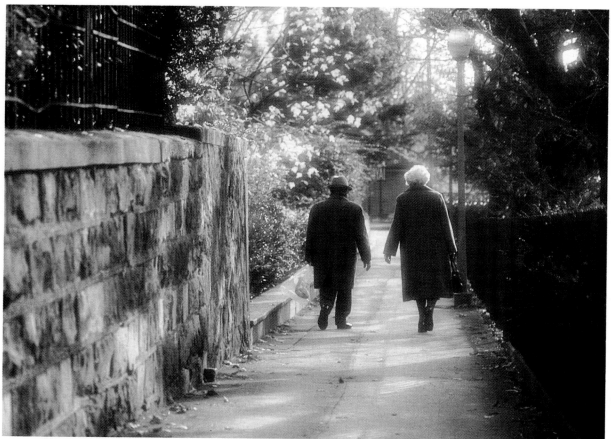

*The loss of a loved one has a profound impact on survivors. The grieving process can last for months or even years, during which time survivors typically pass through a succession of stages.*

# *Getting Through Grief*

*by Laura Fraser*

Hermione Davis, a retired Connecticut social worker with two grown children, knew for more than a year that her husband, not yet 50, was likely to die of a brain tumor. But that didn't make the reality of losing him any easier. "You can know intellectually that someone you love is going to die," she says, "but when it actually happens, it's still a shock."

Although grief is one of the most common of human emotions, most people who haven't gone through it themselves don't understand it very well.

"I don't think most people are aware of the extent of the trauma," says Anne Rosberger, executive director of the Bereavement and Loss Center of New York. "It's mental, it's emotional, it's physical, and it takes your whole being."

Psychotherapists say there is no way to prepare for the full impact of the death of a loved one, or for the ensuing tremors of anger, sadness, and longing that will be felt for years. But there is a growing body of advice on ways to work through grief.

## Pacing the Passage

Grieving is now most often described as a succession of stages, first outlined by Elisabeth Kübler-Ross in her pioneering work *On Death and Dying*. While the stages of grief may be somewhat predictable, our passage through them isn't. Psychologists agree that grief proceeds at an individual pace.

The first state is usually numbness and denial, when it seems as if the death just can't be real and the world feels distorted. "I felt like I was walking through pea soup," says Massachusetts psychologist Judith Souweine, three years after her mother died suddenly at age 63. "I remember not wanting to get up in the morning, not wanting to remember that this had happened."

After the initial shock and denial, mourners may pass in and out of phases of anger, helplessness, depression, guilt, and fear. "I felt absolute rage," remembers Hermione Davis. "It wasn't fair. Why me? Why him?" Such bouts may last for a year or two—or even longer—before the survivor finally comes to a stage of adjustment and acceptance.

"People are often afraid that they're losing control because these feelings are so strong and foreign to them," says John Stephenson, a family therapist in Portland, Maine, and author of *Death, Grief, and Mourning*. Survivors may feel intense guilt for things they failed to do or say to the person who died, or somehow blame themselves for the death, endlessly running over the "what if's." Hallucinations of the loved one, or even suicidal thoughts, are not uncommon. Those who have lost a mate often feel helpless, unable to take on the smallest tasks, or can feel that life isn't worth living.

### Clear Communication

Perhaps the most difficult kind of death for someone to overcome is the death of a child. "We expect our grandparents, and eventually our parents, to die, but we don't expect to outlive our children," says Therese Goodrich, executive director of The Compassionate Friends, a nationwide organization of support groups for bereaved parents and siblings. "The death of a child is out of sync, and it often takes up to five years for parents to start feeling normal again."

Children who lose parents also require special understanding and help, say people who specialize in working with youngsters. Clear communication is the first step. If, for example, children hear that a parent has been "lost," they may wonder when the parent will

be "found." Youngsters often believe that they've caused the death by something they've done or not done, and adults need to explain that they aren't at fault. Children usually heal well from grief, say psychologists, as long as parents and adults don't interfere and tell them how they ought to do it.

For young and old alike, grief can be physical as well as emotional. Peter Niland, an executive assistant for San Francisco's Shanti Project, which works with AIDS-stricken people and their companions, remembers how sick he felt after his lover of 13 years died. "The depression affected me physically, through exhaustion, aches and pains, and an inability to sleep." Appetite loss, headaches, shakiness, indigestion, and heart palpitations are normal. Occasionally, more-serious ailments crop up during bereavement. Studies of widows and widowers have found an increased death rate from cardiovascular disease; those who lose their spouses, it seems, are more likely literally to die of a "broken heart."

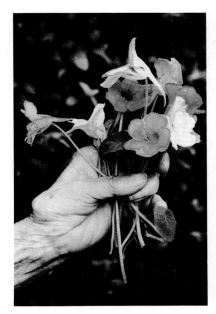

### Continuing Afresh

Most mourners adjust, but that adjustment may come slowly. "I finally came to some accommodation of my husband's death," says Hermione Davis. "I realized this is the way it is, and I'd better work on building a life for myself that doesn't include him. You accept that it's never going to be great, but you discover resources in yourself that you never knew were there." Davis took trips with friends to help her get a sense that her life was continuing afresh without her husband, and she now conducts bereavement support groups to help others who've faced such loss.

The best way to work through grief, say counselors who specialize in the process, is

## Sharing the Burden

Below are just a few of the organizations that either offer regional support groups or can steer you to help in your area. Also check with local hospitals and churches.

**The Compassionate Friends**
Support groups for bereaved parents and siblings. P.O. Box 3696, Oak Brook, IL 60522-3696; 708–990-0010

**Afterloss**
Monthly newsletter focuses on grief recovery. Drawer 599, Summerland, CA 93067; 800–423-8811

**Pregnancy and Infant Loss Center**
Referrals for bereaved families experiencing miscarriage, stillbirth, and infant death. 1421 E. Wayzata Blvd., Suite 30, Wayzata, MN 55391; 612–473-9372

**Parents of Murdered Children**
Referrals to local chapters, plus a newsletter. 100 E. Eighth St., Suite B41, Cincinnati, OH 45202; 513–721-LOVE.

**Elisabeth Kübler-Ross Center**
Workshops; regional bereavement groups. South Route 616, Head Waters, VA 24442; 703–396-3441.

**Theos**
Groups (in both the U.S. and Canada) for those who have been widowed. 1301 Clark Bldg., 717 Liberty Ave., Pittsburgh, PA 15222; 412–471-7779.

**Center for Attitudinal Healing**
Grief groups, including those for children with life-threatening illnesses and their families. Local offices in 50 cities. Head office: 19 Main St., Tiburon, CA 94920; 415–435-5022.

**National AIDS Hotline**
Information and referrals to local counseling groups. 800–342-AIDS.

to sink into it, to grieve fully—allowing yourself and others, including children, time to cry, feel numb, reminisce with friends, be angry, or kick and scream if it helps. The problem is that such grieving isn't openly encouraged in American culture.

"Our culture deals with grief the same way we deal with food," says Robert Ostroff, M.D., an assistant professor of psychiatry at Yale University in New Haven, Connecticut, who works with bereaved patients. "We think we ought to get a nutritious meal in 30 seconds, but the European notion of wearing black for 12 months speaks to the fact that grieving is a long process."

Rituals can help grievers cope, says Kübler-Ross. "It could be a totally nonreligious sharing of a group of human beings, perhaps with some flowers and music and some favorite songs. It is a closure to all the things that were never said and done."

John Stephenson often suggests that his bereaved patients write a good-bye letter to the loved one. "That helps them say perhaps what hadn't been said, and helps resolve unfinished business."

Judith Souweine says that the Jewish ritual of "sitting shivah"—when friends come visit and mourn with the bereaved for a week—comforted her after her mother's death. "What helped was having people who were willing to listen to me and talk to me."

For many people, however, there may be no neighbors who come by. "We don't have the kinds of family customs and culture that support the grieving process anymore," says Ostroff. That's why it often helps mourners to find support groups of people who are undergoing the same kinds of painful feelings. "Grief groups are an unfortunate necessity for communities where there's nobody to talk to about the loss," says Ostroff. Local hospitals, psychologists, and even funeral homes can steer you to a grief group, including those that deal with specific kinds of loss—the death of a child, for instance. Some people are more private and may prefer one-on-one counseling with a therapist.

Even with help, says Ostroff, know that when grief hits, you're in it for the long run. The ancient advice about grief still holds true: "It takes time." And then some.  ◇

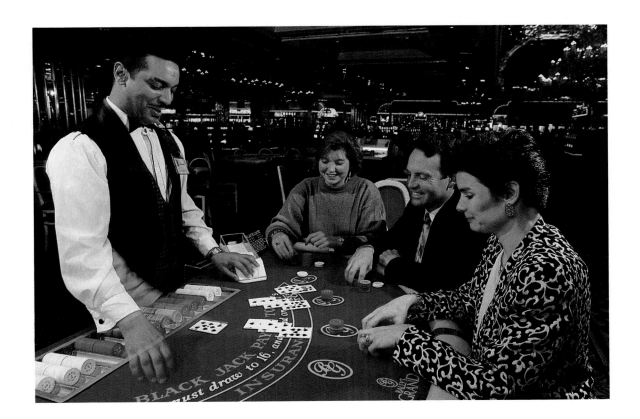

# Is There a Gambler in the House?

*by Sue Berkman*

To the neighbors in her New York City high-rise, she was known as "Helen," or "Mrs. H.," a wealthy widow. To many, she was that nameless "sweet-faced senior on seven"—one of those genteel ladies who dress in hat and gloves to go to the grocery store. But to her fellow travelers to the New Jersey casinos, she was "High-Rolling Helen," whose $500 bets paid off in the form of complimentary meals and lodging, and frequent $1,000 "markers," or IOUs, from the casino managers.

"Helen the Handicapper" could be found at least twice a week at the Yonkers Raceway, studying the racing sheets and placing her bets—not based on intuition, but on well-calculated odds. Meanwhile, some half a dozen lottery-ticket sellers in her immediate neighborhood took in $10 and $20 bills on a daily basis; on days when the prize was high or she "felt a hot streak," Helen would travel around Manhattan by bus, buying tickets wherever she saw a lotto sign. In another reality, Helen was the mother of two grown sons, grandmother of six, and—as she finally admitted—a compulsive gambler.

So much for the old movie images of the "gambling man" as a low-life poker player. Compulsive and problem gamblers (up to 6 million Americans ranging in age from 12 to over 70) are both male *and* female—and they're not so easy to spot. "In real life, compulsive gamblers are regular people— judges, teachers, carpenters, teenagers, and grandmothers, with many outstanding traits," says Valerie C. Lorenz, Ph.D., executive director of the Compulsive Gambling Center in Baltimore, Maryland.

Compulsive gamblers—the word "pathological" is also commonly used—are often highly motivated professionals. They are bright, energetic, outwardly successful people who are hard workers, sometimes to the point of being workaholics. In social situations, they are charming, highly intelligent, and easy conversationalists. Obviously, none of these characteristics would ever mark an individual as a compulsive gambler. "He or she can hide the problem from a spouse or other family members for a long time," says Henry R. Lesieur, Ph.D., an expert on compulsive gambling and chairman of the Department of Criminal Justice for Illinois State University in Normal, Illinois.

Not surprisingly, compulsive gamblers commonly have other addictive behaviors. In one study of an inpatient substance-abuse treatment program, 9 percent were also compulsive gamblers, and another 10 percent showed signs of gambling-related problems. In another inpatient treatment-program study, 47 percent of compulsive gamblers were drug or alcohol abusers.

## High Stakes

Compulsive gambling carries considerable baggage, much of it in the form of physical symptoms. A survey by Dr. Lorenz of Gamblers Anonymous (GA) members and their spouses in Gam-Anon found the following complaints about physical health: 46 percent of the gamblers and 47 percent of their spouses suffered depression; 42 percent and 37 percent had stomach problems; 31 percent and 27 percent frequently felt faint or dizzy; 29 percent and 41 percent had migraines and other types of headaches; 17 percent and 11 percent had high blood pressure; 18 percent and 14 percent had asthma; and 17 percent and 18 percent had backaches.

When compulsive gamblers try to kick the habit alone, they suffer through withdrawal symptoms much like smokers or drug addicts. A study at the Center for Addiction Studies at Harvard University in Cambridge, Massachusetts, found that at least 30 percent of those who tried to go "cold turkey" showed signs of irritability or experienced stomach distress, sleep disorders, higher-

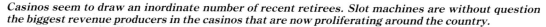

*Casinos seem to draw an inordinate number of recent retirees. Slot machines are without question the biggest revenue producers in the casinos that are now proliferating around the country.*

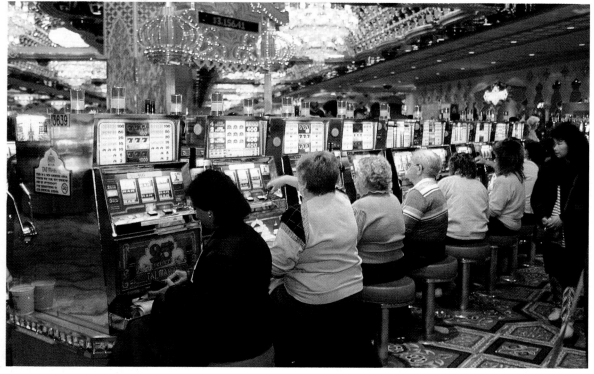

than-normal blood pressure, and a faster pulse. "Whether they're currently gambling or not, the individuals don't associate their medical problems with their addiction," says Dr. Lorenz. They may go to a nurse at work —a visit paid for by the company—and receive advice to "slow down" and "take it easy." They rarely go to their own doctor, because that would consume valuable gambling money. So a minor disorder escalates into a more serious illness that might require hospitalization and even surgery.

Compulsive gambling is socially devastating in other ways. In a study of prisoners, 30 percent were found to be compulsive gamblers, and 13 percent acknowledged that they were in prison because of gambling-related problems. The most common crimes included check forgery (34 percent), civil loan fraud (31 percent), embezzlement and employee theft (30 percent), forgery on business documents (20 percent), tax evasion (19 percent), and tax fraud (12 percent).

At a Gamblers Anonymous meeting in 1993, a small group of men and women shared stories of wasted lives. One, a former graphics designer, told about stealing a purse in a post office. "The old woman just placed it on the countertop while she addressed her envelope. It was a cinch to take it." As he left the building, he looked back and saw the horror and terror on the woman's face, but kept on walking. "I found $500 in the pocketbook, and I really felt like scum. I rationalized that I would have returned it if I knew how. I didn't worry about it very long, though. And soon the money was gone."

## Looking for Markers

Gambling—whether it's card games, bingo parlors, horse or dog racetracks, casino nights, or state lotteries—is not in and of itself a condemnable practice. For many people, it never moves beyond a recreational level. "One major difference between a compulsive gambler and a person who simply likes to occasionally play betting games is a loss of control," says credentialed alcoholism counselor Sheila B. Blume, M.D., medical director of the Alcoholism, Chemical Dependency, and Compulsive Gambling Programs at South Oaks Hospital in Amityville, New York, and clinical professor of psychiatry at the State University of New York at Stony Brook. "A healthy person sets limits; the compulsive gambler cannot. Compulsive gamblers lose the ability and desire to take care of themselves."

Right now, however, even the experts don't agree on how to take care of compulsive gamblers. It's not that gambling is a newcomer to humanity's list of compulsive behaviors; in 1866 Fyodor Dostoyevsky wrote passionately about the lure of gaming in his novel The Gambler, which he wrote to pay off gambling debts of his own. In a 1928 essay, "Dostoyevsky and Patricide," Sigmund Freud analyzed the writer's motives as stemming from unresolved Oedipal conflicts and masturbatory complexes. Freud may not have meant to apply his formulation to all gamblers, or even all compulsive ones, but it nonetheless formed the foundation for long-term individual psychotherapy analysis. "We've come a long way since then," says Dr. Lorenz. Short-term intensive therapy, supported by family counseling and 12-step meetings, seems to work best.

Today two different—and opposing—views question whether compulsive gambling should be considered a disease or simply moral weakness. And the answer will likely have major impact on the funding made available for research, as well as on the thinking of employers who want to fire addicts and insurers who resist paying for treatment.

Some people argue that labeling pathological gambling as an illness tends to excuse such people from being responsible for their behavior. While they agree that it is a problem, they maintain that compulsive gambling is not an illness. Such views are disputed by advocates for compulsive gamblers, who note that since 1980 the Diagnostic and Statistical Manual of Mental Disorders, the widely accepted "bible" of the mental-health field, has listed compulsive gambling as an "impulse control disorder."

The manual, which is published by the American Psychiatric Association, states that compulsive gambling is characterized as a "chronic and progressive failure to resist impulses to gamble, a gambling behavior that compromises, disrupts, or damages personal, family, or vocational pursuits." The manual further describes pathological gambling in terms of its associated features like being overconfident or easily bored, and notes that problem gamblers often are substance abusers and even sometimes have a tendency to be suicidal.

Both clinical and research experience suggest that people who become compulsive gamblers bring to their habit two kinds of motivation: escaping stresses, and overcoming depression, boredom, or loneliness. But no matter what the motivation, the disorder often develops in a similar way. After an average of nine years of controlled gambling, some people begin to gamble pathologically when they become either anxious or depressed in extremely stressful situations. For anxious individuals, gambling provides an emotional escape. Gamblers will say: "I become totally absorbed by playing the slot machine. Nothing else worries me." For depressed people, gambling provides a stimulus. As they put it: "It's like having a 'high.' I'm totally aroused, and nothing bad can touch me." Experts on compulsive gambling point out that underlying anxiety and depression frequently hide behind such overt behavior.

Recent research shows that the key to compulsive gambling may lie in the biology of the brain. A study by Alec Roy, M.D., a psychiatrist now at the University of Medicine and Dentistry of New Jersey in Newark, found that urine samples and cerebrospinal fluid of chronic gamblers show a significant deficiency in levels of a by-product of norepinephrine, a hormone produced by the adrenal glands. Norepinephrine is produced under stress, as in moments of great danger or intense excitement, and has the effect of a strong stimulant. Some brain researchers think that a deficiency in norepinephrine triggers a need to engage in activities like risky, exciting games that will stimulate the brain to secrete more of it. "Compulsive gamblers typically have a long history of depression, anxiety, and low self-esteem. Most gamble to get a rush or a 'high' while in the action, then crash into depression after they lose or stop," says Dr. Lorenz. "To stave off the sense of depression, they go back to the thrill and excitement of the stakes. It's a classic

## Early-Warning Signs

• *Money.* Sudden reduction in regular income is explained away as a late paycheck, error in pay, car repairs, or even a mugging incident. Small valuables may disappear from the home; even household cash may disappear.
• *Personality.* Periods of "hyper" behavior switch to bad moods and back again as winning alternates with losing. Tendency to withdraw and isolate oneself is common, as is a tendency to provoke arguments. Other personality changes include increased nervousness, anxiety, and agitation. First signs of physical abusiveness may emerge.
• *Health.* The stress of risk taking may show up as any of the following disorders, alone or in combination: stomach upset/pains, diarrhea, constipation, overeating, loss of appetite, headaches, insomnia, backaches, heart palpitations, shortness of breath, rapid breathing, stiff neck, chest pain, excessive urination, hives or rashes, dizziness, and numbness in fingers.
• *Work.* Missing work becomes a habit. Even while on the job, preoccupation with gambling leads to missed deadlines, sloppy work, and a high rate of errors. Arguments with superiors are common, as are temper flare-ups with coworkers.

addictive cycle, except that the substance they abuse is money, not drugs."

### The Addictive Cycle
The addictive cycle has three phases: mostly winning, mostly losing, and desperation.

In the winning phase, which is the introduction to gambling and is an enjoyable pastime, gamblers strongly believe in their systems or handicapping abilities. Winning enhances the image of being a big shot, and losing is rationalized as bad luck, a faulty system, or poor advice. Almost half of compulsive gamblers have a big win at this early

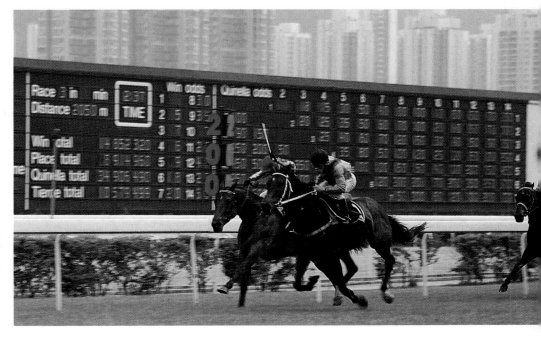

*Many people associate compulsive gambling with horse racing, blackjack, and the like. In reality, though, the truly compulsive gambler will bet on everything from football scores and election results to the next day's high temperature.*

point in their careers. And though they lose frequently, the losses are easily recouped through further gambling or short-term loans from friends and family. At this point, borrowing money doesn't hurt relationships (see the sidebar at left).

In the losing phase, sometimes called "the chase," gamblers need to counter the inevitable increased losses, not so much to uphold financial responsibility, but to salvage self-esteem. At this stage, gamblers negotiate larger personal loans and bet on credit, using borrowed money to try to break even. Typically the losses and borrowing are hidden from others, as is the increased time spent in gambling. Some gamblers even go into the gambling business in other ways as proof to themselves that they are professionals. The losing phase may continue for decades; the greater the access to money, the longer the involvement with the action, until all viable options are reduced. This is when lies and theft escalate.

The desperation phase begins when gamblers grasp at any and every means of getting even and paying off debts. By now a full-time obsession, gambling becomes a total emotional drain; depression and a sense of panic ensue with the realization that punishment may be near from illegal activities, coupled with the knowledge that the action will cease if credit dries up. Their former lives and values are lost in the degradation of their addiction. Family, friends, and colleagues shun them when they need help the most; they are isolated and devastated.

"Only four solutions remain: suicide, prison, running away—typically to Las Vegas or some other gambling haven—or looking for help," says Dr. Lesieur.

### Win or Lose? It's a Long Shot

The recovery process also involves three phases: the critical phase, rebuilding phase, and growth phase. The first, or critical, phase finds the compulsive gambler at rock bottom, in a hopeless state, complete with suicidal thoughts. He or she may face arrest, divorce, and an emotional breakdown. Even when they have hit rock bottom, compulsive gamblers often resist seeking help because they are afraid of treatment. But sometimes, with the urging of a close relative or friend, the gambler is able to experience an honest desire for help, and turns to Gamblers Anonymous or a professional inpatient or outpatient treatment program. In the early recovery stages, the gambler begins to think clearly, to make sounder decisions, and to regain some hope that the cycle will be broken. This is when the gambler decides to stand up to the demons and stop betting.

In the second phase, the gambler develops new interests, regains some self-respect, and accepts weaknesses as well as strengths. Plans are made for repayment of debts to creditors, and there is increased hope that legal problems will be resolved.

Finally, the growth period begins when the preoccupation with gambling decreases. The former gambler knows how important it is to face problems promptly and not try to solve them through addictive behavior. Giving, understanding, and appreciation of self and others means that recovery is under way.

"Gambling has never been a highly visible problem in the addiction-treatment world," says Dr. Blume. "Most compulsive gamblers never get in touch with a good treatment program. Their first difficulty is denial. Compulsive gamblers don't consider their habit a treatable disease." One patient who was hospitalized after an attempted suicide later confided that he had spent virtually his entire confinement on the phone with his bookie.

In addition, few substance-abuse professionals screen for gambling problems or are prepared to treat them. Seven years ago, Dr. Lesieur and Dr. Blume developed the South Oaks Gambling Screen (SOGS), which is now used by mental-health professionals as a pencil-and-paper test or a structured interview.

There are about 40 treatment programs specifically for gamblers in 14 states; in addition, many chemical-dependency programs screen for gambling. These programs rely heavily on individual, group, and family counseling in which patients and their families are educated about the disease and taught to combat denial. They are usually persuaded to join 12-step programs such as GA (for the gambler) and Gam-Anon (for families).

A study by Dr. Lesieur and Dr. Blume was the first to evaluate combined treatment for chemical dependency and compulsive gambling. Researchers followed 72 of 119 compulsive gamblers for 6 to 14 months after hospitalization—19 who considered gambling the main problem, 17 who considered alcohol or drugs the main problem, and 30 who regarded both as serious problems (the remainder could not be definitive). All three groups improved substantially in all areas of their lives with the combined treatment program. Ninety-four percent of the patients contacted had fewer gambling problems after treatment, and 64 percent were no longer gambling at all. Patients who attended GA had the best long-term results.

## Legal Betting: Big Business

"The pendulum seems to be swinging toward an increase in the acceptability of gambling, with both church and state promoting it," notes Dr. Blume. During the past two decades, many types of gambling have become legalized in this country. Forty-eight of the 50 states now permit gambling of some kind; in some places, it has become big business. A Gallup poll in 1989 showed that 80 percent of all Americans have gambled at some time, and nearly one-third gamble at least once a week. According to *Gaming and Wagering Business Magazine,* more than $329 billion was wagered legally, $40 billion wagered illegally, in 1992 in the United States. The total is more than $1,000 for every person in this country. The industry's take was about $32 billion (an annual growth rate of about 11 percent over the past decade); if this were concentrated into a single corporation, it would be among the top 15 in the country.

But if revenues increase with legalized gambling, so do the problems. And, paradoxically, states that allow substantial gambling provide little public support for programs aiding compulsive gamblers. Only eight have made funds available. One solution is evident, at least to mental-health experts: "All states should follow the lead of Iowa and Texas, which dedicate a portion of their lottery revenue to public and professional education, research on pathological gambling, and the treatment of compulsive gamblers," says Dr. Blume. Not that she thinks it will happen anytime soon. "When it comes to compulsive gambling, society has a blindfold on." Dr. Lorenz agrees: "Communities and governments are fighting drug addiction and alcoholism, but encouraging gambling. It doesn't make any sense."  ◇

**Help Begins Here**
Gamblers Anonymous (self-help with group support), P.O. Box 17123, Los Angeles, California 90017. 213-386-8789.

Gam-Anon (support groups for spouses of compulsive gamblers), P.O. Box 257, Whitestone, NY 11357. 718-352-1671.

National Council on Problem Gambling (information and treatment resources), 445 West 59th St., New York, NY 10019. 1-800-522-4700.

Compulsive Gambling Center, (information and treatment resources), 924 E. Baltimore St., Baltimore, MD 21202. 1-800-332-0402.

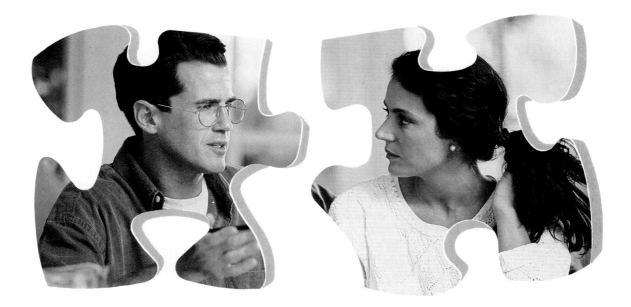

# The Growing Controversy Over Gender Psychology

*by Preethi Krishnamurthy*

Tom and Mary are lost. Circling around aimlessly, the couple is trying to find a friend's house. While Mary urges Tom to ask a passerby for directions, Tom insists that he can find his bearings without anyone else's help. Meanwhile, Tom claims that Mary can't make sense out of a simple road map. Sound familiar? According to some psychologists, incidents like this one may be the result of inherent gender differences.

Gender psychology is a relatively new branch of psychology. Although gender differences have been recognized since Adam and Eve, documented studies of gender psychology began to be published only in the late 1950s. Later, during the burgeoning women's movement of the 1960s and 1970s, gender differences were played down, as differences seemed to undermine women's fight for equality. For a while, gender psychology seemed unfashionable.

Nowadays the subject sparks great controversy. Feminists often fight the attempts of psychologists to prove gender differences. They argue that studies on gender differences only serve as fodder for those who wish to deny women equality. Nevertheless, studies revealing gender differences, from the fairly insignificant to the relatively colossal, abound.

The field of gender psychology encompasses a broad spectrum of experts, from linguists to sociologists and education experts. Yet these researchers from such seemingly diverse fields are working toward a common goal: to understand the significance of the language men and women use and the connections they make about their world. Identi-

> *Are gender differences a matter of biology or of the way we are raised?*

fying gender differences and the role they play in every aspect of personal and business relationships can help men and women account for, adjust to, and learn from each other's styles.

## Caring versus Justice

Imagine the following scenario: John can't afford a lifesaving drug for his dying wife, whom he loves. Should he steal the drug from the druggist? This hypothetical question and others like it are common tools for assessing the basis of an individual's system of morality. By comparing the answers of women and men, researchers are able to evaluate the presence or absence of gender differences.

One prominent researcher believes that the entire moral systems of men and women

**DIFFERENCES THAT ARE ALL IN THE HEAD**

**Frontal lobe**
More women focus their language skills in the frontal lobe, while more men focus language skills in the parietal lobe.

**Parietal lobe**

**Corpus callosum**
A thick bundle of nerves that connects the brain's right and left hemispheres. Often larger in women than in men, possibly allowing for greater crosstalk between the hemispheres.

**Hypothalamus**
Associated with sexual behavior. A group of neurons in the anterior hypothalamus was found to be larger in heterosexual men than in homosexual men or women.

**Spinal cord**

are different. Carol Gilligan, Ph.D., a professor in the department of human development and psychology at Harvard University's Graduate School of Education in Cambridge, Massachusetts, has published a breakthrough work on the differences in women's morality, titled *In a Different Voice* (Harvard University Press, 1982). By using hypotheti-

cal scenarios like John's, and by interviewing men and women about real moral choices they faced at different stages of their lives, Gilligan began to see a great difference between the moral systems of men and women. Men seem to be much more concerned with abstract concepts of justice, which they apply logically to case after case. For instance, a man might argue either that John should steal the drug, based on the fact that human life is sacred, or that he should not steal the drug, based on the fact that stealing is wrong. Women, on the other hand, are more likely to develop moral systems based on caring. They tend to try to solve conflicts so that no one will be hurt. A woman might argue that John should steal the drug because he loves his wife and wants to save her.

Gilligan believes women view the world as a network of caring, connected individuals, while men view the world hierarchically, attempting to define their position within the hierarchy. Of these two moralities, Gilligan says, "While an ethic of justice proceeds from the premise of equality—that everyone should be treated the same—an ethic of care rests on the premise of nonviolence —that no one should be hurt."

Of course, Gilligan is not implying that all women have a caring morality or that all men have a justice morality. Researchers recognize that gender psychology generalizes, and that it therefore can't always be applied to a specific man or woman. However, in Gilligan's view, the majority of men and the majority of women base their moral judgments on different reasoning.

Other experts disagree. Kathleen Galotti, Ph.D., the chair of the psychology department at Carleton College in Northfield, Minnesota, conducted a study showing that women's and men's moral reasoning is in fact remarkably similar. She asked a group of college students about the factors that influenced their decision making when faced with a moral dilemma. The students, answering in writing, shared much of the same reasoning, regardless of gender. Galotti labeled themes as stereotypically masculine or feminine, yet still found that both men and women relied on both feminine themes, such as "what others would think or feel," as well as masculine themes, such as "legal issues." The only real difference was that many more men than women identified "reasoning systematically" as a basis for decisions. Galotti's research could not identify any major gender differences in moral reasoning.

Galotti explains that these contradictory results are just good science. "The way research proceeds is to have differences in opinion, and then to have people ask why these differences exist. The lack of consensus is a healthy thing. If you had everyone agree, that would show that something is wrong." Galotti later adds, "What I'd like to see in the future is an assessment of the similarities and of the socialization factors that contribute to the differences. We're [currently] really drawn to look at the differences and to make inferences from them."

### Cognition: Are Men More Mathematical?

Throughout history, many societies have considered women incapable of pursuing research in mathematics or even of solving the simplest calculations; indeed, only recently has mathematics become an occupational field open to women. Now that more and more women are taking advanced mathematics courses, however, many researchers are noticing differences between male and female mathematical performance, particularly on standardized tests, such as the Scholastic Aptitude Tests (SATs) required for college entrance.

SATs: just the mention of these gruesome tests conjures up memories of panic and dread for millions of Americans. Since their conception, researchers have been interested in the so-called "gender gap" associated with the SATs in particular, and standardized tests in general. Boys have always outperformed girls on the math portions of the SATs, often by a large margin. Until the 1980s, girls on the average received higher scores on the verbal section than boys. Are these differences due to actual discrepancies in male and female capabilities, or are they a result of society's attitude toward women in mathematics? Questions like this have for years prodded researchers into finding answers, with varied results.

A variety of theories has been proposed to explain this gender difference. One is that gender-specific language and gender bias contribute to the relatively poor performance of girls on the math section, and to their sometimes superior performance on the verbal section. For instance, mathematical word problems that have a male main character may help boys identify with the problem, so that their solutions are reached more quickly and are perhaps more accurate. Also, on the verbal section, reading-comprehension passages may be geared toward stereotypically "female" pursuits such as shopping for groceries, thereby allowing girls to grasp the point of the passage more quickly and perhaps more accurately. Another possible explanation for the gender gap is that girls are made to believe—either by their parents or by their teachers, or by both—that math is for boys. Yet another current theory is that girls and women inherently excel at verbal tasks, while boys and men are naturally better at mathematical tasks. Does this smack of sexism? Perhaps, but some believe it is the most convincing explanation for the SAT gender gap.

*Men tend to view the world hierarchically, while women see things as interconnected.*

In the midst of the uproar over gender inequality on standardized tests, Alan Feingold, at the time a researcher at Yale University in New Haven, Connecticut, showed in 1988 that male and female average scores on a test similar to the SATs—the DAT, or Differential Aptitude Test—have been converging. Until 1980 females did better than males on three portions of the test: spelling, language, and clerical speed and accuracy, all of which can be classified as verbal tests. However, the differences between male and female performance in these three

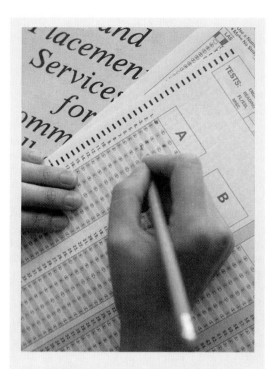

## 1993 National Scholastic Aptitude Test (SAT) Profile

Ever since the Scholastic Aptitude Test (SAT) was introduced in 1926 for college-bound high-school seniors, the average scores for girls have been consistently lower than the scores for boys. As the statistics below show, 1993 was no different. Some hypothesize that males solve problems using analytical, deductive reasoning while females tend to approach these same problems with a more innovative, open-minded approach that a multiple choice test cannot measure.

**Male:**

| | |
|---|---|
| Total number of test takers: | 495,086 |
| SAT Verbal Average Score: | 428 |
| SAT Math Average Score: | 502 |

**Female:**

| | |
|---|---|
| Total number of test takers: | 549,379 |
| SAT Verbal Average Score: | 420 |
| SAT Math Average Score: | 457 |

*Source: The College Board*

dial-reading programs in elementary schools, which generally helped boys overcome reading problems. Unfortunately, the gender gap is still present in mathematics. Another recent study shows that girls actually do better than boys on most classroom mathematics tests, and that girls actually earn better grades. However, as the table at left shows, girls are still outperformed by boys on the math SATs.

One explanation for this apparent anomaly is in the realm of spatial cognition, or mental images of three-dimensional figures. Much research leads to the conclusion that men do in fact possess more natural ability to picture such images in their minds and to rotate them mentally. The physiological reasons for this advantage are as yet unknown; however, this may be the reason for the stereotypically male complaint that women cannot read maps. Maps are in fact two-dimensional representations of three-dimensional structures; if men actually do possess a greater inherent ability to deal with spatial mental images, there is little doubt that many men would be better map-readers than many women.

On the other hand, one recent study seems to reveal that it is the directions attached to spatial problems, not the spatial problems themselves, that determine the male-female differences in performance. Matthew Sharps, Angela Welton, and Jana Price, all from California State University at Fresno, published a study in early 1993 that questions the results of earlier studies documenting gender differences in spatial problems. The team of researchers presented the same problem, which involved mentally rotating a picture of a three-dimensional object, to groups of men and women, using different directions. When the directions emphasized the spatial, mapping nature of the problem, men clearly outperformed women. When the directions were more general and did not let on that the problem was in fact spatial, men and women performed equally well. Some other studies have found that men and women actually do perform equally well on spatial tasks, but that men do them more quickly. Finally, a few studies show that there is no difference between men's and

subjects decreased between 1947 and 1980. It seems that boys have been catching up. Feingold theorizes that the reason may be attributed to the increased emphasis on reading skills in the classroom and to more reme-

women's capability in terms of spatial problems requiring mental imagery.

For now at least, the actual causes of superior male performance on mathematical standardized tests are unknown; most likely, however, the reasons are a composite of currently circulating theories involving societal, biological, and even gender-bias causes. In addition, mathematical problem solving requires a number of fairly diverse skills. It is difficult to isolate which skill or skills, if any, accounts for better male performance. Even a relatively limited area such as spatial cognition presents controversy. While some studies reveal gender differences, others clearly do not.

Melissa Hines, Ph.D., assistant professor in the department of psychiatry and biobehavioral sciences at the University of California at Los Angeles (UCLA), proposes that these contradictory results "may relate to how you define a sex difference. When I say there is a sex difference, I'm not saying how it comes about, whether it's innate or societal. Some people misunderstand what it means to say a sex difference. If you look at all kinds of mathematical areas, you find that girls perform better in some areas. If you look at other specific areas, you find that boys perform better. If you look at understanding mathematical concepts, you find that [boys and girls] perform equally well. People are looking at different things, so are coming to different conclusions. [Gender differences] are not as general as they appear to be when they get out into the public opinion," Hines concludes.

### Linguistics: Networks versus Hierarchies?
"Even if they grow up in the same neighborhood, on the same block, or in the same house, girls and boys grow up in different worlds of words," explains Deborah Tannen, Ph.D., in her best-selling book *You Just Don't Understand* (Ballantine Books, 1990). Men and women often claim they don't understand one another. But is this a result of different speaking styles, or just a general complaint? As many linguists and psycholinguists address this question, the results are sometimes contradictory. Some linguists seem to see fundamental differences in male and female speech, while others see little or no disparity.

Tannen, a linguist at Stanford University's Center for Advanced Studies in the Behavioral Sciences in Palo Alto, California, is among the proponents of relatively vast male-female linguistic differences. Tannen believes that men and women view many of the same situations in entirely different lights, and that linguistic differences are the result of these distinct perspectives.

Like Carol Gilligan, the advocate of moral differences, Tannen, too, believes that men

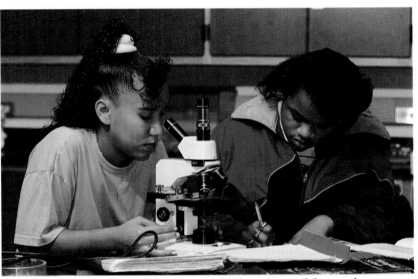

*Some experts contend that young girls may be steered away from careers in science and mathematics by parents and teachers influenced by gender bias.*

view the world hierarchically, while women see things from a perspective of interconnection. Her research seems to show that men are constantly gauging their place in the hierarchy by seeing themselves in relation to others. They are always either "one up," higher up on the ladder, or "one down," lower down in the hierarchy. Women, on the other hand, tend to see networks and webs of equals; relative importance is minimized, and connection with others is stressed. This, in Tannen's view, is the cause of Tom and Mary's argument in the car. Whereas Tom doesn't want to ask for directions for fear of being "one down" in relation to the direction giver, Mary doesn't see asking for help as a way of losing face.

Tannen's studies also note differences in the speaking styles of men and women. The same network-versus-hierarchy problem presents itself in speech. Men speak more in public, because, as speakers, they are seen as "one up." Women, however, speak more in private, because they can better build connections to others that way. In addition, men tend to be more argumentative while speaking, whereas women tend to shy away from confrontation because it disrupts the possibility of developing intimacy and interpersonal connection. Finally, Tannen has found that women tend to interrupt each other more often, while men prefer one speaker at a time.

*Identifying gender differences may improve many aspects of male-female relationships.*

In stark contrast to Tannen's research, a group of Belgian linguists found that male and female speech patterns hardly differed at all. Agnesa Pillon, Catherine Degauquier, and Francois Duquesne of the University of Mons-Hainaut in Mons, Belgium, placed 20 men and 20 women in random pairings of one woman and one man, and asked them to discuss a particular topic. Both men and women equally shifted the conversation, and started it up again after pauses. Perhaps surprisingly, the men were not more argumentative than the women; likewise, the women were not more emotional or personal than the men. This small study concluded that linguistic differences, at least in the case of a mixed-gender pair, are minimal.

Linguistic gender differences fall prey to the same lack of definition that besets moral and cognitive gender differences. Some experts argue for differences, while others argue for similarity. So creating a gray area is left up to individuals, as the experts themselves seem to rely on black-or-white explanations of gender linguistics.

Gender psychology is a growing field in which consensus is a rarity. Contradictory studies, however, are not a result of bad science. Psychological experiments are extremely difficult to conduct, in part because factors that seem to be insignificant often have a great influence on the outcome. For instance, when tests for linguistic gender differences are performed, the results may be entirely different for an all-female group and a group of both males and females. The mixed-gender group may in fact blend the styles of both genders, resulting in what seems at first glance like gender similarity. More research is necessary to determine the effects of factors like the composition of study groups, and to enlarge the study groups for more accurate results.

Although many studies suggest either definite gender differences or overwhelming gender similarities, no one is willing to bet why. Differences may be caused by societal and environmental factors, as in the case of parents unconsciously pushing boys toward math and science, and girls toward the humanities; genetic and physiological factors, such as the different brain lobes where male and female language skills are centered; and other factors like gender-specific language on standardized tests. All, none, or a combination of these factors may in fact be responsible for gender differences, if they exist. However, few experts are willing to embrace a definitive explanation.

The field of gender psychology boasts numerous studies, many with conflicting conclusions. But as researchers refine their methodology and broaden our understanding of human experience, many misperceptions of male and female personality will be discredited. The results will have far-reaching consequences affecting the way children are raised, the development of male and female self-esteem, and, of course, the daily interactions that tend to define relationships in all arenas of life. ◇

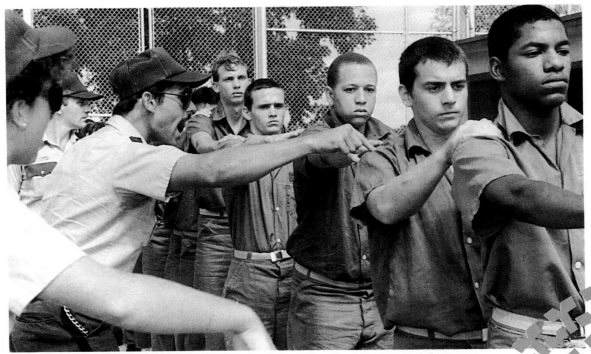

*The harsh dose of prison life provided by shock-incarceration boot-camp-style programs is sometimes just what's needed to set a young offender back on the right track.*

# BOOT CAMPS FOR YOUNG CONVICTS

*by Donald Cunningham*

"Sir, motivation, sir! Zero, one, two, three, four . . ." So it goes, as prisoners in a correctional boot camp in Jessup, Maryland, count off during a session of jumping jacks. One inmate, losing his balance and moving out of sync with the others, is scathingly upbraided by the instructor, and, for everyone, the exercise begins again: "Sir, motivation, sir . . ."

Such is the routine at experimental military-style prison camps in more than 30 states today. It has been 10 years since Oklahoma and Georgia launched the first shock-incarceration programs (the official name), in which young first-time offenders engage in brief, grueling programs of discipline, physical labor, and education. Currently New York maintains the largest population of shock-camp prisoners—more than 1,500. Georgia

has the most camps, nine, with more under construction. Yet, as the number of programs has increased, so has skepticism about what some people call merely a fad.

Politicians especially have supported the growth of shock-incarceration programs. One version of the 1993 federal crime bill even called for nearly $3 billion to fund expansions of the camps. The reason? Shock camps are less expensive to build than are traditional prisons, and prisoners spend less time there, sometimes trading a sentence of many years for a few months of shock incarceration. Many boosters of the camps cite an intuitive rationale and support for the concept, because the shock programs stress hard work and discipline. In theory, shock incarceration promises all things to all critics: hope of rehabilitation and less chance of back-

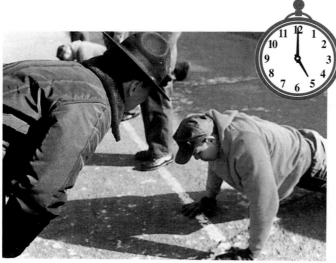

*The rigid discipline begins at dawn. At a camp in New York state, the early-morning routine includes push-ups and other calisthenics.*

sliding into criminal behavior; the penalty of hard labor; and cost savings. In reality the results are mixed.

### A Response to Crime

Shock-incarceration programs grew in response to the increasing number of young criminals—especially drug dealers—in the early 1980s. At the same time, prisons had become more crowded, and judges grew more inclined to choose the option of parole for first-time offenders. The shock programs were meant to address such problems by offering new, less costly prison space. It was also hoped that the shock element would reduce recidivism, or relapsing to a life of crime, by changing the habits of young criminals—again easing overcrowding in prisons.

Those qualifying for the programs typically range in age from 16 to 25, and have been convicted of nonviolent or drug-related crimes. They have traded prison sentences of a few years for a three- to six-month stint in a shock camp. Many prisoners do not qualify because of their health or for other reasons. And many in the programs do not finish and are returned to traditional prisons. In New York, for example, recent tallies found that about 37 percent of inmates failed to complete the programs; in Florida the failure rate approaches 50 percent.

The programs vary from state to state: some emphasize education and rehabilitation; others emphasize punishment. All programs feature a basic regimen of hard physical labor and discipline. At most camps, prisoners attend workshops to develop personal skills and self-esteem, deal with substance-abuse or other problems, and earn high-school-equivalency diplomas. Several states include programs for women. The programs are designed to instill values of respect, orderliness, punctuality, and hard work in streetwise young criminals unaccustomed to the rigors of a law-abiding society or a 9-to-5 workday.

### State-to-State Variations

In South Carolina the Wateree River Correctional Institution recently doubled the size of its shock-incarceration program, to about 200 beds. Its inmates, ranging in age from 17 to 24, have been convicted of nonviolent crimes such as drug dealing, burglary, and various misdemeanors. They have traded away prison terms of up to eight years for an average 90-day stay in the shock camp.

Wateree's program avoids demeaning language on the part of instructors. Instead, they employ "voice commands" that are loud and stern, but not humiliating. During the first month of incarceration at Wateree, inmates are not allowed to speak to one another, and are forbidden visitors and canteen privileges. To speak, to ask for water, even to request bathroom privileges, an inmate must raise his hand.

At Wateree the daily schedule begins at 5:00 A.M. sharp, when an inmate jumps out of bed and stands at attention. In 30 minutes,

*Much of an inmate's day involves heavy labor. Inmates in the Midwest helped sandbag during the summer floods in 1993.*

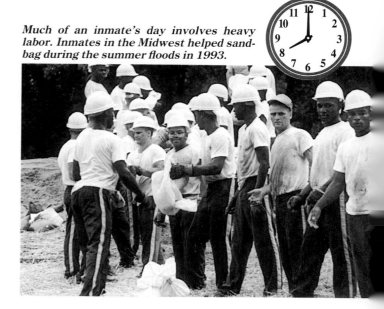

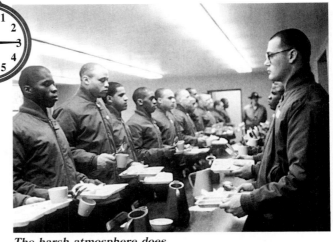

he showers, shaves, and makes his bed in a careful, precise fashion. Before eight o'clock, he has dressed, performed calisthenics, been inspected, and eaten breakfast. Then he begins eight hours of hard labor—usually a communal project such as digging fence posts, raising a structure, or clearing brush. If he is slow or moves out of place, he does push-ups. At 4:15 in the afternoon, the inmate begins two hours of classes. At 6:15, he marches to the dinner hall. Beginning at 7:00 P.M., there is one hour of supervised study, one hour of free time, and one hour of cleaning the living area. At 10:00 P.M., the lights in the living area are turned out.

At the Toulson Correctional Boot Camp in Jessup, Maryland, inmates awaken at 4:00 in the morning. An hour of physical training precedes breakfast. The morning includes classes and more exercises. After lunch, inmates perform four hours of physical labor. After dinner, there are three hours of physical training, a flag ceremony, and cleanup. Lights are turned out at 9:00.

The program at Toulson lasts six months. The inmates are young, first-time offenders, and many serve part of their sentence in a state prison before joining the shock program. In early 1992, Maryland introduced a follow-up support program, in which graduates gather once a week to nurture continuation of their newly acquired discipline and self-esteem. One Maryland parole officer said his staff can easily distinguish regular parolees from boot-camp graduates by the latter's more respectful, positive attitude.

New York, whose population of shock-camp inmates is the largest in the country, claims the biggest cost savings as well—some $300 million in a recent six-year period (a number that does not take into account the incidence of recidivism). Begun in 1987, the state's program contains the usual training, drills, calisthenics, and physical labor. Each week, one full day and two evenings are devoted to education. Other evenings offer mandatory classes, substance-abuse treatment, and counseling. A follow-up program known as After Shock provides counseling and supervision for graduates.

At Camp REAMS, a shock facility at Ohio's Southeast Correctional Institution, the lan-

*The harsh atmosphere does not relax at dinnertime. At meals, inmates march to their tables and consume their food in silence.*

*The evening regimen includes supervised study time. High-school dropouts can work toward an equivalency certificate.*

guage is not pretty. Within the first few days of prisoner orientation, one might overhear something like, "All right, you pigs, maggots—get over here at attention!" REAMS is an acronym for Respect, Education, Attitude, Motivation, and Success.

Georgia developed its first shock-incarceration programs in 1983. Since then, Georgia's programs have expanded more than those in other states, thanks in part to one of the concept's most enthusiastic supporters—Governor Zell Miller, a former Marine.

Georgia officials estimated that in 1990 their average daily cost per inmate in shock incarceration was less than half the cost per inmate in the general prison population. In 1992 the Georgia legislature allotted $14.3 million for expansion of the state's shock camps. The bill specifically prohibited television and air-conditioning in the camps.

## Measuring Success and Failure

Analysts gauge the success of shock-incarceration programs by a number of factors, including cost savings, reduced recidivism, and positive changes in the behavior or char-

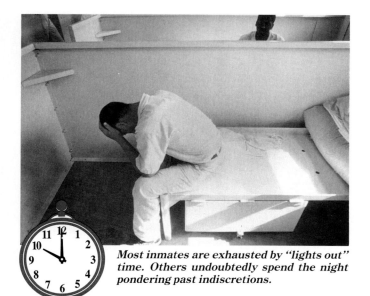

*Most inmates are exhausted by "lights out" time. Others undoubtedly spend the night pondering past indiscretions.*

acter of inmates. Recidivism is a key factor: it relates both to costs and to the character of the inmates. All factors seem difficult to measure satisfactorily, and measurements vary widely from state to state. Perhaps for such reasons, the debate about shock incarceration continues to be dominated by strong skepticism and strong boosterism.

In the late 1980s, Dale Parent, an analyst at Abt Associates Inc., in Massachusetts, performed a study of nine shock programs for the U.S. Department of Justice. He found that, in general, shock camps are less expensive to run than maximum-security prisons. That fact loses some importance when one considers that many shock-camp inmates would have been placed in much cheaper parole programs were it not for the shock-camp option. On the other hand, for communities wishing to eliminate parole for many first-time convicts, shock incarceration represents a new but smaller cost—especially when compared to traditional incarceration.

Parent found that in some states, rates of recidivism for shock-camp graduates can actually be higher than those for regular prisoners (in Oklahoma, 50 percent versus 28 percent after 29 months). The reverse is true in other states, although generally the difference is not wide. Georgia measured recidivism for shock-camp graduates at 42.7 percent—compared to 51.4 percent for regular inmates.

Doris MacKenzie of the National Institute of Justice studied shock-incarceration programs in Louisiana. She concluded: "When you balance all costs, there was a savings for the state of Louisiana." The state saved 154 prison beds and $1.6 million in one year as a result of shock incarceration. Per-day costs in these camps were higher than per-day costs in regular prison; however, confinement was much shorter—the population was comprised of inmates who would have served one to five years otherwise. MacKenzie found no evidence of overall reduced recidivism resulting from shock incarceration.

An equally important issue is the effect of shock incarceration on inmates. Does it change them for the better? All programs seek to instill a regard for discipline and other virtues. Do such traits persist following completion of the programs? Can they ever be measured? Some critics note that whereas military boot camps strip away a recruit's identity and rebuild it as a component of a team, prison boot camps probably fail to perform the latter task.

Some critics question the need for battering and demeaning inmates. They worry that this treatment may instill resentment in youths already prone to volatility. And no evidence has established that "shock" therapy is any more effective than a strict, no-nonsense approach.

Governor Miller of Georgia has said, "Nobody can tell me from some ivory tower that you take a kid, you kick him in the rear end, and it doesn't do any good." Yet, equal levels of recidivism after shock and regular incarceration might be interpreted as a measure of a relative failure of shock programs to benefit prisoners. Detractors also cite abuse and the potential for abuse in shock programs. There have been a few exercise-related deaths in the past, which might have been avoided. Stricter health restrictions exist today.

Most shock-incarceration programs are just beginning or are only a few years old. Although an effective design has not been found, the strategy has potential. Perhaps in the future, some states will create a mix of work, discipline, and education that greatly reduces recidivism and holds down costs. The huge sums of money that federal and state governments continue to set aside for shock programs will give the states an opportunity to show whether that can happen.  ◇

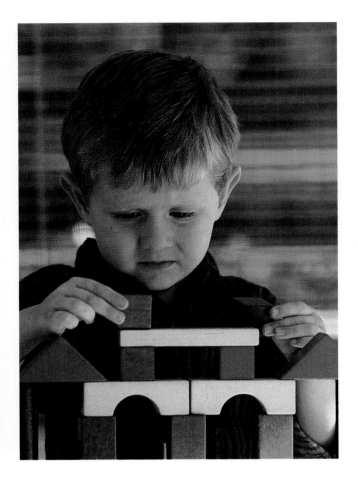

# A CHILD'S THEORY OF MIND

*by Bruce Bower*

I f you think kids say the darnedest things, get a load of what they think.

Consider a group of preschoolers shown a box that they all agree appears to contain candy. Each child gets a chance to fling open the receptacle, but only a stash of crayons greets their hungry glares. If asked by an experimenter what someone else will think the box contains upon first seeing it, four- and five-year-olds typically grin at the trick and exclaim, "Candy!"

They realize, in their devilish way, that the shape and design of the box at first create a false belief.

Yet most three-year-olds react entirely differently to the trick box. After falling for the sweet deception, they insist that a newcomer will assume crayons lie within the container. If an adult enters the room, peers into the box, and does an obvious double take, three-year-olds still maintain that the grown-up expected to find crayons. What's more, the same youngsters assert that they, too, initially thought the box held crayons.

Of course, three-year-olds cherish cantankerous and contrary remarks, but further experiments indicate that a deeper process orchestrates their explanations of the world. Observe, for instance, preschoolers given some toys purchased at a novelty store: a large sponge shaped and painted to look like a rock, a "sucker" egg made of chalk, and a green cardboard cat covered by a removable red filter that makes it appear black. Give them plenty of time to examine the objects. Most four- and five-year-olds separate each object's real qualities from its apparent attributes; they note, for instance, that the sponge only looks like a rock.

But those obstinate three-year-olds find such subtleties about as appealing as going to bed early. In their minds an object possesses either real or apparent characteristics, but not both at the same time. For instance, some assert that the phony rock looks like a sponge and really is a sponge, while the cat looks black and really is black.

These findings emerge from research conducted over the past decade to examine how children reach an understanding of the mind's trappings, such as beliefs, desires, intentions, and emotions. Some investigators contend that this hybrid of developmental and cognitive psychology explores the ways in which children construct "theories of mind." Others argue that the research illuminates the origins of "folk psychology" or people's shared assumptions about how the mind works.

*Between the ages of three and five, children undergo a fundamental shift in the way they think.*

## A Fundamental Shift?

Whatever terminology they use, scientists generally agree that knowledge about mental states and attitudes changes substantially throughout childhood. Debate revolves around a number of clashing explanations of how and why that change takes place. "There's a genuine argument now over whether a fundamental shift occurs in children's understanding of their own and others' minds between ages 3 and 5," says John H. Flavell, a psychologist at Stanford University and an early explorer of how preschoolers understand thinking.

The March 1993 *Behavioral and Brain Sciences* contains two opposing reviews of work on children's understanding of the mind, and 60 written comments from an international group of investigators.

More than 50 years ago, Swiss psychologist Jean Piaget launched the study of how youngsters conceptualize mental life. He argued that infants use a few basic reflexes, such as sucking objects that enter their mouths and following moving objects with their eyes, but extract no other meaning from the environment. Preschoolers make themselves the center of the universe, in Piaget's theory; they fail to grasp that other people have different viewpoints and different sources of knowledge. A full appreciation of mental states as experienced by oneself and others blooms in later childhood and adolescence, Piaget held.

Today researchers contend that more goes on in the heads of babies and young children than Piaget imagined. "Theory-of-mind" advocates argue that infants possess a primitive sense of being like others; soon thereafter, children assemble a succession of progressively more sophisticated predictions about the types of thought that coordinate behavior in particular situations. This process resembles the accumulation of knowledge through theory testing in science.

In 1978 investigations into children's theories of mind got a major boost from a controversial article in which two researchers suggested that chimpanzees theorize about mental states. To test this assertion, scientists began to look at whether chimps and children attribute false beliefs to others. Chimps showed little talent for viewing the world from another's misleading perspective, but children at different ages yielded results that spurred continued research.

Some investigators now suggest that an innate brain mechanism allows even very young children to begin theorizing about mental states. Others view the child's emerging understanding of the mind as a by-product of a maturing brain that manipulates many types of information in increasingly complex ways.

*The gradual process by which a child's mind evolves is revealed to some extent by observing the child at play. A three-year-old boy, for example, revels in the art of finger painting (left). Two years later (right), the same boy uses abstract thinking to work on a puzzle.*

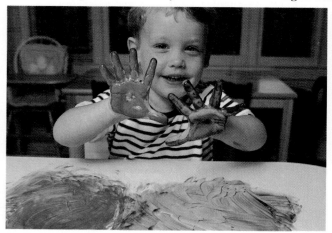
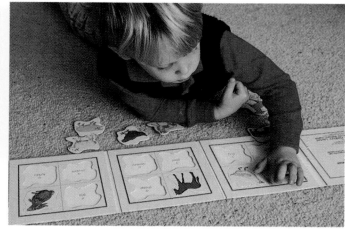

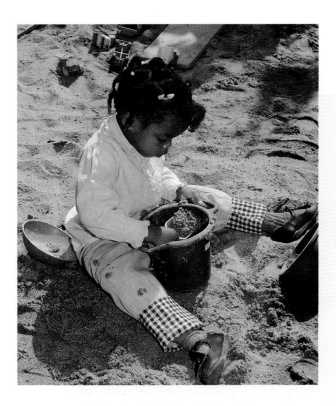

## Don't Just Sit There, Think Something

Children know much about the mind by age 4, but their conception of how people think still diverges sharply from that of older children and adults, according to a report in the April 1993 issue of *Child Development*. Beginning around age 7, youngsters tend to conclude that mental activity goes on continuously in a waking mind. Younger children, in contrast, assume that the mind switches on when it has a job to do, and switches off at the conclusion of a task, leaving the mental landscape blank.

A four-year-old who attributes complex meaning to beliefs and other mental states, as proposed by "theory-of-mind" researchers, at the same time fails to realize that people lead continuous inner lives and experience a "stream of consciousness," contend John H. Flavell, a psychologist at Stanford University, and his colleagues.

In one trial conducted by Flavell's team, groups of 20 children at ages 3, 4, and 6 to 7 years, as well as 20 adults, stated whether they believed a female experi-

menter entertained any thoughts or ideas in three situations: waiting quietly in a chair facing a blank wall, looking at pictures on the wall, and attempting to explain how someone got a big pear into a small glass bottle. Participants indicated the absence of thought by selecting a drawing of a woman's head underneath an empty "thought bubble" (commonly used to indicate the thoughts of cartoon characters), and signaled the presence of thought by choosing a portrayal of a woman's head under a thought bubble containing three asterisks.

Warm-up tests established that all of the participants viewed the asterisks as representing ongoing thoughts or ideas of the observed female experimenter.

Only one of the three-year-olds attributed mental activity to a waiting person facing a blank wall. That number increased to four in the four-year-olds, 11 in the six- to seven-year-olds, and 19 in the adults. In contrast, at least 13 members of each age group granted thoughts to a person who was observed looking at pictures on the wall or trying to explain the pear-bearing bottle.

In further trials with four-year-olds, most of these youngsters contended that people can voluntarily empty their minds of all thoughts and ideas for a few minutes and that the mind of a waiting person "was not doing anything."

And in unpublished results, Flavell's group finds that not until about age 7 do children consistently recall thoughts they just had while contemplating a problem.

Preschoolers may seldom reflect on their own and others' thoughts, and probably experience confusion or difficulty when they try, Flavell suggests. Prior studies directed by Flavell suggest that at around age 7 kids realize that one thought triggers another in a chain reaction, and that a person's facial expression may contradict inner thoughts. By this age children also realize that some psychological states linger indefinitely, such as worries that a monster will emerge from the night.

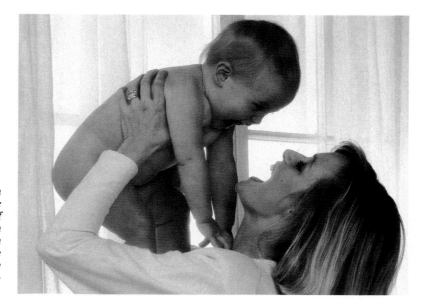

*At a very early age, a child begins to mimic the facial expressions of the people around him or her. It takes much longer, however, before a child can perceive the meaning behind an expression.*

Another school of thought regards commonsense notions about mental life as socially and culturally learned tools for dealing with others, rather than as theories for making predictions about people.

And a final account emphasizes intuition as the driving force behind children's take on the mind. In this view, preschoolers first imagine having the desires or beliefs of another person, and then mentally simulate what that person would do and feel.

### The Theory Theory

Alison Gopnik, a psychologist at the University of California, Berkeley, champions an influential version of the theory-of-mind approach known as the "theory theory." Individuals gradually construct commonsense psychological beliefs as a way of explaining themselves and others, according to Gopnik. On the basis of their experience, children theorize that invisible mental entities, such as beliefs and desires, exist and operate in lawful ways, she contends. Youngsters modify or discard a favored theory if it encounters too many difficulties or continually leads them astray in social situations, just as scientists drop or modify a theory that cannot account for or predict key phenomena, the Berkeley psychologist posits.

"The same mental capacities that children use to understand the mind have been applied to science by adults. It's not that children are little scientists, but scientists are big children," she says, chuckling at the implication.

Gopnik presents a rough outline of what researchers know about the development of an understanding of the mind. Even infants display a vague notion of internal psychological states, she asserts. For example, studies find that babies deftly mimic adult facial expressions and gaze in the direction they see others looking.

From around 18 months to 3 years, children learn to distinguish between mental and physical events, Gopnik notes. They know the difference between, say, an imagined dog and a real dog, and begin to engage in pretense and make-believe games. Their talk includes words for perceptions, such as "see," "look," and "taste"; and for emotions, such as "happy," "love," and "want." By age 3, most also use words such as "know," "think," and "remember."

In Gopnik's opinion, three-year-olds retain a fascination with "silly" states that stand apart from the real world, such as dreams and make-believe. They also assume that beliefs and other mental states apprehend the world directly, just as their eyes see whatever lies in front of them. They do not assume that a person holds a belief about the contents of a box; in the three-year-old's theory, the person's belief corresponds to what the box holds. Thus, the typical youngster says the box contains candy when assessing its appearance. But the same child sheds that assumption upon seeing its contents, and acquires a belief that the box has always held crayons and that other people know that.

A theory of mental states as direct conduits to reality, rather than as representations of what may or may not exist, also sometimes causes children to confuse appearance with reality, as in encounters with spongy rocks and chalky eggs.

Further evidence suggests that three-year-olds assign either total knowledge or absolute ignorance to mental states, Gopnik says. In other words, they fail to appreciate that belief comes in degrees. For instance, in contrast to four-year-olds, three-year-olds show no preference for information offered by people who express certainty about what a box contains versus people citing doubts about what the box holds.

### Engaging in Pretense

Some investigators argue that three-year-olds know enough about false beliefs to attempt to deceive others. A child at that age who breaks a lamp may, when asked by his or her mother if he or she touched the lamp, quickly utter, "No." But Gopnik maintains that researchers cannot yet say whether the denial signals a conscious attempt to manipulate mother's beliefs or a learned strategy for avoiding punishment, devoid of any deeper understanding of why that strategy might work.

By age 4 or 5, children come to the conclusion that people form beliefs and other mental states *about* the world, Gopnik holds. These youngsters entertain notions of false belief, distinguish between real and apparent qualities of the same object, and recognize changes in their own beliefs, she says.

Moreover, five-year-olds usually understand that individuals may perceive an object in different ways depending on their line of sight. They also recognize that beliefs dictate a person's emotional reactions to

*As a sense of right and wrong evolves, a child may become consumed with guilt for minor misbehavior.*

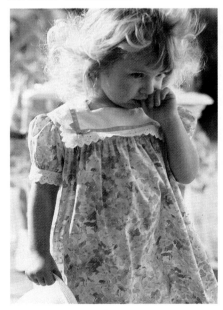

particular situations, such as an adult's expression of surprise at discovering crayons in a candy box.

"By five years of age, children have acquired a remarkable understanding of the mind, in many ways quite like that of adults, and certainly very different from that of two- or even three-year-olds," Gopnik contends.

Although adults generally believe that each person uses direct knowledge of his or her own mental states to make educated guesses about how others think, research with children suggests otherwise, she adds. At any given stage of development, children make the same inferences about their own minds and those of other people, Gopnik argues.

When confronting false beliefs, she points out, three-year-olds make errors about their own immediately past beliefs, such as saying they thought the box contained crayons all along, and they commit a similar blunder in claiming that a newcomer believes the box holds crayons.

In contrast, three-year-olds perform much better when dealing with "silly" mental states that bear no relation to the real world. For example, in one study directed by Gopnik, three-year-olds knew they had first pretended that an imaginary glass contained hot chocolate, and then had imagined that the same glass was full of lemonade. Children at this age also realize that other people engage in pretense and may change the details of an imagined situation.

Arriving at an adult-like, abstract account of thought requires a child to continually tinker with and sometimes replace theories about how the mind works, Gopnik says. Other psychologists currently direct investigations aimed at shedding further light on these theories of what the mind perceives as a child ages.

In an ironic twist, relatively stable theories of mind rapidly become second nature after age 5, and foster the false impression that we directly experience our own mental states, rather than making well-practiced inferences about what we believe, want, and feel, Gopnik asserts. Master chess players experience a similar warping of perception, she says. After years of practice, their consideration of numerous potential moves during a match occurs so quickly and effortlessly that they report only a sensation of reacting to the competing forces and powers on the chessboard, rather than making a step-by-step analysis of the proper move.

### Brain Mechanisms

Other researchers argue that a child's ability to theorize about mental life depends on a specialized brain mechanism that exerts its influence by around age 2, when children begin to use pretense. Contrary to Gopnik's proposal, four-year-olds probably do not overhaul their assumptions about mental states, argues Alan M. Leslie, a psychologist at the University of London in England. Instead, he says, their new treatment of false belief and other concepts reflects a maturing capacity to parcel out different information in their minds.

*Children have a strong tendency to make sense of their own actions by telling stories about those deeds.*

For instance, unlike many three-year-olds, four-year-olds also realize that an out-of-date photograph—say a picture of candy in a cupboard that is now bare—represents a past state of affairs that has changed.

Leslie and his colleagues propose that young children easily slip into and out of pretend play because the brain's "theory-of-mind mechanism" allows them to grasp that people hold invisible attitudes about the veracity of a fictional state of affairs. Hence, even two-year-olds understand that if Mother pretends a banana is a telephone, she won't serve the telephone for lunch and call up Father on the banana.

The same brain mechanism allows three- to four-year-olds to understand that a person behaves according to potentially misleading beliefs, hopes, or other attitudes held about people and objects, Leslie asserts.

Autistic children provide an example of what happens when apparent brain damage destroys the theory-of-mind mechanism, he contends. Studies conducted by Leslie and University of London co-workers Uta Frith and Simon Baron-Cohen indicate that autistic youngsters fail to develop any rules of thumb for understanding how mental states cause behavior. Autistic children cannot conceive that they or others hold false beliefs, and they find it difficult to understand deception, according to the British investigators.

As a result, symptoms of autism revolve around the absence of imagination, an inability to communicate with others, and a poverty of social skills, Leslie suggests.

### Powers of Imagination

Philip D. Zelazo of the University of Toronto and Douglas Frye of New York University, both psychologists, take a different approach. They hold that a four-year-old's altered conception of mental states depends on the emergence of a general ability to reason first from one perspective and then from another, incompatible, perspective.

One experiment conducted by Zelazo and Frye required children to place cards in various locations according to their colors, and then sort the same cards according to their shapes. Three-year-olds succeeded at the first set of rules, but could not immediately switch to the alternate rules; four- and five-year-olds performed well at sorting cards both by color and by shape.

Other investigators doubt that common-sense notions of the mind spring either from specific theories or a more general versatility at manipulating information.

Instead, children possess a powerful innate tendency to make sense of their own and others' actions by telling stories about those deeds, argues Jerome Bruner, a psychologist at New York University. Myths, oral stories, books, and other cultural influences on family and social life shape the ways in which children arrive at a personal understanding of belief, deception, and the rest of mental life, he asserts. Bruner expands on this notion in his book *Acts of Meaning* (Harvard University Press, 1990).

If Bruner's argument is correct, children in the United States and Sri Lanka, or in other markedly contrasting cultures, should report striking differences in their assumptions about the mind. To date, virtually all evidence regarding children's understanding of the mind comes from Western cultures, Gopnik points out.

Another explanation of folk psychology rests on a child's powers of imagination. Three-year-olds have trouble imagining mental states that contradict their own current mental states, and thus exhibit difficulty with false-belief tests, holds Alvin I. Goldman, a philosopher at the University of Arizona in Tucson. By age 4, children can imagine having the beliefs and desires of another person; they then mentally simulate that person's resulting feelings and behaviors, Goldman argues.

Paul L. Harris, a psychologist at the University of Oxford in England, agrees. In some studies, three-year-olds accurately report

*Building blocks make good toys because they stimulate abstract thought processes and play upon a child's emerging sense of order.*

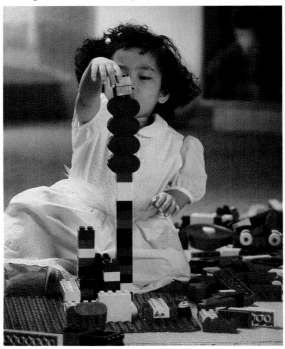

their psychological experience and understand that mental states refer to the real world, according to Harris. When asked to visualize an imaginary object, three-year-olds understand the direction to "make a picture in your head," and describe the mind as a container that at times displays pictures of nonexistent things, he notes.

Children apparently adopt such metaphors as a way of capturing their inner psychological experiences and improving their mental simulations of how others think, Harris asserts.

In addition, he says, three-year-olds perform much better on false-belief tasks when an experimenter presents a situation in words rather than in actions. For instance, an experimenter may tell three-year-olds that an object that apparently belongs in one box has been secretly transferred to another box, rather than showing them the transfer. The children then look in both boxes to verify the transfer. Compared with same-age counterparts who only observe the transfer, these youngsters are much more likely to realize that an uninformed newcomer will guess the object's location incorrectly.

A verbal description makes it easier for three-year-olds to imagine the object in its initial location and to ignore the knowledge that they saw the object in an unexpected box, Harris holds.

Still, Gopnik argues, the presence of an underlying theory best accounts for the wide range of understanding about the mind achieved by children around age 4. What's more, considerable research already suggests that adults often remain unaware of the unconscious mental states that direct their attitudes and judgments, adding to the likelihood that children also lack direct access to their own mental states, and must construct theories to explain mental life, she points out. Unfortunately, much remains unclear about the origins of theories and the reasons for their change in childhood as well as in science, Gopnik acknowledges.

"The scientist's ability to learn about the world is still almost as mysterious as the child's," she maintains. "Nevertheless, reducing two mysteries to one is an important advance, and a great deal more than we usually achieve."  ◇

# Housecalls

by Stephen G. Underwood, M.D.

**Q** *My six-year-old son has terrible temper tantrums. My husband and I have tried ignoring the tantrums, sending him to his room, and even spanking him. It's easy enough to ignore a tantrum at home, but what should we do when he explodes in public?*

**A** If your son has frequent and severe losses of control at that age, you may want to at least consider whether he should be evaluated or whether you might want to seek some counseling on skills to help you handle the situation. In a two-year-old, such regular fits are more the norm, but a six-year-old should have developed more control. In judging your son's needs, a therapist will want to know how often the tantrums occur, to what extent, and what circumstances trigger the fit.

When he acts out angrily in public, the challenge is for you to immediately provide an example of the type of self-control you are trying to instill in him. For example, smacking him will probably just make the problem worse. Removing him from the environment can help, as can "time-outs." Misbehavior and the need for discipline in public may feel very embarrassing for the parent, but try to remember that it may not be as disruptive to others as it seems.

Before you go out, you may want to talk to your son about what behaviors are best and what behavior will bring about an abrupt end to an excursion or cause him to otherwise lose privileges. The most effective discipline sets the choices and lets children decide between them, and also rewards and reinforces good behavior with praise.

---

**Q** *Is everything discussed with a psychologist or psychiatrist considered absolutely confidential? Can their records be subpoenaed for use in court?*

**A** Laws vary from state to state, but, in general, information divulged to such professionals is considered totally confidential and cannot be revealed except by consent of the patient. Courts, though, can subpoena a psychologist or psychiatrist to testify. In such cases the law typically permits these professionals to answer broad questions about their patients—how long was the patient in therapy, what was his or her level of function, etc.—without considering it a breach of confidentiality. In court, therapists are in a difficult position, because revealing too little or too much could place them either in contempt of court or subject to a lawsuit by the patient.

---

*A parent with a child who is having a temper tantrum in public faces the awkward dilemma of applying discipline immediately or of abruptly removing the child from the "tantrum environment."*

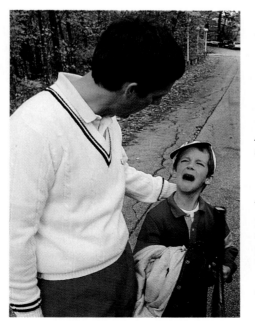

**Q** *My grown daughter's therapist recently told her that she had suppressed the memory of her father (my husband) sexually abusing her when she was two years old. My husband denies it, and I find it impossible to believe. Can psychologists really evoke such memories?*

**A** One must be extremely cautious about interpreting childhood memories that may have long been suppressed. Deciphering recollections of childhood 20 or 30 years later is difficult, particularly if the individual was very young when the supposed event occurred.

If abuse happens briefly in a nonaggressive or nontraumatic way, the young child may largely forget it. Experienced therapists can usually identify the person who has been clearly and repeatedly abused, but pursuing traces of a possible one-time event may cause more harm than benefit for the patient and family.

People who are in therapy for a long time become highly subject to suggestions by the therapist, especially about something as much in the news as sexual abuse. Thus, a therapist who convinces a patient of a highly tentative recollection can be doing a great disservice.

---

Q **My husband and I are considering placing our one-year-old daughter in a day-care center while we work. What are the latest findings on the effects of day care on young children?**

A Many consider the upsurge in the utilization of day care in recent history to be a huge social experiment, the effects of which will not be fully apparent for decades. A fair amount of evidence, though, seems to indicate that day care per se is not harmful, and may even give children a developmental advantage in certain skills, such as socialization and communication. Factors in the current debate include:
• Quality of the day care. Quality has to do with adherence to state regulations, ratio of adults to children, qualifications and personality of caregivers, the physical environment, nutrition, and the types of activities that the center provides for the children—all factors that may vary widely.
• Stability in the child's environment. Children do best with a few faces as their *primary* caregivers. Stability facilitates a sense of security. Finding a day-care center where the child is assigned to, at most, a couple of adults as primary caregivers is probably important. It does not help the child to be transferred often between different day-care centers.
• The amount of nonparental care the child receives. Day-care opponents argue against nonparental care for preschoolers. Long day-care days of 8 or 10 hours or more can certainly be tiring. All agree that how nurturing the parents are when with the child is critical.
• Age at which the child is in day care. Some feel that the supposed detriment of day care is directly related to how young

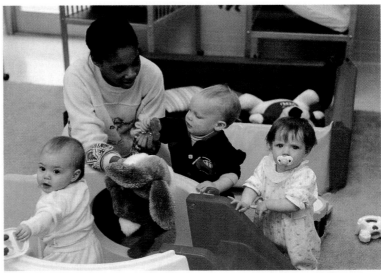

the child is, maintaining that babies should be cared for at home, and that day care is not best for children, at least up to age 3 or 4 (after which separation anxiety lessens). On the other hand, infants readily accept care from many people, and toddlers, in their own way, are already demanding group socialization.

All of these factors are intertwined, and depend on the personality of the child, parents, and the day-care workers.

*Current thinking holds that most children in day care gain an advantage in socialization and communication skills compared to their counterparts who are reared exclusively at home.*

---

Q **I have heard the drug Prozac referred to as a miracle drug in treating depression. Is this true? Does the drug commonly cause any adverse reactions?**

A Prozac is one of a new generation of antidepressants, and it has rapidly become the most widely prescribed antidepressant in the country. Although Prozac is very effective, no drug is perfect. When this one works—as it does for many people—it works well, often producing a dramatic improvement in a few weeks.

Prozac has relatively few serious side effects, in comparison to older antidepressants. Occasionally patients experience nausea or other gastrointestinal problems, as well as headaches, a fidgety feeling, or other reactions. The brief scare that Prozac caused a higher suicide rate in certain patients has been disproved.

---

*Do you have a psychology question?*
Send it to Editor, Health and Medicine Annual, P.O. Box 90, Hawleyville, CT 06440-9990.

# Practical
# News to Use

**See also:**
Individual articles in the second half of this book, arranged in alphabetical order, for additional information.

As people take new responsibility for their well-being, they discover that there are numerous steps they can take to prevent illness, injury, and premature death. Shunning tobacco and illegal drugs, limiting alcohol consumption, eating properly, exercising regularly, avoiding safety and environmental hazards, having timely immunizations and medical checkups—actions such as these go a long way toward ensuring good health.

The alternatives can be deadly. For instance, according to the Mid-America Research Institute, a driver has a 40 percent probability of dying in a crash at 55 miles per hour; at 65 miles per hour, the probability jumps to 73 percent. However, in 1987, because many drivers weren't obeying the 55-mile-per-hour speed limit, the U.S. Congress allowed states to raise the speed limit on rural interstates to 65. Forty states did so. The result: people drove even faster than before. In 1992 those 40 states had 348 more deaths on their rural interstates than in 1986, despite increases in the percentage of cars that had air bags and other safety features.

In contrast to more-lenient speed limits, momentum for smoking bans in public buildings, offices, and restaurants has increased as the risks of environmental tobacco smoke (passive, or "secondhand," smoke) become irrefutable. In 1993 the U.S. Environmental Protection Agency (EPA) concluded that environmental tobacco smoke is a human-lung carcinogen, responsible for an estimated 3,000 lung-cancer deaths annually among U.S. nonsmokers. The EPA also notes that the smoke causes serious respiratory problems for infants and young children. Michael Siegel, M.D., of the Centers for Disease Control and Prevention (CDC), reports that waiters and bartenders have a 50 percent greater risk of getting lung cancer than other people; his analyses showed that levels of tobacco smoke in restaurants were 1.5 times as high as in homes with at least one smoker; smoke levels in bars were 4.4 to 4.5 times as high as in residences.

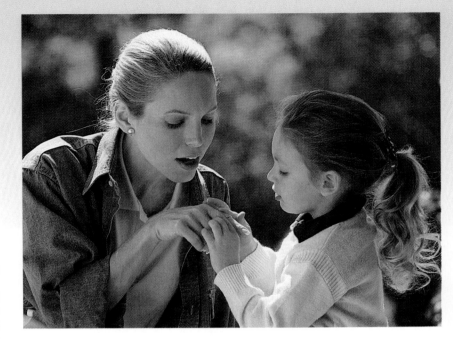

Sometimes medical experts disagree on the value of procedures and behaviors. Although there is general agreement that having mammograms every one to two years reduces breast-cancer death rates among women over 50, experts are divided over the value of mammograms to younger women. The National Cancer Institute (NCI), saying that studies fail to show clear benefits to women under 50, dropped recommendations that these women undergo regular mammograms. The American Cancer Society, however, recommends that women in their 40s have mammograms every one to two years, and that women over 50 have them annually.

Another problem occurs when a behavior has conflicting effects. Evidence indicates that moderate alcohol intake protects against heart disease. But scientists at Johns Hopkins report that people who have more than seven drinks a week are 4.6 times more likely to have a particular type of eye cataract, called posterior subcapsular cataract, than nondrinkers. Also, what's good for the gander may not be good for the goose. Although alcohol protects women's hearts as well as those of men, it also increases the risk of breast cancer. NCI research indicates that women who drink moderately have a breast-cancer risk 40 to 100 percent higher than women who do not drink.

Much of the progress made during the 20th century in reducing incidences of infectious diseases resulted from improvements in basic hygiene, food production and handling, and water treatment. But Americans have recently been reminded that pathogenic contaminants of food and water supplies are still around. Early in 1993 an outbreak of a virulent strain of the bacterium *Escherichia coli* occurred in the western United States when people ate contaminated hamburgers that had been undercooked; three children died, and 600 people became severely ill. The strain, 0157:H7, was first linked to human illness in 1982, and its importance as a human pathogen appears to be increasing.

Several months later impure water made national headlines when the protozoan *Cryptosporidium* sickened at least 183,000 people and contributed to six deaths in the Milwaukee, Wisconsin, area. The parasite apparently entered Lake Michigan in farm runoff, then passed through a water-treatment plant while employees were in the process of testing a new sanitation chemical.

*There are many steps that people can take to prevent illness, injury, and premature death.*

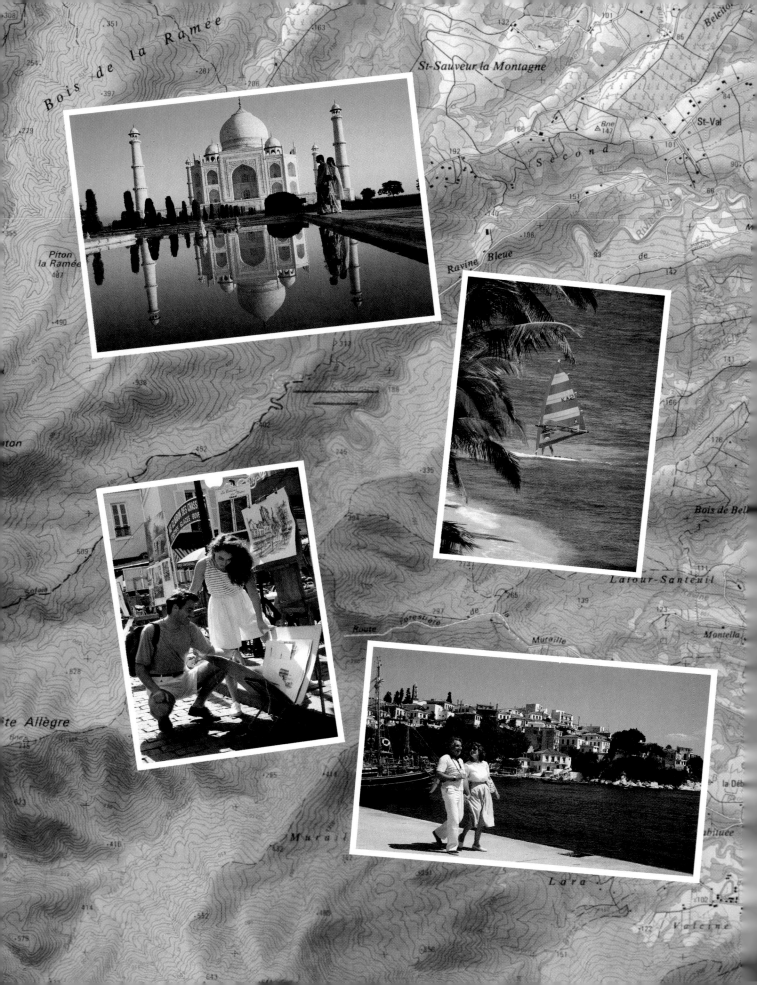

# THE HEALTHY TRAVELER

*by Marcy O'Koon*

Seasoned travelers do not pass up the adventure and reward of a trip abroad simply out of fear of getting sick. Instead, they learn about the potential health risks associated with their destination. Then they take appropriate precautions to increase their odds of returning home healthy. Such travelers know that it is better to return with souvenirs and photographs than with some exotic infection.

## The Variables of Risk

For any given trip, a traveler usually faces only a handful of health concerns, concerns determined mostly by destination, length of stay, and planned activities. The industrialized countries of Canada, Britain, Western Europe, Australia, Japan, and Scandinavia are all considered low risk for many—but not all—diseases. The developing countries of Asia, Africa, and Latin America are considered high risk. A number of other destinations fall somewhere in between.

People who stay for an extended period in one general area tend to suffer more travel-related health problems than those who make brief visits. The more-frequent and longer contact with the local population raises the opportunity for communicable diseases. And after awhile, long-term visitors often neglect to consistently practice preventive measures.

Even spending less than a full day in the great outdoors, in either rural or wilderness areas, raises the risk of certain diseases, particularly those transmitted by insect bites. It also means a greater chance of developing problems related to sun exposure or extreme temperature.

A host of other variables can raise or lower the level of risk as well. Those who are sexually active while abroad take a chance of acquiring a sexually transmitted disease, particularly in areas of Asia and Africa where the rate of infection with the human immunodeficiency virus (HIV) may be high. People traveling with an organized tour tend to be at a somewhat lower risk of health problems, largely because they are more likely to be given instruction in preventive measures.

Your health status before the trip begins must also be taken into account. The very young, the very old, pregnant women, and people with diabetes, heart disease, weakened immune systems, and other chronic health problems are, of course, at greater risk than is the average traveler.

## A Range of Health Concerns

By far the most common health problem afflicting international travelers is traveler's diarrhea (TD). The U.S. Centers for Disease Control and Prevention (CDC) in Atlanta, Georgia, estimates that between 20 and 50 percent of people who visit other countries suffer an episode of watery bowel movements, exacerbated by abdominal cramps, nausea, urgency, bloating, or malaise that typically lasts four to six days before clearing up on its own. Some extreme cases last up to a month, however. TD results from the gastrointestinal tract's reaction to unfamiliar strains of bacteria introduced via drinking

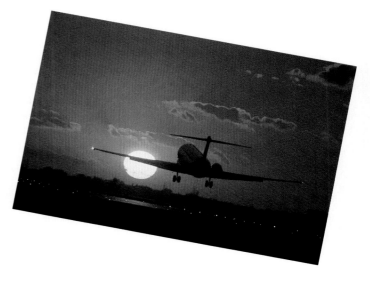

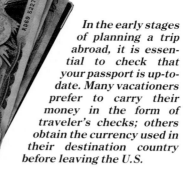

water or contaminated food. Various organisms, such as salmonellae and shigellae, can cause TD, but the most common bacterial culprit is known as *E. coli.*

In certain countries a mosquito bite can cause more than just an itchy red bump. A single bite from an infected mosquito can transmit any of dozens of diseases, including malaria, yellow fever, dengue fever, filariasis, and Japanese encephalitis, some of which can prove fatal, especially if diagnosis and treatment are delayed. Insects other than mosquitoes that transmit disease through their bites include blackflies (river blindness); sand flies (leishmaniasis); tsetse flies (African sleeping sickness); fleas (bubonic plague); the reduviid bug (Chagas' disease); and ticks (Lyme disease, typhus, relapsing fever).

No matter how pristine fresh stream water, lake water, or unchlorinated swimming water appears, contaminants may abound, and can infect people who drink it with hepatitis A and various gastrointestinal diseases. Other diseases, such as schistosomiasis, are introduced to the body through the eyes, ears, nose, or directly through the skin.

*When one goes abroad, health concerns vary according to destination, length of stay, and activities.*

The climate can cause conditions with symptoms ranging from merely uncomfortable to fatal. A skin rash, sometimes called prickly heat, is a minor problem, but heatstroke is much more serious. Exposure to intense sun can cause a painful sunburn or sun poisoning. Cold weather can cause frostbite of any exposed extremities as well as hypothermia, a dangerous drop in body temperature, which can result in shock and heart failure.

Abrupt arrival at locations 6,000 feet above sea level or higher can cause altitude sick-

*In the early stages of planning a trip abroad, it is essential to check that your passport is up-to-date. Many vacationers prefer to carry their money in the form of traveler's checks; others obtain the currency used in their destination country before leaving the U.S.*

ness. This condition results from the reduced atmospheric pressure, which makes it difficult for the lungs to obtain sufficient oxygen from the air. Symptoms include headache, nausea, and fatigue. At altitudes 10,000 feet or higher, the condition can cause dysfunction of the lungs and swelling of the brain—sometimes with fatal results.

## Before You Go

Perhaps the greatest influence on any traveler's degree of health risk is behavior. "The behavior you practice as a traveler is much more significant than the incidence of disease in the country you are visiting," says Roz Dewart, chief of the traveler's-health section for the CDC. "If you are going to a cholera-infected country, whether you get sick or not is determined more by your behavior than by the fact that you are surrounded by cholera-infected people."

The behavior that will keep you healthy begins at home about 8 to 10 weeks before your departure. First, see your family physician or a travel-medicine specialist for a general health checkup and to discuss your plans. If you are pregnant, over 40, have signs of heart disease, or have some other temporary or chronic health condition, find out what sort of special precautions are necessary, as well as what limitations on activity would be prudent during your trip. If you are on medication, be sure your supply will last the length of your trip.

Kenneth Dardick, M.D., a travel-medicine specialist with Connecticut Travel Medicine in Storrs, Connecticut, suggests asking your doctor for a one- to three-day supply of an antibiotic in case you contract a case of traveler's diarrhea. "It's proven that antibiotics can be effective within the hour," he says.

For every prescription you will be carrying with you, have your doctor write a letter on business stationery stating the reason for the medicine, appropriate dosage, and any information that would be useful in case of emergency. Keep your prescription medication in its original pharmaceutical container. These measures will help you avoid the suspicion of customs or border guards on the lookout for drug peddlers.

Depending on the degree of health risk in the region you'll be visiting, your doctor may suggest one or several of the following vaccines: Japanese encephalitis, rabies, typhoid (an oral vaccine), hepatitis B, meningococcal, pneumococcal, tetanus/diphtheria, measles, rubella, mumps, or polio. You probably received several of these immunizations in childhood, but may need some booster shots. You should also be sure to receive the latest influenza vaccine.

Before granting entry, a few countries require a certificate showing you have had a yellow-fever vaccine. The yellow-fever vaccine has a limited distribution, so you may need to visit one of the 500 or so travel clinics that stock it to receive your inoculation.

Keep in mind that a required vaccine is also meant to protect the local population from you and other travelers who might introduce to local people a disease against which they have no immunity. Similarly, the local population may be immune to a number of other diseases to which outsiders are vulnerable and should be vaccinated against. The vaccines or prophylactics (preventatives) for these diseases are often termed "recommended," yet are considered essential in certain situations. Antimalarial medication (in pill form) is a good example of an important prophylactic that is termed "recommended," but not required, for travelers to tropical climates.

### Insurance

Before departure, you should also check with your health-insurance company to determine whether your current policy covers health care outside the United States, and what the restrictions and procedures are. Certain poli-cies require precertification, or prior approval for surgeries and treatments. Some companies will pay the health-care provider directly upon your discharge from a hospital; others require the policyholder to pay and then be reimbursed later.

After you discover the areas where your standard health coverage falls short, you might want to investigate supplemental traveler's health insurance. Some benefits to look for: direct payment; transport, in case you should, say, break a leg in a remote location and need an emergency airlift to a hospital; repatriation, which means that after you are stabilized, the policy covers the cost of your flight home for further treatment or surgery; and family transportation, which means your nearest relative can be flown to your bedside.

### Jet Lag, Motion Sickness, and More Fun

You've heard that "getting there can be half the fun"? That saying may prove to be a cruel joke if you tend to suffer from jet lag, motion sickness, or altitude sickness. Fortunately, jet lag, though common, is only mildly debili-

*The thin air at high altitudes can have a dramatic effect on the stamina of a person accustomed to lowland living. It is best to gradually ascend to destinations higher than 6,000 feet.*

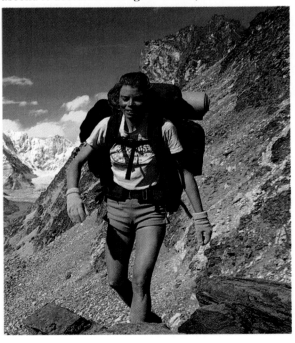

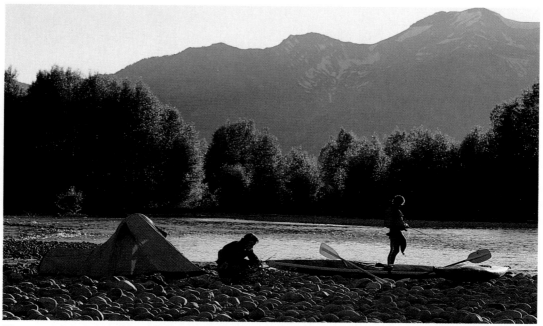

*Many people who fall ill abroad do so from drinking contaminated water. Even in the United States, people should be very wary of drinking from lakes and rivers, no matter how pristine they look.*

tating. When people fly across three or more time zones (east to west or vice versa), their body clock can have trouble adjusting to the local time in their destination. Symptoms include fatigue, insomnia, and irritability.

The best cure for jet lag is taking time to adjust. To help it along, Dardick says travelers should adjust immediately to the current time. "If it's breakfast time in that city, don't go to sleep." In addition, he says, "If you fly east, you should spend time outdoors in the morning sun, and if you fly west, you should spend time in the afternoon sun. Exposure to sunlight at the right time of day resets your internal clock."

Although numerous preventives or cures for jet lag have been touted, none have proved effective in scientific studies. Complex diets during the week prior to departure, various regimens of light therapy to reset your body clock gradually, and a multitude of other folk remedies are probably ineffective.

Dardick says ongoing, but not-yet-released, studies are showing that a pill form of melatonin helps the body's clock adjust to local time. This may be the jet-lag cure of the future, he says.

The best ways to reduce the symptoms of jet lag, according to Dardick, are to drink lots of water on the flight and to avoid consuming too much alcohol and coffee, which exacer-

bate the process of dehydration in your body. Water consumption increases urine production, which in turn forces you to walk about the aircraft. Dardick notes that "You will feel much better when you arrive if you've walked the aisles and stretched a few times during the flight."

The repeated and enduring motion of any moving vehicle, be it a car, ship, train, or airplane, can cause some people to feel nauseated, break out in a sweat, and sometimes vomit. Self-care includes keeping your head still to help the balance mechanism in the inner ear stabilize somewhat, closing your eyes, looking straight ahead when your eyes are open (looking at the horizon if you are on the deck of a ship), and not reading.

If you are prone to motion sickness, your doctor may prescribe one of several medications that prevent or help ease symptoms. According to Dardick, the leading choice is Transderm-Scop, a patch worn behind the ear that allows a motion-sickness drug to gradually pass through the skin.

To prevent altitude sickness, it is best to gradually ascend to destinations higher than 6,000 feet. Ideally, you should gain no more than 1,000 feet per day, and sleep at the intermediate levels. Flying directly to a city such as La Paz, Bolivia, which is at nearly 12,000 feet above sea level, makes a gradual adjustment impossible. As a rule, land-based travelers are better able than fliers to make such a gradual ascent.

Youth and physical fitness are no deterrent to altitude sickness. Depending on your planned rate of ascent, your doctor might recommend one of two drugs that help diminish your chances of getting altitude sickness. A high-carbohydrate diet can also help by stimulating breathing, which, in turn, increases your blood's oxygen level. Treatment of mild altitude sickness consists of resting for several days before ascending further. The more severe forms cause shortness of breath and a cough from fluid collecting in the lungs. Such cases require immediate, rapid descent to lower altitudes and medical attention.

### Precautions on Location

Once you reach your destination, two of the most important behaviors requiring modification are drinking and eating. Indeed, food and water are perhaps the most common means through which travelers acquire bacterial, viral, and parasitic diseases.

Unchlorinated tap water or water that originates in an area of substandard sanitation should not be ingested in any form. In other words, do not drink it directly, do not use it as ice to cool a drink, and do not brush your teeth with it. Drinks made with boiled water are safe, as are commercially bottled beer, wine, carbonated soft drinks, and carbonated water.

This set of instructions may sound simple enough, but there are all kinds of pitfalls that trap tourists. Do not drink bottled water that has not been opened in front of you. Sometimes bottles are saved from previous guests and refilled with tap water in the restaurant kitchen. If your drinking glass or beverage has come into contact with ice, removing the ice does not make that glass or drink safe, because bacteria can be transferred to the container or liquid at the instant of contact.

If you are staying in a first-class hotel, you may have easy access to bottled water. You may even find it supplied in your room for brushing your teeth. Other situations may make it necessary for you to sanitize your own water supply. There are various methods for accomplishing this. Boiling your water is the most reliable method for making it safe to drink. The water needs to simply reach a

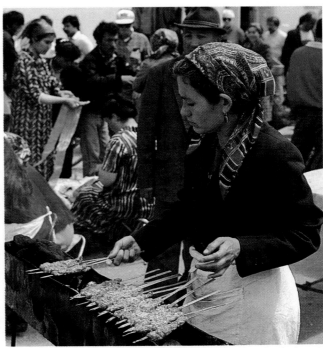

*Persons traveling to exotic locales may eat food that is cooked in unfamiliar ways or that comes from sources of questionable cleanliness. Prudent travelers always request their meat well-done.*

boil and then be allowed to cool (do not use unsanitary ice to hurry it along!). The taste of water that has been boiled can be improved by adding some salt or pouring it back and forth several times from one sanitary container to another in order to aerate it again.

A heat source is not always available, so certain situations may call for one of the two alternative methods of disinfection: filtering or chemical. Portable filters use either microfilters that can screen out parasites, larvae, and possibly bacteria, depending on the fineness of the filter. Dewart says that the

CDC does not recommend filters because there have been insufficient studies to verify their effectiveness.

Chemical disinfection can be accomplished with either iodine or chlorine (tablets or liquid). These commercial chemical products come with specific instructions regarding dosage and time required for disinfection to take place, requirements that vary according to the temperature and original condition of the water. If no other method of sanitation is possible, allowing water that is uncomfortably hot to the touch to cool to room temperature may suffice.

Eating requires the same rigorous attention as drinking. Never eat raw food or shellfish, including salads and uncooked vegetables. Eat only fruits that you peel yourself, such as bananas. Pass up unpasteurized milk and milk products, such as

Swimming in anything but a well-maintained, chlorinated pool is risky and should be avoided. Fresh- or saltwater bodies may be polluted with human sewage, animal feces, or urine, making it both unpleasant and potentially hazardous to your health. Do not be misled if the locals regularly swim there— they may have developed some immunity over the years. If you must swim in such water (if you are hiking, for example, and have to cross a deep stream), keep your head above water and your eyes closed to splashes, if at all possible.

Preventing insect bites is an integral part of disease prevention in tropical countries. As mentioned earlier, mosquitoes, flies, and various other insects are often vectors, or transmitters, of viral, parasitic, and bacterial diseases. A multipronged approach offers the best protection because any one method may

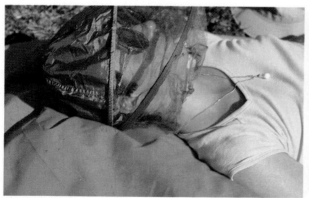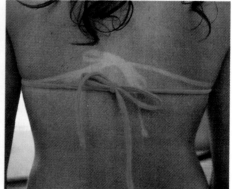

*Tropical climates introduce a host of potential problems. Campers are advised to use mosquito netting when they sleep (left); sunscreen is a must for all outdoor activities.*

cheese and ice cream. It is safe to eat food that has been *thoroughly* cooked and is still hot when it is served to you. If the food has sat at room temperature, say on a buffet, it may not be safe to eat, unless it is thoroughly reheated to kill any bacteria that may have proliferated on it. As with water, your best efforts to avoid unsafe foods can be thwarted. Watermelon seems to be a safe fruit because of its thick skin, which is not eaten. Some watermelons, however, are injected with water in order to increase their weight for market.

not be 100 percent effective. Keep in mind that certain insect species tend to feed, or bite, at certain times of the day. The *Anopheles* mosquito, which transmits malaria in Africa, for example, feeds from dusk to dawn, so remaining indoors at night is a first-course strategy.

Clothing and mosquito netting (at night) make formidable physical barriers to most insects. Wear loose clothes (insects can bite through thin, clinging material) and long-sleeve shirts tucked into long pants to reduce access to exposed skin. Further precautions, such as tucking pant legs into socks or ankle-high shoes, also help protect you from insect bites.

Some studies have shown that protective clothing combined with repellents can confer nearly 100 percent protection. Chemical repellents for skin and clothing should be used consistently. Spray or wipe a deet-based repellent on all exposed skin about every four hours, sooner after heavy sweating, swimming, or bathing.

Insect repellents come in various deet concentrations. The most widely recommended level is 30 percent. Higher concentrations may be toxic. Skin-So-Soft, a cosmetic lotion, and citronella, a plant essence, have reputations as effective alternatives to chemical repellents. However, such anecdotal reputations are scientifically unconfirmed. Considering the seriousness of malaria, yellow fever, and other insect-transmitted diseases, experts urge travelers to use the proven deet-based products.

Your clothing itself can help repel—and kill —biting insects if it has been treated in the wash or sprayed with a peremethrin solution. Peremethrin's repellent properties can last through several launderings. Mosquito nets should also be treated with a peremethrin product. In addition, unless your sleeping quarters are air-conditioned or tightly screened, you should spray the room with an insecticide before bedtime.

*The very young, the very old, and people with chronic illness are at the highest risk when traveling.*

The prevention of HIV and other sexually transmitted diseases (STDs) while abroad requires the same measures as in the United States. Infection with the HIV virus can occur in only a few ways: through sexual activity, blood contact (via blood transfusion, the use of contaminated needles for, say, drug use or tattooing, or the use of unsterilized dental tools), and birth from an infected mother. The best method of protection from HIV is avoiding high-risk behaviors. Abstain from sex unless both you and your partner have been recently tested for HIV and are monogamous. Refuse to use

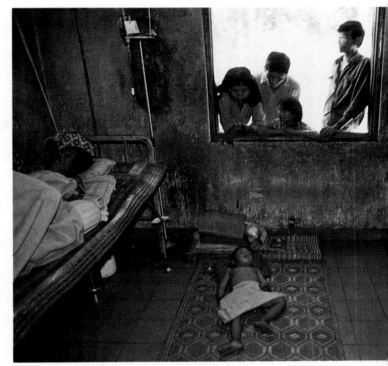

Health-care facilities in foreign lands frequently do not meet the standards of American hospitals and clinics. It may be wise to contact the nearest American embassy in case of severe illness.

or be treated with anything but sterilized dental tools, and unused, disposable needles. Avoid a blood transfusion in countries without adequate HIV-screening techniques, unless your life is in imminent danger.

Even though latex condoms are not 100 percent effective, the CDC recommends using them with partners whose status in regard to sexually transmitted disease is unknown. Remember, you cannot necessarily tell who has HIV or another STD by looking —or even asking. People with chlamydia, gonorrhea, venereal warts, hepatitis A, B, or C, genital herpes, syphilis, or HIV may be asymptomatic. People can be infected by the HIV virus for as long as five years before symptoms appear. Always use a latex condom; a diaphragm and spermicidal jelly may offer further protection, says the CDC.

If you should have any sort of health problem in the year after your return to the United States, be sure to see your doctor. Some of the more exotic diseases and infections may not occur to your doctor as a cause of your symptoms without adequate information about your trip.                                    ◇

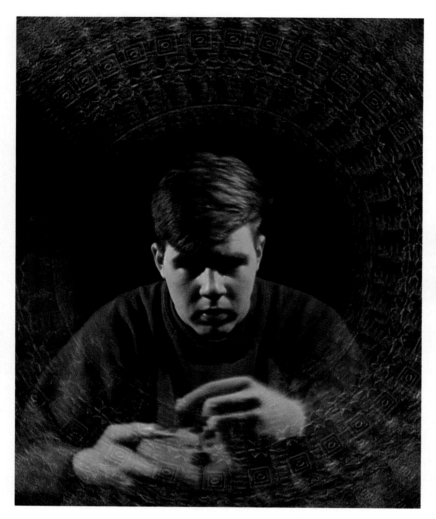

# VIDEO GAMES:
## *Victim or Villain?*

*by Joseph C. DeVito*

I t's 1:34 A.M. in John Farrell's apartment, but he's far from asleep. The room is dark and quiet save the music wafting from his compact-disc player and the tapping of his fingers on a Nintendo controller. His eyes focus dead ahead, heavy-lidded from lack of sleep, and yet somehow able to trace every movement on the television screen.

John isn't thinking of the bag of chips at his feet or how tired he'll be at school the next day. All he knows is that if the Pittsburgh Steelers are to make the play-offs in his Super Tecmo Bowl game, he's got to score a touchdown now. It may be another hour before he packs it in, but he'll retire satisfied—a champion.

Like millions of other Americans, John Farrell is a dedicated video-game player. But can this entertaining diversion turn into a dangerous obsession?

## Why Do People Play Video Games?
Like most devotees, John will tell you he likes video games because they're fun. "Playing a few games is a good way to pass time, especially when my friends are hanging out," John says. "Besides, it gives me a chance to be a pro-football star, something I could never do in real life." Like most expert players, John usually dominates the computer, unless, as he claims, "it cheats."

Jonathan Bloomberg, M.D., a psychiatrist specializing in child development at the Rockford Memorial Hospital in Rockford, Illinois, sees video games as a way players can empower themselves. "For kids, mastering a game gives a sense of control in an environment that's free of adults," Dr. Bloomberg says. "They see the results of their actions immediately on the screen, so there is instant gratification."

Children also like the repetition inherent in video games. "Who doesn't enjoy a second chance," Bloomberg asks, "to go back to a bad decision and do better?"

Players are attracted to computer graphics that can flash millions of colors in seconds, and to the intricate plotlines of games based on hit movies like *Aladdin, Home Alone,* and *Terminator 2.* Fans vary in age, although the core market is males between the ages of 10 and 20. Most enjoy the challenge of moving from level to level as their skills improve. Programmers realize this, and thus make the games captivating but not too frustrating.

### From the Game Room to the Living Room

Computer games have been around for almost 20 years, although few would recognize their low-tech ancestors. Pong, a game based on squash, tennis, and hockey, consisted of little more than black bars moved vertically to propel a small ball. Advances in programming brought improved graphics and innovative "joystick" hand controls. Soon arcades began replacing their pool tables and pinball machines with refrigerator-sized games that attracted players of all ages and a steady diet of quarters.

Colorful and full of beeps and whistles, hits such as Space Invaders and Asteroids let players fire rockets and lasers at an assortment of otherworldly enemies. Pac Man, a game in which a smiling yellow ball consumed energy dots and fluorescent ghosts, inspired "Pac Mania" T-shirts, a breakfast cereal, and even a novelty song, "Pac Man Fever."

Seizing on the video-game craze, Atari, Coleco, and others began marketing home systems that spawned a multibillion-dollar industry. The most popular home games are made by Nintendo, whose 1992 sales topped $4.7 billion. "The original Nintendo Entertainment System [NES] is still the least expensive model [$40 to $80], and the easiest to learn," says Perrin Kaplan, the corporate-communications manager for Nintendo.

There are an estimated 36 million 8-bit NES units in American households. The company has also introduced the 16-bit Super NES, a unit with improved sound and graphics, and is developing a 64-bit 3-D machine known as Project Reality.

Other systems include Sega Genesis and NEC's TurboGrafX, which offer improved sound and graphics, but cost more and have fewer games. Both have optional compact-disc attachments that contain several times the memory of traditional units and can be used with home audio/visual equipment. Several companies offer hand-held units that can play adapted versions of popular home and arcade games.

### Beyond Child's Play

Incredibly, some research has shown video games to be more than just high-tech toys. Because they improve hand-eye coordination, Chicago's Illinois College of Optometry and other hospitals use games to treat "lazy eye" and other vision problems in young people. The motor skills and visual response needed to play video games have helped in the rehabilitation of brain-trauma and stroke victims to stimulate impaired abilities. Game playing also has a positive mental-health impact on cancer patients, and has been effective in reducing side effects of chemotherapy.

In addition to dexterity, games can develop problem solving. Educational games like Hidden Agenda put the player in the role of president of a fictitious South American country, where he or she must decide foreign and domestic policy. Similar games with historical and environmental themes are far from the typical arcade fare, but share elements of strategic planning and logic skills.

Joe Cook, Jr., director of the Paige Academy in Roxbury, Massachusetts, uses 20 game systems installed at the private elementary school to see how, and what, children learn from game play. Studying those who are just developing their physical and social skills has uncovered extraordinary things.

*For some, video games are an entertaining diversion; for others, they are an obsession.*

"The games help younger children understand cause-and-effect relationships," Cook says. "At first, they must look at the control pad the whole time, and don't make the connection with what's occurring on the screen." When the children see how the combinations

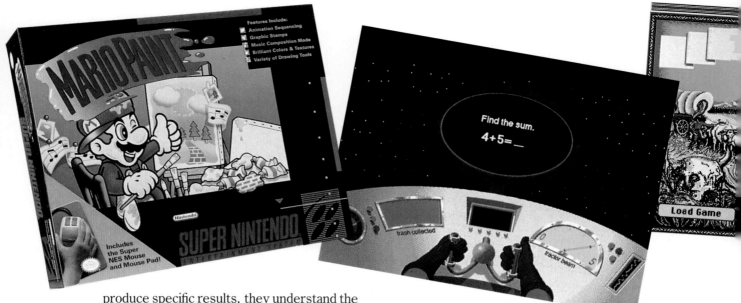

produce specific results, they understand the workings of controls in general.

Children soon realize that timing is important, as most game activities require responses that seize the moment. For those who are only beginning to understand the differences between "now," "before," and "later," playing improves their grasp of time and spatial relationships. Puzzle and search games foster development of planning and methodology. "The students responded well to games where they had to search for an object in different locations," Cook adds. "It was like being in a book where they were able to control the story line."

The Paige Academy has rules prohibiting toy guns and simulated gunplay on the playground, an attitude that carries over to the

*The stir that accompanied the release of "Mortal Kombat" (below) and other violent video games led manufacturers to self-impose a rating system on their products.*

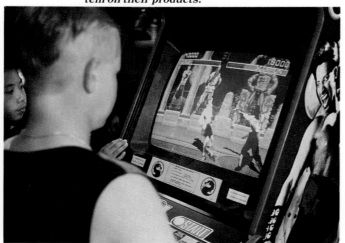

video games. "Games like Ninja Gaiden were helpful because they had many combinations, but our focus is on nonfighting games," Cook says. Nor are games that show women as the weaker sex tolerated. Even with this gentle approach, the courtesies and rules the children develop are surprising.

"They don't distract each other while they're playing, and offer advice on how to defeat the computer," Cook says. "The students share the secret codes and techniques they've learned to help each other overcome the difficult parts of the game." Sometimes the children make judgment calls, withholding the secrets from players who aren't advanced enough in their play, while others wish to figure out the tricks by themselves.

"Many teachers discredit video games, but they do fit with our changing ideas of what learning and education mean," Cook says. "It's an interactive method that genuinely interests the children, providing a good introduction to technology." In fact, some older Paige students delved into programming, creating games of their own. "There's also a good deal of related reading material the children dig into, such as manuals, instruction guides, and magazines," Cook adds.

Perrin Kaplan agrees. "In moderation, video games teach good coping skills, perseverance, and persistence to victory," she says. Nintendo is interested in how video games can be used to teach, and the company participates in numerous studies. Nintendo recently gave a $3 million grant to the Massachusetts Institute of Technology (MIT) to finance a study of how children learn.

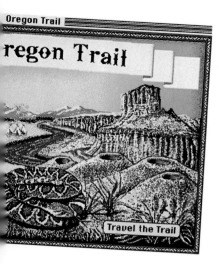

Oregon Trail

*For many children, video games help make learning fun. Art, math, and history are just a few of the subjects that are now approached in the video-game format.*

### When It's No Longer Fun and Games

Aside from sore eyes and fingertips, there are no physical afflictions caused by video games. The American Academy of Pediatrics does recommend that play be limited to no more than 1 to 2 hours each weekday. An exceedingly tiny segment of the population, however, suffers from a rare type of epilepsy known as photosensitivity, in which seizures can be triggered by flashing lights. Although fewer than 1 percent of epileptics suffer from this condition, game cartridges and systems list warnings in their operation manuals.

Controversy arises from the content of video games, which many consider to be too violent. Look into your local arcade, and you're likely to find Street Fighter, Lethal Enforcer, and Mortal Kombat as the most popular attractions. When Mortal Kombat flashes its "finish him" command, the victor can choose deadly martial-arts moves, electrocution, or a variety of other gruesome ways to annihilate an opponent. Mortal Kombat's programmers used sensors attached to a martial-arts expert, recording and digitizing his motions so they could be faithfully re-created on-screen. While teenagers and adults may recognize this as fantasy, what about younger players?

Judy Primavera, Ph.D., a professor of psychology at Fairfield University in Fairfield, Connecticut, sees repeated exposure to games that reward violent behavior as numbing. "There are no cookbook answers," she cautions, "but the studies seem to echo what we've seen with television. Repeated exposure to violence desensitizes children, and reinforces a value system that has violence as the preferred response."

Primavera claims that children who live with violence in their schools, neighborhoods, and families are especially at risk. "The normal stopgaps in people that keep anger from exploding into rage might not exist in kids that grow up in fear," she says. "By combining TV's realism with an interactive component, it's as close as you can get without actually doing it."

"Games like Mortal Kombat can harm younger children because they haven't developed an understanding of the world," says Parker Page, founder of the Children's Television Resource and Education Center and author of *Helping Children Survive Video Games*. His organization translates the clinical data from studies into programs that parents can implement and understand.

"In moderation, there's nothing wrong with game playing per se," Page says. "But parents must be aware of the lessons the games teach."

Psychologists are concerned, but the studies alone are inconclusive. Although a 1989 report by the National Coalition on Television Violence classified 80 percent of video games as portraying harmful violence, there is no clinical study that finds an absolutely definitive link between video games and any type of negative behavior.

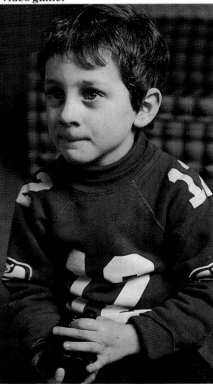

*Many parents become alarmed when they see their child transfixed by a video game.*

Dorothy Singer, Ph.D., a psychologist with the Yale University Family and TV Research Center in New Haven, Connecticut, agrees that while the research is important, it is rather difficult to interpret. "The problem with studies is that it is very hard to separate video-game players from TV viewers, who often comprise the same audience," she says. "Studies have indicated an increase in aggressive behavior in watchers of action-oriented programs, but it's hard to find a pure sample of game players who don't also view these shows."

Proponents argue that aggression alone is not always a negative, and aggressive behavior is, in fact, a necessary component of competition. Game players may become more aroused because of the stimulation the games provide. A 1981 study pointed out that since children manifest their aggression against objects in a game instead of each other, they are "simply playing."

Because parents are growing ever more concerned, Nintendo has produced a guide titled "Everything You Always Wanted to Know About Video Games . . . But Were Afraid to Ask Your Kids." The colorful pamphlet offers parents advice on regulating playtime, using games as a reward for chores and homework, and the importance of discussing how the games work and their content with your children. Also listed in the guide is Nintendo's self-regulating code, which prohibits, among other things, sexually suggestive or

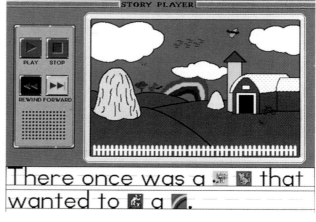

*The "Kids Keys" game (below) helps familiarize children with the alphabet. "Kid Works 2" (above) encourages youngsters to write their own stories. Video games have also proved to be a valuable tool for special-education teachers (left).*

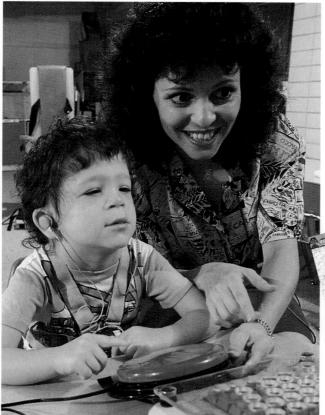

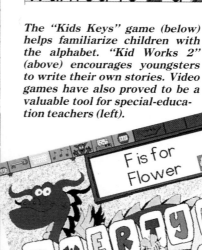

explicit content, excessive violence, negative stereotypes, or references to cigarette smoking, drugs, or alcohol.

Now that the notorious Mortal Kombat game is available to home audiences, manufacturers are struggling to meet the fans' expectations without incurring the wrath of advocacy groups. The game's violence is cartoonish but extreme: Heads explode, blood flies freely, and losers can be decapitated or impaled upon a bed of stakes. The home versions quickly sold out, thanks in part to a $100 million marketing plan that utilized movie trailers, giveaways, and TV commercials depicting swelling crowds of teenagers chanting "Mortal Kombat!" in the streets.

The Sega home cartridge carries the MA-13 rating, labeling the game as appropriate for those 13 or older. A secret code must be entered to access the blood and lethal moves of the arcade version, but is easily obtained through retailers, other players, and game-advice telephone services. The Nintendo version does not contain the more violent moves or graphic death scenes.

"There's a struggle in the industry between moral responsibility and profits because the manufacturers know violent games are still the big sellers," says Page. "But the most important influences on a child's life and values are still the parents, and the research is clear on that."

### For Fans, the Play's the Thing

Your local arcade may provide a different perspective. Sheena Muscato, a manager at Time Out, a game arcade in a suburban Connecticut mall, puts little stock in concerns over violence. Time Out's games range from the mild (the Simpsons and Wacky Gator) to the wild (Lethal Enforcer and Fatal Fury) and, of course, Mortal Kombat.

Speaking with the world-weariness of a 19-year-old who dispenses quarters to the masses, Sheena believes "those complaints are stupid. You see a lot more dangerous things on TV, and those are real."

Chuck Krausz, age 22, likes Mortal Kombat's realistic graphics, but doesn't believe that the games affect the players. "You could win a game of Monopoly," he says, "but that doesn't mean you've got $8 million." His slight build exaggerated by baggy clothes, Chuck hardly resembles a thug. He remains calm and collected, even as his character, Rayden, launches lightning bolts at his opponent's skull.

"It's fun to see what different moves you can do," Chuck says over the game's electronic whoops and war cries. "I guess there are better things I could do with my time, but I could also be out doing drugs," he adds. "I'd say this is somewhere in between."

Keith Leniart, age 18, heads for the video-game arcade several days a week. "It took about $40 before I could beat the computer, but now I'm good enough to get respect in most arcades," he says proudly. Despite his aptitude with the character Kano (finishing move: tears beating heart from chest), Keith's appearance is also more beatnik than roughneck. While he relishes the fighting technique of the game, he has no interest in learning martial arts. "That has nothing to do with playing the game," he insists.

"The regulars for the martial-arts games are 'new wavers,'" says Sheena, gesturing toward the shaggy heads surrounding the game, "and most of them are vegetarians." She looks around again. "If they don't eat animals, how violent can they be?"

Like the students at Paige Academy, the competitors at Time Out have developed their own code of chivalry. Some moves, while allowed by the computer, are considered inappropriate. They are often unspoken, even though players often compete against total strangers.

In one game the throwing of chairs is frowned upon. "Sometimes you'll throw one by mistake," Chuck says, "so you let the guy you're playing get a free shot to make up for it." While some players will have a tantrum when they lose, Muscato reports that she has never seen a fight in the arcade.

Perhaps Keith offers the most telling commentary on video games, violence, and the competitive spirit. "If you beat someone really bad, don't rub it in," he cautions, "especially if he's bigger than you." ◇

*For some kids, mastering a video game gives them a sense of control in a world free of adults.*

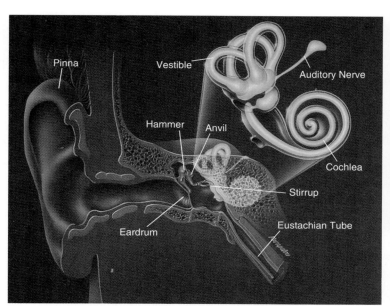

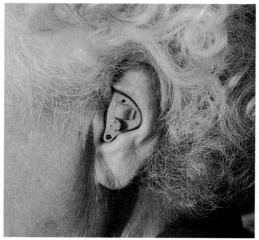

*The structure of the ear allows us to hear. For the hard of hearing, hearing aids can help amplify sounds. The degree of hearing loss determines whether the hearing aid is worn internally or externally.*

# HEARING ENHANCEMENT

*by Donald Cunningham*

More than 25 million Americans suffer some sort of hearing loss, from slight impairment attendant upon early aging to profound deafness caused by a variety of factors. Eighty percent of these cases of hearing loss represent permanent and irreversible damage. Yet in most instances—including many of the 2 million Americans who are profoundly deaf—impaired hearing can be enhanced with devices or surgery.

Many of the hearing-impaired do not take advantage of measures for enhancement, often citing vanity, cost, and inadequacies of the technologies as the reasons. This picture may change soon, especially now that rapid improvements in hearing-enhancement technologies and strategies are emerging.

And just in time. Americans are, on average, getting older. A large segment of the population is heading into the later years, when hearing impairment becomes common. As early as the mid-fifties, age-related hearing problems can begin. By age 65, more than one-third of Americans suffer from some degree of hearing impairment. That figure rises to a formidable 50 percent for Americans who are 85 years old.

Strategies for combating hearing loss include personal electronic devices that amplify sound (hearing aids); speech processors connected to implanted electrodes, which bring stimuli to the inner ear (cochlear implants); surgery to correct problems within the ear; and external amplification devices. Researchers have made improvements in all areas.

### Hearing Aids

Hearing aids are devices that shape and amplify sound waves before they pass into the inner ear. These devices have traditionally bolstered the hearing of people whose ears have lost some of their ability to conduct sounds. Today sensitive and powerful hearing aids benefit people with milder hearing loss as well as those with more profound loss associated with neural pathways.

In normal hearing, sound waves enter the ear and hit the eardrum, which conducts the sound through the middle ear by small, oscillating bones. The bones transmit vibrations to the cochlear fluid of the inner ear. This moving fluid stimulates the series of fine hairs lining the cochlea; these hairs in turn stimulate nerves that send messages to the brain. Over the years, accumulating damage to the cochlear hairs causes gradual hearing loss. Today's powerful hearing aids can stimulate the remaining intact hairs of the cochlea.

Older, analog hearing aids continue to be big sellers. They use continuous electronic signals that change in ways that imitate the sound-pressure waves approaching the ear, and then create amplified versions of the original sounds. Analog devices now come in improved versions containing digital chips that better control parts of the operation. One new aid has a computer chip that causes faint sounds to be amplified more than loud sounds. It can conceivably help people whose ability to hear faint sounds has diminished, yet whose ability to hear loud sounds has remained intact.

A stubborn problem with analog hearing aids is the difficulty—or impossibility—of fine-tuning their operations to the user's personal characteristics and to the sound experience. This problem is compounded by the fact that an electronic circuit that amplifies speech but not noise has yet to be invented.

New digital hearing aids represent an improvement on their analog counterparts. These devices convert sound pulses to digital information that can more easily be tuned or programmed before sending pulses into the ear. Users can potentially adjust the aids to respond to certain frequencies, volumes, noises, etc. But there are drawbacks. Digital hearing aids are expensive (up to $3,000), require more power to operate, and are larger and bulkier. Their improved performance has yet to be demonstrated fully.

New programming aspects of hearing aids include multiband control, in which the spectrum of sound is broken into segments, and those segments are processed individually and sent to the ear. Users have sensitivities to certain loudnesses, frequencies, and combinations of the two. Multiband processing helps to equalize different portions of the complex spectrum of speech so that the listener receives smoother, more-understandable sounds. A problem with multiband processing is that it necessarily excludes many of the details of speech.

About 20 percent of users, especially children, wear behind-the-ear hearing aids, which feed sound into the ear through a small tube. More popular are in-the-ear hearing aids, which sit in the opening to the ear. Thanks to advances in molding technology, in-the-ear aids can now block extraneous noise more efficiently. A third form of hearing aid, in-the-canal, is further miniaturized so that it can sit in the ear canal. Although it is more aesthetically pleasing, the in-the-canal hearing aid is difficult to service because of its size.

*In most cases, impaired hearing can be effectively enhanced with electronic devices or surgery.*

## Cochlear Implants

For severely deaf people, for whom hearing aids yield no significant improvement, cochlear implants offer hope. Implants do not restore normal hearing, nor do they approximate normal hearing. Instead, they produce, in response to sounds, neural stimuli in the inner ear that users can learn to interpret as a new hearing vocabulary.

With an implant a formerly deaf person can suddenly hear environmental sounds such as ringing telephones and running water. With recent advances, such as multichannels and improved processing, implants are even leading to some recognition of speech. This is especially important for children born deaf because speech recognition affects their ability to speak and learn.

The first cochlear implant was developed in the 1960s. Mostly because of high cost and strict qualifications for recipients (who must

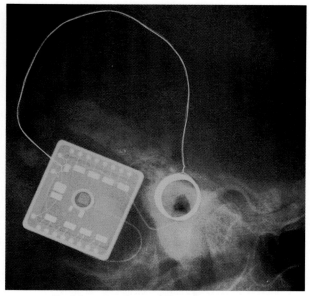

*Cochlear implants (X ray above, embedded in the ear) produce, in response to sound, neural stimuli in the inner ear that users can use to interpret as a new hearing vocabulary.*

demonstrate a potential to benefit from an implant more than from a hearing aid), the number of implants in use has grown only very slowly. Today in the United States, fewer than 3,000 people have received cochlear implants. Yet hundreds of thousands of adults and children are potential candidates for implants.

A cochlear implant comprises three components: a fine metal electrode, which is surgically inserted into the spiral-shaped cochlea of the inner ear; a processor/synthesizer of speech and sounds, which is usually worn on a belt or other clothing; and connectors—wires, plugs, receivers—between the two pieces of hardware. Recent advances include longer electrodes that can stimulate cochlear nerves in complex ways, and flexible sound processors that filter desired aspects of sounds before sending them to the electrode.

An example of an early version of a cochlear implant is the House device. Approved by the Food and Drug Administration (FDA) in 1984, it is now used by about 1,000 people, but is no longer prescribed. The House device has a 6-millimeter electrode that is inserted into the cochlea. A single channel of sound sent by radio waves from a processor to the electrode stimulates a small number of nerves feeding the cochlea.

Examples of an improved generation of implants are the Nucleus device, with a 25-milli-meter electrode, approved in 1985, and the Ineraid device, with a 22-millimeter electrode, approved in 1989. The former is used by about 1,300 people; the latter, by fewer than 200 adults thus far. The digital speech processors of these two devices perform what is called "feature extraction," filtering desired aspects of speech and environmental sounds. These devices also use four separate sound channels, allowing for stimulation of cochlear nerves in helpful patterns along the longer electrodes.

New advances in the processors yield wider ranges of pitch and loudness, reduced noise, and overall better sound. Users can replace old processors with new, improved models without having to replace implanted electrodes. One new device, which won FDA approval for use in children aged 2 through 17 in 1990, features 22 sound channels.

Although the trend is toward the use of many channels in order to process complexities of sound, especially speech, multichannel devices are bulky and expensive. Single-channel devices have the virtues of small size, lower power requirements, and lower cost. For such reasons a new single-channel implant that improves on the sound of older single-channel devices has been developed and awaits FDA approval. This device is small enough to be worn entirely on the head.

Cochlear implants strongly enhance a user's ability to read lips. The latest implants allow the user to recognize some words, especially when they are parts of sentences. As a result, some users can communicate with familiar callers on the telephone. This involves having the implant user query the caller with questions that elicit simple responses—for example, yes and no.

Cochlear implants can revolutionize the lives of people who lack the ability to hear. But the small number of devices implanted so far is testimony to the downside of the technology. In addition to high cost, other negative aspects include: (1) problems and side effects of surgery—for example, damage to nearby nerves; (2) malfunctioning of the implant; (3) extensive adjustment and therapy required to attain optimal use of the device; and (4) the inability of the implant to provide real hearing.

## Other Types of Correction and Assistance

At this point, damaged fine hairs of the inner ear cannot be repaired or replaced, making hearing aids and implants necessary. But the middle ear is a different story. The tiny bones of the middle ear, which transmit sounds to the inner ear, often are damaged by infection, tumors, and physical trauma. Because of the accessibility of the middle ear, surgery to insert artificial bones or transplant healthy bones is straightforward and now routine.

Another category of hearing enhancement comprises what are known as assistive listening devices—external devices and strategies that work alone or in conjunction with

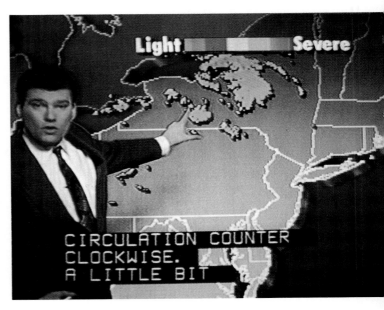

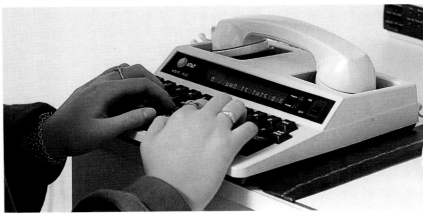

*Deaf people have benefited from new technology that compensates for their hearing loss. Closed captioning (above) allows the hearing-impaired to better follow a television broadcast. Profoundly deaf people can use special communication devices (left) to transmit messages over telephone lines.*

hearing aids. Perhaps most familiar is television captioning. Closed captioning refers to captioned text of televised dialogue that is transmitted along with the entire television program, and which appears on the screen only with the aid of a decoding device. Today some 500 hours of weekly televised programming contains closed captioning. The Television Decoder Circuitry Act of 1990 mandated that, by 1993 all television sets 13-inches and larger sold in the United States have a built-in decoder. Captioning also is available on many prerecorded videos, such as rental movies and educational tapes.

Infrared and FM waves are now used in different systems that deliver amplified sound to earphones or hearing aids of listeners in concert halls, theaters, and lecture halls. A simpler, hard-wired device consisting of microphone, amplifier, and earphone, can be used in cars or the home.

New videophones allow the hearing-impaired to exploit lipreading to communicate over telephone lines. Profoundly deaf people can also use the Telecommunications Device for the Deaf (TDD), which transmits messages over special telephone lines.

Advancements in assistive devices and technologies are ongoing. Hearing aids and implants are continuing to develop better sound with less noise. Telephones and other external amplification devices continue to be more user-friendly for the hearing-impaired. In the future, surgery or chemical therapies might lead to the replacement of damaged cochlear hair cells. Such advances ensure that the hearing-impaired will continue to move into the world of normal hearing.    ◇

# SEXUAL HARASSMENT: What is the Law?

*by Marcy O'Koon*

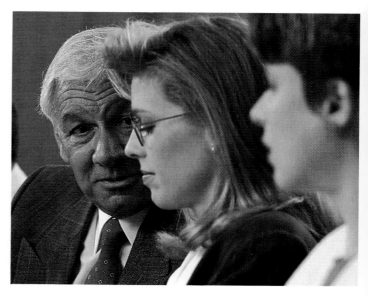

Though few people *support* sexual harassment, there are plenty who do not understand the prohibitions against it. They believe that nowadays a man cannot compliment a female coworker on her appearance, and that dating a coworker has become a federal offense.

That's not true, says Renee Evridge, director of 9 to 5's National Job Problem Hotline in Cleveland, Ohio. "No one ever called our hot line and said, 'I'm being harassed. My boss said he liked my new haircut.' A compliment makes you feel good about yourself; harassment doesn't," she says.

"Now, if that boss loads his comment with innuendo, telling you that you look hot or sexy, or backs you physically into a corner and whispers it to you, that sounds like harassment, not a compliment," says Evridge. The law does not address consensual relationships between coworkers. Maybe it is against company policy, but that's not sexual harassment, she explains.

"When you have a group of people working together for some time, there's bound to be some sexual banter. If everyone is comfortable with it, that's fine," says Evridge. Harassment begins when someone becomes uncomfortable, which is usually the harasser's intention.

Harassment's underlying purpose is almost always power, not passion, says gender-studies specialist Susan Marshall, associate professor of sociology at the University of Texas in Austin. While some cases of harassment involve obsessed Romeos, like the case of a man who would not quit writing bizarre love letters to his coworker, most sexual harassment has very little to do with romance.

## Legal Landmarks

Although it's a good bet that gender-based on-the-job harassment has been going on since ancient times, the legal concept is quite young. Congress passed the Civil Rights Act of 1964 and Title VII of the Act laid the groundwork for prosecution of sexual harassment by making it illegal to discriminate against a person on the basis of sex, race, religion, or national origin.

A number of cases of sex discrimination (the term "sexual harassment" was not coined until 1975) had been tried and lost in the early 1970s. But in 1976 a court ruled for the first time in favor of a sexual-harassment plaintiff. The court agreed that a woman had been discriminated against when her boss fired her for rejecting his sexual advances.

In 1980 the Equal Employment Opportunity Commission (EEOC), the federal agency created to enforce Title VII, formally issued guidelines concerning sexual harassment to clarify the law as it had developed.

While sexual-harassment claims are based on Title VII, the legal definition and understanding of sexual harassment consists of the decisions that have been made on a case-by-case basis in the courts. In each case a judge makes an interpretation of the intent of Title VII, building upon precedents set in other court decisions and applying them to the circumstances of this one. And, of course, higher courts can overturn the decisions of lower courts, changing the precedent and thus the direction of the law.

So in 1986, when the Supreme Court heard *Meritor Savings Bank v. Vinson,* a landmark was set. Bank employee Mechelle Vinson claimed that over a three-year period, her supervisor, Sidney Taylor, groped her in front of other employees, followed her into the ladies' room, exposed himself to her, and on several occasions raped her in the bank's vault. Vinson lost in a federal district court when the judge concluded that her relationship with Taylor was voluntary and that the problems between them were personal. The appeals court overturned that ruling, saying that the "hostile environment" at work caused her to submit to her supervisor's assaults. The Supreme Court agreed.

This "hostile environment" ruling established a second type of sexual harassment. The first, and less common type, is *quid pro quo,* a Latin term meaning "this for that." In a *quid pro quo* case, the boss offers an employee something such as a raise or a promotion or the right to keep a job in return for a sexual favor.

In November 1993, Supreme Court Justice Sandra Day O'Connor, writing the majority opinion, said that a person does not have to have a nervous breakdown before gaining the protection of federal law. In this case, Teresa Harris, a manager at a truck-leasing company, endured two years' worth of gender-demeaning comments from her boss. In addition, her boss, Charles Hardy, would drop objects on the floor and ask her to pick them up, he would ask her to fish coins from his front pocket, and he once asked her, in front of other employees, if she had slept with someone to get a new account. As a result, Harris resigned.

The appeals court decided that Hardy's comments and actions were not enough to "seriously affect" Harris's "psychological well-being." Directing the appeals court to reconsider the case, the Supreme Court not only reaffirmed the 1986 hostile-environment ruling, but added that a victim does not have to experience "severe psychological injury" in order to have a case.

### Taking Action

Women like Teresa Harris (or men, because they, too, can be victims of sexual harass-ment) usually deal with each incident as if the problem—or the harasser—were going to disappear tomorrow. But these situations can worsen, and preparing now for the worst-case scenario is wise.

Whether you simply want the harassment to stop or are considering filing a lawsuit, the steps you should take are the same. How far you have to go to find resolution depends on what happens at each stage of the process.

1. Confront your harasser. Sometimes the simplest way to end the harassment is to tell the perpetrator to stop it. An important criterion in the EEOC guidelines and in the relevant case law is that the physical or verbal abuse be unwelcome. If someone's behavior or comments are unwelcome and offensive to you, let the person know in direct terms: "I do not want to hear about your private sexual escapades," or, "Please do not touch me."

2. Put the message in writing. If a simple "please stop" does not bring the result you desire, write a letter reiterating the fact that the behavior is unwelcome, and keep a copy of the letter for yourself. Evridge suggests sending a certified letter and saving the receipt, so there can be no doubt later that the person received it.

3. Talk to someone. Discussing the situation with a friend can not only provide you with moral support, it can be helpful if later you need to provide witnesses in court.

4. Keep a log. Early on, begin keeping notes detailing what has happened, when it happened, where it happened, your response, who saw or heard the incident, whom you told about it and what you said. Do this for each and every encounter.

Evridge says that victims who have tape-recorded encounters with the harasser have had an easier time winning their cases. They have used microcassette recorders and hidden them in their purses or pockets, or clipped them to their waist.

5. Keep records. If your job might be in jeopardy, keep a work diary to establish that you have done your job competently. Also keep copies of work evaluations, and record positive comments received from supervisors, coworkers, and clients.

6. Initiate a formal complaint within the company. If harassment continues, you may

need to look inside the company for help. This may mean going to your supervisor (not if he or she is the harasser, of course) or to someone in the human-resources department. Many companies now have sexual-harassment policies and procedures that you can use to guide you.

## The Accused

Unless the alleged harasser finds his or her own attorney, there is no one watching out for the rights of the accused, says Betsy Plevan, a New York City attorney and partner with Proskauer, Rose, Goetz, & Mendelsohn who handles employment litigation.

If the employer determines, for example, that a supervisor was indeed sexually harassing an employee, that supervisor may be fired. In less extreme situations, the harasser may simply receive a warning, be demoted, or be transferred to another office.

The company's management does the investigating and determines how the situation will be resolved. Because the employer is ultimately liable if the case goes to court, and because the employer risks bad publicity and a lot of expense, the internal investigators must act on its behalf, rather than on the behalf of the accused. In court the employer has to prove that it responded appropriately to the complaint and that it attempted to remedy the situation, or else it will be held accountable.

The accused should be allowed to tell his or her side of the story, says Plevan. The alleged harasser may say the accuser is lying. The accused may claim ignorance as to the offensive nature of his or her behavior, apologize, and promise never to do it again. Or the accused may deny everything.

Plevan advises people who are accused to cooperate with the investigative process. If you are guilty, she says, your best bet may be to resign.

7. Go to the EEOC or your state human-rights agency. If the company fails to resolve the situation to your satisfaction, you may opt to seek a solution outside. If there are fewer than 15 employees in the company, your legal remedy will be found through your state's fair-employment laws and/or through a civil case in the courts. The local field offices of the EEOC handle cases when there are 15 or more employees.

### Do You Have a Case?

When you are being sexually harassed, you know it. You do not have to consult any authority for confirmation. If you are seeking a legal remedy, however, you have to abide by legal definitions and restrictions.

The EEOC definition reads: unwelcome sexual advances, requests for sexual favors, and other verbal or physical conduct of a sexual nature constitute sexual harassment when submission to or rejection of this conduct explicitly or implicitly affects an individual's employment; unreasonably interferes with an individual's work performance; or creates an intimidating, hostile, or offensive work environment.

Keep in mind that in a *quid pro quo* case, one instance can be deemed sexual harassment, but in a hostile-environment case, the harassment must be ongoing.

Because both state laws and the EEOC have limitations on how long a person can wait before filing a claim, you should act promptly to first end the harassment, and later, if necessary, to file a formal charge. The EEOC requires the claim be filed within 180 days of the harassment, or within 300 days if you have first filed a state claim.

After an EEOC investigation, the plaintiff receives a right-to-sue letter. This letter may say that there is or is not a case; however, it gives you the right to pursue further action, if you wish, through the civil-court system with your own attorney.

No one can go straight to court with a sexual-harassment case without first going through a state agency or the EEOC. Evridge says these agencies are set up to weed out ineligible cases and arbitrate settlements for eligible cases, taking most of the burden off the overcrowded court system. ◇

# The Essence of Color "Blindness"

*by Gode Davis*

One Easter Sunday when he was 6, Nathan Bryant, now 25, participated with several other children in a penny hunt, searching for copper pennies against a brown dirt background. "Adults scattered pennies everywhere in a small, concentrated area. All the other kids found bagfuls. I found just a single penny, when someone dropped it, and had to be consoled by my parents. 'You'll find more next time,' they said, but I never would," he recalls.

The next year, Bryant discovered why. "We had a color-guessing exam at school, with colors buried in a jumble of gray dots to form numbers. I couldn't distinguish red, green, purple, or blue."

Due to a genetic defect passed on to him from his carrier mother, Bryant and his two brothers (but *not* his sister) inherited the most common form of color blindness, or, more accurately, color-vision deficiency: the inability to distinguish red, green, purple-violet, or some combination of these colors. Usually inherited but occasionally acquired, red-green and blue-yellow color deficiencies affect approximately 8 percent of the world's males and perhaps 1 in 200 women; as few as 1 in 100,000 persons are actually color-blind, able to perceive only black-and-white and perhaps a few hues of gray.

Showing an artistic bent early, Bryant tended to color the sky brown or a horse green. Selecting his own clothes by age 14, "I'd look for a blue shirt and come home with a pink one," Bryant says. Sometimes he'd be the butt of parlor games. "They'd ask me to name colors, then laugh at my answers," recalls Bryant. He describes "hell" for a color-blind person as "having to sort a giant basket of mismatched dark-colored socks." He can never tell when he's sunburned. "I think I'm getting a great tan," Bryant says.

Leon Ward, 68, confuses greens and browns. But he can still distinguish between two colors if one has a high-density pigmentation. As a result, Ward wasn't aware of his color-vision deficiency as a child. As a young adult, he discovered his visual weakness while working with litmus paper in a university chemistry lab. "I couldn't tell what the green litmus paper changed to; in fact, I couldn't even tell if it was green in the first place," says Ward. A Korean War "desk-job" veteran, Ward's color-vision weakness had shut him out of the Army Rangers and the Marines, his preferred military options, because "I couldn't pick out camouflaged G.I.'s, or even see the camouflage," Ward says.

*Color-vision deficiency can often be diagnosed through special visual tests. For example, in the circles at left and below, people with normal color vision can see the numbers 32 and 63; those with red-green blindness see no numbers at all.*

According to Anthony Adams, O.D., Ph.D., a professor and dean at the University of California School of Optometry in Berkeley, and world-renowned authority on color-vision deficiencies, all color-vision weaknesses can be traced to how the human eye perceives the visible-light spectrum.

## Life Without Color: Monochromatic Vision

Some people, called monochromats, are totally color-blind. Lacking cone receptors—or at least functioning ones—monochromats find different segments of the visible-light spectrum indistinguishable—probably seeing only in black and white and a few gray shades. Fortunately, the defect is extremely rare, affecting somewhere between 1 in 40,000 and 1 in 100,000 persons of either sex in virtually identical proportions.

"Vision specialists know they see in monotones, but we're unsure how colors actually appear to them," says Anthony Adams, O.D., Ph.D., at the University of California School of Optometry in Berkeley. Because our eyes' cone receptors produce a day vision and sharp vision as well as color vision, most persons with monochromatic vision can be blinded by daylight, and must wear dark glasses to distinguish objects outdoors in the daytime; the world perceived by most monochromats tends to be a fuzzy place in which objects can't be seen clearly, lacking focus and details.

While the origin of most monochromatic vision is congenital, in a few cases the defect can be caused by vascular accidents such as hemorrhages or other direct traumas to the brain. In these extraordinarily rare cases, enough cone receptors may survive intact for the monochromat to perceive a colorless world in sharp focus—a most unusual visual phenomenon.

### Newton's Spectrum

In 1660 Sir Isaac Newton passed a beam of sunlight through a prism and discovered that the refracted light fans out into the colors we now refer to as the visible spectrum: red, orange, yellow, green, blue, indigo, and violet (purple). Although most people share a common appreciation for the mixtures of light along the spectrum we call "colors," some suffer from a reduced sensitivity to various segments of the color spectrum.

In the normal eye, light stimulates special light-sensitive cells in the retina called rods and cones. The rod receptors are crucial for night vision, but their contribution to color vision is negligible. The cone cells, however, are divided into three classes. Each class is sensitive to different parts of the visible spectrum, and a specific light wavelength will induce a unique pattern of response from the cone cells. When light hits the cone cell, it causes a structural change in pigment contained within the cone, which in turn causes the cone to emit an electrical impulse that is sent to the brain. As these signals from the three classes of cone cells are transmitted, they are blended so that the brain perceives all the colors of the spectrum.

Most cases of color-vision deficiency are caused by an inherited defect of one or more classes of cone cells, or an abnormality or reduced number of cone cells.

"The result of a missing or impaired cone-receptor type is a reduced version of the colored world, making some colors appear different to normal-sighted persons while appearing the same to someone who is color-deficient," says Adams.

People with normal color vision are trichromats, able to utilize three primary colors—red, green, and blue (or violet)—in matching all the colors on the visible-light spectrum. Persons with a mild to moderate reduction in red- or green-color sensitivity also use three colors to match a given color, but the proportions they perceive tend to vary from the norm. Thus, a subject with a decreased sensitivity to red will require more red in the "mix" to match a given color.

While Ward could be a borderline trichromat actually matching inadequate amounts of green, he's more likely a "green-weak" dichromat—utilizing only two primary colors to match all the hues in the color spectrum. (Bryant is almost certainly a "red-weak" dichromat.) As a rule, dichromats experience confusion of reds, browns, olives, and golds; pastel pinks, oranges, yellows, and greens will look similar; and purples are confused with blues. "When I wore olive-drab fatigues in the Army, I didn't realize *what* color they were," says Ward. Despite their difficulty in distinguishing colors, even severely affected dichromats tend to be normal in other aspects of their vision.

People utilizing only a single primary color to match the hues of the color spectrum are called monochromats. Because they lack functioning cone-type receptors and are able to perceive only black and white and shades of gray, these persons are genuinely color-blind, and often are afflicted with other eye disorders, such as light oversensitivity; rapid, involuntary movements of the eyeball; and low visual acuity.

### Inherited or Acquired?
Most color-vision defects are sex-linked genetic disorders. Constant in type and severity during a person's life, they are passed on primarily to male offspring through the defective recessive gene of the mother.

"The trait has occurred to the males in our family for five generations," says Bryant.

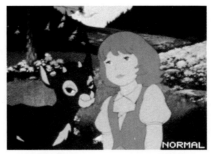
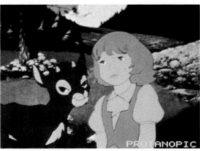
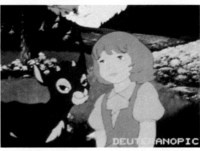
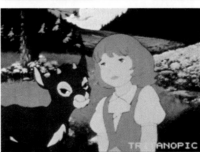

*The top image shows what a person with normal color vision perceives. The other images show how people with various types of color-vision deficiency perceive the same scene. A protanopic person is said to be "red-blind"; a deuteranopic person is said to be "green-blind"; and a tritanopic person is said to be "violet-blind."*

Inherited color-vision deficiency can occur as a consequence of several genetic combinations. Females have two X chromosomes, so if they inherit one affected X, the normal one dominates, and they will have normal color vision, but will become carriers of the defect. A male, however, has a Y chromosome inherited from his father and an X inherited from his mother. If the inherited X chromosome is affected, the boy will be color-vision-deficient. A carrier mother has a 50 percent chance of passing her defective X chromosome to each child; the boys receiving the affected X will be color-vision-deficient, and the girls will be carriers. An affected father's son will have normal color vision, since he passes the Y chromosome to a son, and all of his daughters will be carriers, since they receive their father's affected X chromosome. Carriers reported to have mild symptoms comprise the majority of the women who have color-vision deficiency; otherwise a female needs to inherit an affected X from each parent to get the congenital defect.

In less frequent instances when the brain itself or cone receptors in the retina are damaged due to accident or disease, color vision can also be adversely altered in normal-sighted persons. Such acquired losses affect the sexes equally, but comprise fewer than 10 percent of all color-vision-deficiency cases. Acquired color-vision defects may be of the red-green or blue-yellow varieties, the latter being more frequent. The defect may also be mixed (i.e., red-green- *and* blue-yellow-weak). While inherited color-vision deficiencies affect both eyes equally, acquired color-perception losses may affect just one eye, or affect one eye more than the other.

When this atypical color-loss condition is diagnosed, it can indicate a more serious condition. In 1987, for example, at Kent County Memorial Hospital in Warwick, Rhode Island, a kindergarten-aged outpatient was examined by an ophthalmologist. Found to have normal color vision in the right eye and defective color vision in the left, he was subsequently referred to a neurologist, and then to a neurosurgeon for removal of a tumor at the base of the pituitary gland.

### Color-Smart Traffic Lights

In 1931 the International Commission on Illumination adopted standards for signal lights to aid color-vision-deficient persons in distinguishing the red from the green light other than by position. Green traffic lights around the world have been implanted with a subordinated blue color, and red lights may have some orange overtones.

"I don't see a green traffic light; I see a blue one," says Ward. Bryant ordinarily sees an orange-hued "red" traffic signal, but because the engineered color can't be created at caution or single flashing red signals, "Sometimes I get to a light and can't tell the difference between red and yellow, and so must make a complete stop," he says. Since the engineered color can be masked by distance and darkness, Ward has driven *through* the orange-hued "red" traffic lights at night. "They look like streetlights to me until I'm practically through the intersection," he insists.

*Color-deficient vision affects about eight percent of the world's males.*

Hunting caps and vests in the United States were also changed from red to orange in the 1950s with the color-vision-deficient population in mind.

### Occupational Limitations

Until 1965 persons with color-vision deficiency were barred from careers in electrical engineering. "That's the year they changed the color codes in resistors and wiring to accommodate the color-vision-deficient," says Donald Milne, O.D., an optometrist based in Salt Lake City, Utah. Many other careers (e.g. interior decorator, commercial pilot, law-enforcement officer, firefighter) require accurate color discrimination, and so remain closed—sometimes for excellent reasons. "In Europe a train accident was attributed to a color-vision-deficient signal switcher," notes Adams. Other jobs require color coding, and the use of color monitors is becoming prevalent. Mild color-vision deficiencies may be no hindrance to some jobs requiring accurate color discrimination, and sometimes a color-vision-deficient person can learn to compensate.

### Detection and Treatment

Children should be screened for color-vision deficiencies prior to enrolling in kindergarten. Prompt detection helps minimize emotional consequences that can adversely affect a child's budding self-esteem. "Children may feel stupid for not knowing their colors," Milne says. Other children experience anxiety in an attempt to conceal their color-vision handicap. "Even as adults, my brothers won't admit to being color-blind," says Bryant.

Color-vision-deficient children have special educational requirements. For instance, the extensive use of colors in early-childhood education may be helpful to the child with normal color vision, but such aids as colored chalk, colored lettering, and color coding can be detrimental to the color-vision-deficient child. Older students can be alienated by colored maps as well as colored computer monitors.

Although no cure exists for inherited color-vision deficiency (occasionally an acquired color weakness is correctable), various attempts have been made to improve color vision with the use of prisms, lights, and filters. One such filter is the X-Chrom lens—a single red contact lens worn over one eye to help color-deficient persons distinguish between red and green. ◇

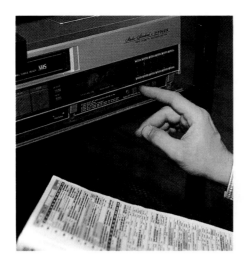

# ERGONOMICS

*by Elizabeth McGowan*

"I was on a radio talk show once, and a man called in and said, 'I'm an expert engineer and I design guided missile systems for a living.' Then he went on to tell me how he couldn't program his own VCR," recalls Dr. Donald Norman, a psychologist, engineer, and professor emeritus, University of California, San Diego. "VCRs that are impossible to use have become a national joke." The reason? Designers of these and other modern "conveniences" have put form before function, and have lost sight of the people for whom they are designing.

It's the rare consumer who hasn't been humbled by a product purportedly designed to make life easier. Ever tangled with a digital watch that requires 10 steps to set? A computer program so complicated it makes the pencil and legal pad look fast? Or how about an espresso machine so obstreperous that every morning starts with a cup of instant?

If specialists like Norman have their way, user-hostile machines will land in the same historical junkyard as the Edsel. Norman, who is the former director of the Institute for Cognitive Science at the University of California, San Diego, and now conducts user research for Apple Computer, is part of an expanding scientific school determined to bring "people" back into the technology equation. Though they come from a variety of disciplines, including psychology, sociology,

*Products designed ergonomically are often considered "user friendly." Below, an engineer incorporates ergonomic principles into the design of an electric mixer. VCRs (above) represent one of the many household products and devices notorious for a lack of ergonomic elements.*

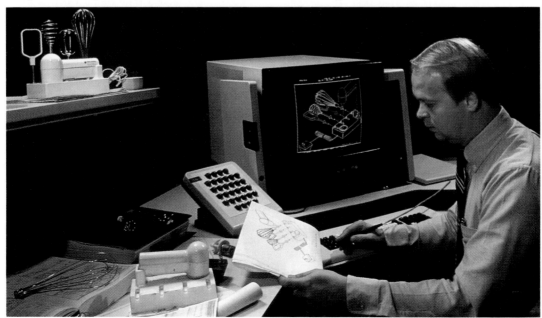

engineering, physical therapy, occupational therapy, education, physiology, and architecture, what these specialists all have in common is a focus on "human factors," also known as "ergonomics."

### Ergowhat?

Ergonomics—a word that derives from the Greek *ergon* ("work") and *nomos* ("natural laws")—"is a science that addresses human performance and well-being in relationship to jobs, equipment, tools, and the environment," explains Marilyn Joyce, president of the Joyce Institute, an ergonomics consulting and training firm in Seattle, Washington.

According to the Human Factors and Ergonomics Society in Santa Monica, California, there are approximately 6,000 ergonomists in the United States, specializing in the research and design of products and facilities to suit human needs. Although it isn't exactly a household word—ergowhat? is the typical response ergonomists get when they tell others what they do for a living—ergonomic expertise is present to some extent in almost every aspect of life—from the home and the workplace to the cars people drive and the sports equipment they use.

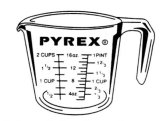

*A looped handle makes a measuring cup (top) difficult to use. An open-handled design (above) makes good ergonomic sense.*

### Ergogenesis

Since the Stone Age, humans have been adapting their tools and living and work quarters to suit their needs. But it wasn't until the dawn of the Industrial Revolution that the effort to study the relationship between people, machines, and methods of work resembled anything like science.

In the 1880s Frederick W. Taylor, a steel-factory foreman, declared that "the greatest obstacle to harmonious cooperation between workman and management lay in the ignorance of management as to what really constitutes a proper day's work for a workman." He set out to educate his bosses and to prove

his theory by conducting studies on his co-workers. One of the things Taylor discovered, which today is an undisputed tenet of ergonomics, is that the amount of work a person can do in one day is directly correlated to the length and frequency of rest periods. Today Taylor is widely acknowledged for his application of scientific method to industry, and for his recognition of the psychological components that influence the human capacity for production.

If Taylor is considered the father of scientific management, Frank and Lillian Gilbreth might best be described as the mom and pop of time-motion studies. Following their marriage in 1904, Lillian, who was trained as a psychologist, and Frank, who had an engineering background, joined forces with a lofty goal: to make the world a more efficient place.

Frank Gilbreth had a genius for developing commonsense solutions to make work less fatiguing and more productive—for example, creating a scaffold that could be adjusted to the most comfortable worker level; designing benches to hold a worker's tools so the worker didn't have to bend; and constructing worktables of the proper height both for the task and for the worker's body size.

The Gilbreths also pioneered the use of cameras for micromotion analysis. The data they gathered were used to create wire models that could be manipulated to demonstrate proper task movements to workers. The Gilbreths authored several groundbreaking books, including *Fatigue Study, Motion Study for the Handicapped,* and *The Psychology of Management,* and developed the therblig (an anagram of Gilbreth) system of categorizing hand movements—still a standard motion-and-time-analysis technique.

Though their emphasis came down more on the side of production than human physical well-being, the Gilbreths and Taylor laid some of the foundation upon which ergonomics is built. But it wasn't until the onset of World War II that the science came into its own. As weapons of destruction became increasingly sophisticated during the war, military leaders started to notice a disturbing pattern of accidents attributed to human error. In response, alarmed military chiefs recruited teams of physiologists and psychologists to study human tolerance and abilities. Their mandate: to create guidelines for the

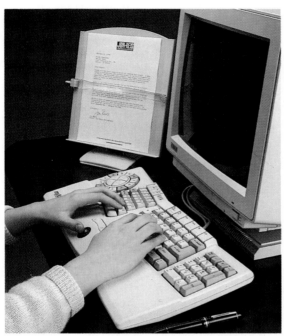

New computer keyboards have a decidedly unusual but nonetheless ergonomic design intended to reduce repetitive stress injuries.

engineers who were designing the equipment. Among the results of ergonomic studies conducted during World War II: the G suit, which guards aircraft pilots against oxygen loss at high altitudes, a refined version of which is still used by the military's Top Guns.

Consideration of human factors is now standard procedure in military design, although technology still sometimes leaps ahead of human ability. For example, in 1988 the U.S.S. *Vincennes* mistakenly shot down an Iranian airliner, killing 290 civilians. The

error has been blamed in part on difficult-to-read computer-monitor displays and information overload: in the short time the cruiser crew had to react, the crew members were not able to correctly interpret all the data they were receiving.

The postwar era saw the formalization of human factors as a scientific specialty, and the application of human factors to nonmilitary arenas. The Human Factors Society was founded, and ergonomics departments were developed at universities across the United States. As pilots returned to civilian life, elements of military-cockpit design found their way into commercial aircraft, and, a little later on, into car dashboards. Manufacturers of other stripes also began to see the benefits of ergonomic design: if their products were easier to use, they'd sell better.

## Ergonomically Correct

As the VCR example at the beginning of the article illustrates, ergonomics has not been totally embraced by the design and engineering community—some designers regard ergonomic considerations as antithetical to pleasing aesthetics, to say nothing of an infringement on their artistic license. Still, over the years the science has gained considerable, if sometimes grudging, respect. Today companies like Kodak, Xerox, and the Big Three car manufacturers have incorporated human-factors departments into their product-development laboratories, designing products with ergonomic input at all stages. Apple Computer's Dr. Norman, the author of *The Psychology of Everyday Things* and *Things that Make Us Smart,* cites Xerox for its whole-hearted and very successful commitment to ergonomic design. "Xerox has worked very hard to make

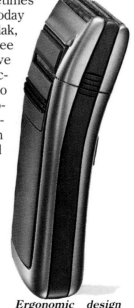

Ergonomic design makes this electric razor easy to hold.

their copiers easy to use and very easy to service. The real problem with copier machines," he explains, "is when the paper jams. It's almost impossible to stop paper jams.

"What Xerox discovered is that even though they can't stop the paper from jamming, they can make the problem easy to fix. Inside the machine, it looks very open, very colorful, big numbers, 1, 2, 3. It's very easy to decipher. Even someone who's never seen the machine can fix a paper jam."

Whether the product is cars or copiers, a fundamental of the ergonomic process is to

*A gooseneck spout and lever handles not only make kitchen work easier, they add a contemporary flair to the faucet set's overall design.*

define the user's needs and to follow a structured program of scientific method to assure that a product meets those needs. Ergonomists believe they should work with the designers from the beginning to ensure that what consumers need is what they get.

In product design, ergonomists offer an immense range of input, including data on the physical dimensions of the human body; sociological statistics; and psychological consid-

erations. Ergonomists also conduct and analyze field studies. In designing a new car steering system, for example, an ergonomist might go out on the highway and observe how real-life drivers actually grip the wheel—and figure out how engineers might make a wheel that works better with the human body. For a more controlled situation, ergonomists might conduct a laboratory study, videotaping real-life users working with a product prototype.

When Corning wanted to find out how its redesigned Pyrex measuring cup measured up, for example, the company gathered a group of housewives who spent a lot of time cooking. In a laboratory kitchen, the women used several variations of the cup to boil water, pour, make pudding, and, of course, to measure. After putting several designs through the culinary obstacle course, the testers told the designers which handle configuration they thought was most comfortable and practical—which handle, in other words, was most ergonomically correct. Corning was happy it followed the housewives' suggestions. Sales for the already well-selling cup increased by 150 percent.

When a Joyce Institute ergonomist helped Microsoft design an innovative new mouse, he took several detours before getting to the user-testing stage. He started by analyzing competing mice to see if and where they were flawed. "Next he looked at how the hand and wrist operate, and at the interface between mouse and computer screen," explains the company's Marilyn Joyce. Based on that information, the ergonomist suggested how high the mouse should be to support the wrists, and how wide for hand comfort. Then designers built a prototype. After several refinements the product was ready to be tested by users. It passed the exam, and finally hit the stores in April 1993, its sales projections burnished by awards for good design.

## Repetitive-Motion Illness

With the recent avalanche of repetitive-motion-illness claims and lawsuits, many aimed at manufacturers of video-display terminals (VDTs), Microsoft isn't the only company conducting stringent ergonomic assessment of its products. Indeed, it is in the arena of health and safety that ergonomics has made the biggest splash, at least in consumer perception. Why? Carpal-tunnel syndrome, the much-headlined repetitive-motion illness. According to the U.S. Bureau of Labor Statistics, repetitive-motion illnesses accounted for a whopping 62 percent of workers'-compensation claims in 1992. That's up from 50 percent in 1988, and only 18 percent in 1981. Less publicized but just as much an ergonomic issue, back injuries come in second on the workers'-compensation list, accounting for approximately 20 percent of labor cases.

Repetitive-motion and back injuries are notorious in industries like meatpacking and auto assembly, where, until recently, heavy lifting, bending and twisting, and the use of high-vibration tools were considered an inescapable part of the job. But in this age of the electronic office, these injuries, once the province of factory workers, are invading the traditionally "safe" white-collar world. According to all the ergonomic experts surveyed for this article, VDTs are the major culprits. Unlike the office workers of yesteryear, who did a variety of tasks like photocopying, phone work, and typing, today's VDT operators sit in front of terminals for hours at a stretch, taking few breaks and repeating the same motion all day.

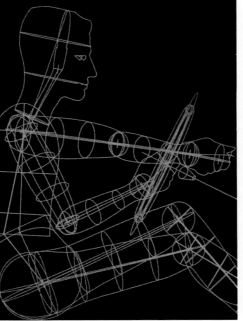

*Automotive engineers draw from a variety of sources to create the computer simulations needed to ergonomically design a safe and comfortable car interior.*

Stanford University professor David A. Thompson underscored the repetitive nature of such jobs in a recent article for *Safety and Health* magazine: "If a person spends six hours of a workday keying at 50 words per minute, that's 108,000 keystrokes a day, half a million strokes a week, 27 million strokes a year. And that's just the minimum proficiency level to get hired for a keyboarding position."

Thompson estimates that the average VDT worker exerts about 8 ounces of force per keystroke. "From an engineering standpoint," he says, "that's 25 tons of force per day flowing through the fingertips of a high-end user. . . . It's no wonder wrists are breaking down."

Common injuries caused by repetitive trauma include carpal-tunnel syndrome, a compression of the median nerve as a result of repeated bending of the wrist; tendinitis, an inflammation and swelling of the tendons of the hands, wrists, or arms; and tenosynovitis, an inflammation of the synovial sheath housing the tendon, usually occurring in the hands and wrists. All can result in permanent nerve damage if not addressed early on. In some cases, surgery is required to relieve the pain, although there is some debate among doctors about its effectiveness.

Meanwhile, VDT manufacturers are working fast to refine their products before there's no one left able to use them. Several new keyboard designs allow the wrists to work in a more natural, turned-slightly-inward position, and voice-operated systems are also in the works. Wrist rests are also hitting the market in several designs and colors.

Although VDT users have gotten the most publicity, repetitive-trauma-illness victims come from all professions and walks of life. At this writing, Kathleen Roe, a dental hygienist and the former president of the Dental Hygienist Association of New York State, is midway through a two-month disability leave from her job, due to a work-related combination of carpal-tunnel syndrome and osteoarthritis. "I'd be at work, and by the middle of the day, the pain would be excruciating," Roe recalls. "It got worse and worse, until I finally realized that it wouldn't go away on its own."

Initial treatment for her condition consisted of anti-inflammatory medication and steroid shots. She now wears wrist splints and has found vitamin $B_6$ helpful in reducing the pain. Still, there are many days when she has trouble holding a bar of soap, and when doing the dishes requires monumental effort.

Unlike wrist and hand dysfunction, eye problems, another modern-age ailment, seem to be more easily reversible. "Studies have shown that between 75 and 80 percent of VDT workers have eye-related complaints like dry eyes, or blurry and double vision," says James Sheedy, Ph.D., chief of the VDT Eye Clinic at the University of California at Berkeley. Few VDT-related eye problems are permanent, he says, and most can be

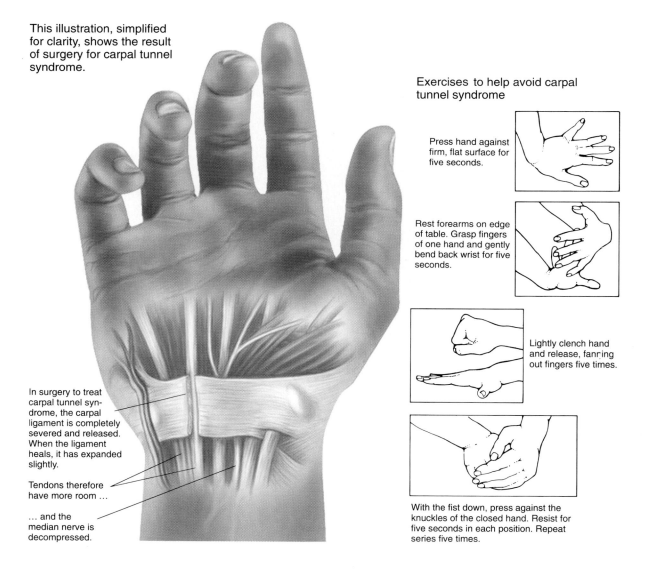

This illustration, simplified for clarity, shows the result of surgery for carpal tunnel syndrome.

In surgery to treat carpal tunnel syndrome, the carpal ligament is completely severed and released. When the ligament heals, it has expanded slightly.

Tendons therefore have more room ...

... and the median nerve is decompressed.

Exercises to help avoid carpal tunnel syndrome

Press hand against firm, flat surface for five seconds.

Rest forearms on edge of table. Grasp fingers of one hand and gently bend back wrist for five seconds.

Lightly clench hand and release, fanring out fingers five times.

With the fist down, press against the knuckles of the closed hand. Resist for five seconds in each position. Repeat series five times.

## Make Your Office Ergonomically Correct

**Neck** positioned upright and relaxed.

**Shoulders** relaxed and in lowered position, with the chest area open.

**Back** upright, or slightly forward from the hips, maintaining the natural curve of the lower back.

**Elbows** positioned at a right angle, with forearms parallel to the floor.

**Wrists** in a neutral position, with no flexing up or down.

**Knees** slightly lower than hips.

**Chair** backrest adjusted so that lower back is fully supported and at proper height to permit feet to rest on floor.

**Head** positioned 18 to 30 inches from the screen.

**Screen** positioned at eye level or slightly lower.

**Fingers** relaxed and gently curved over keyboard.

**Keyboard** flat to align wrists at or just below elbow level.

**Feet** should rest firmly on the floor, slightly forward until knees are at a 90 to 110 degree angle. There should be 3 to 6 inches of legroom between lap and desk or keyboard tray.

---

"cured" by adjustment of room lighting and computer-screen glare, and taking regular rest breaks.

Backs are also suffering—VDT operators often sit hunched over the keyboard in whatever chair happened to come with their desk when they were hired. The key to fixing the problem is a chair and a workstation that can be ergonomically adjusted to the user's body —a 95-pound, 5-foot woman should not be sitting in the same-height chair as a 350-pound, 6-foot-plus man.

Though office-worker health problems have received the lion's share of consumer-news coverage—due perhaps to the fact that repetitive-motion-illness statistics are high among journalists who spend long days at the computer terminal—factory workers are also hurting themselves in record numbers. In the meatpacking industry alone, there were 36,000 cases of repetitive-motion illness in 1992. And according to the Occupational Safety and Health Administration (OSHA), back injuries alone cost American industry an estimated $16 billion per year.

## Applying Ergonomics Early

Good ergonomic practices can prevent many of these injuries from happening in the first place. Many companies, including Ford Motor Company and L. L. Bean, have instituted proactive ergonomics programs for their workers, with much success.

In 1983 Ford teamed up with the University of Michigan's Center for Ergonomics in an attempt to address workers' complaints and to lower their injury rate by redesigning equipment and tools, and by changing work procedures. Led by Don Chaffin, Ph.D., a professor of industrial engineering, students interviewed workers and videotaped them doing their jobs. They also surveyed medical records for statistics on jobs causing the most injuries. Observations were augmented by work in the lab—students devised computer simulations to determine which jobs caused unnecessary body stress.

The many student-suggested changes that have been implemented in Ford plants include: raising conveyor belts to reduce bending; using hoists to cut down on manual lifting; installing bins that tilt so workers don't have to reach down into them to get the parts they need; and attaching pistol grips on tools to prevent "trigger finger." The joint venture, originally projected to last only four years, has been a hit with both workers and management, and is now an ongoing program.

Like Ford and many other companies throughout the United States, L.L. Bean first recognized in the 1980s that it had a cumulative-disorder problem. As Ted Rooney, the Maine company's manager of employee safety, puts it, "It's not the type of thing that jumps up and bites you. It's a slow process, and we spent most of the 1980s trying to figure out what the problems were and where they were coming from."

L.L. Bean met the challenge by designing an ergonomics program with the help of the Joyce Institute. Today ergonomics is as integral to L.L. Bean's corporate identity as is

*Ford Motor Company's assembly lines are ergonomically arranged to reduce the amount of bending a worker must do to perform a task.*

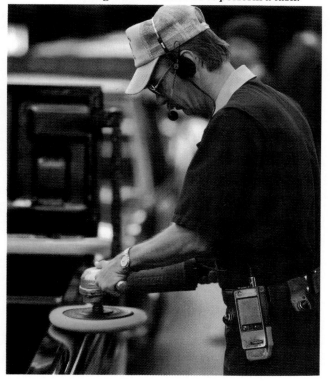

their mail-order catalog. Explains Rooney: "We try to pick up problems real early." As in any effective ergonomics program, L.L. Bean tackles each situation on an individual basis. Solutions may involve rearranging a workstation, providing task lighting, redesigning the day's work routine (i.e., scheduling one type of task for a few hours and then switching to another). The key to developing ergonomic solutions, says Rooney, is employee involvement.

As standard company-wide procedure, L.L. Bean also requires VDT operators to take mandatory, paid work breaks, and it encourages employees to visit on-site physical therapists during company time to take care of ailments.

Does the program work? Although Rooney declined to give figures, he did say that the rate of injury was significantly reduced, and that both workers and management are happy with the results.

Companies like Ford and L.L. Bean have recognized that healthy workers are more productive workers. But according to Rani Leuder, president of Humanics Ergosystems, Inc., an ergonomics consulting firm in Encino, California, many other companies don't address ergonomic problems until they have no choice. As she puts it, "Sometimes they wait until they are being sued or their worker's compensation is so outstanding they can't stand to look at it."

And if a lawsuit doesn't coerce companies to address ergonomic issues, maybe a big fine will do the trick. In December 1993, OSHA announced that a much-awaited, long-delayed ergonomics-standards proposal will be ready by October 1994. The proposed standards will be subject to a comment period and public hearings before they are finalized.

Companies looking to get a jump on the soon-to-come standards would be wise to take the advice of the experts, who warn not to expect ergonomics to be a quick fix, a health-and-safety magic bullet.

As L.L. Bean's Ted Rooney, borrowing a quote from L.L. Bean president Leon Gorman, explains this user-friendly field, "Ergonomics is just a day-in, day-out ongoing, never-ending, unremitting, persevering, compassionate type of activity." ◇

# Electrolysis: Getting to the Roots

*by Sue Berkman*

"You should be women, and yet your beards forbid me to interpret that you are so." While these words from Shakespeare's *Macbeth* might strike some as amusing, others find no humor in them. Abnormal hair growth is a reality for as many as 10 percent of all adult women—and it's no laughing matter.

Doctors use the word *hirsute* to refer to excessive hair growth on an adult body, and the condition is by no means unique to women. Quite the contrary, many men have abundant hair on their upper lips, chins, chests, backs, abdomens, arms, and legs. And while women are typically more likely to consider hirsutism a cosmetic liability, men may be self-conscious about heavy beards that necessitate shaving twice a day; thick, woolly hair on their backs; and tufts of hair that emerge from their ears and nostrils.

The use of electric current to permanently remove unwanted excess hair, a procedure known as *electrolysis,* began over a century ago. In 1875 a St. Louis ophthalmologist, Charles Michel, became the first known practitioner of electrolysis when he treated ingrown eyelashes by using a needle to destroy the follicles. Today, while countless other methods of removing excess hair are in use —razors, tweezers, bleaching solutions, waxing kits, depilatories—electrolysis (albeit more refined and sophisticated than Dr. Michel's technique) remains the *only* way to banish unwanted hair forever.

### Hair by Hair

Most electrologists and people who seek treatment refer to the process as electrolysis; however, there are, technically, two dif-

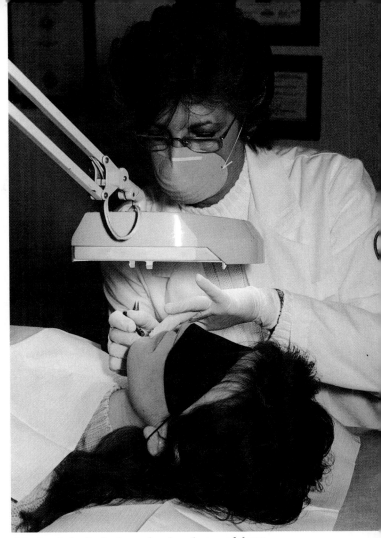

*A trained electrolysis professional can safely remove excess unwanted hair on the body using a fine-needle probe that carries an electric current to the hair follicle.*

ferent techniques. The *galvanic* method uses a direct electric current to induce a chemical change within the hair follicle. This procedure produces the chemicals hydrogen gas and lye, which usually destroy the follicle. *Thermolysis* uses a high-frequency electric current to damage the bulb and make it unable to produce new hairs. In both techniques a very fine electric needle called a probe is inserted into the follicle to carry the current. The loosened hair is then removed with a tweezer. "In most instances the two techniques are used simultaneously, thereby destroying the hair follicle in two ways," says Trudy Brown, a Certified Professional Electrologist (CPE) and president of the International Guild of Professional Electrologists in High Point, North Carolina.

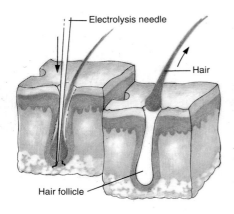

Electrolysis needle

Hair

Hair follicle

*The electrolysis needle is inserted into the hair follicle to destroy the root of the hair. The pain of the procedure may be lessened somewhat with an anesthetic cream.*

To remove hundreds of hairs on an upper lip, for example, a client may need to undergo months of treatment, with each session lasting 15 to 30 minutes. For less sensitive areas, such as the arms and legs, the sessions may last one to two hours. "The professional electrologist tailors the treatment program to the individual client," says Brown. Certain factors determine the number and length of treatments required, such as the number of hair follicles contained in the area of treatment, the sensitivity of the skin, the particular area to be treated, and the methods of hair removal previously undergone by the patient. Patients should ask for a treatment schedule on the first consultation.

No matter how short the session or light-handed the electrologist, there is no such thing as painless electrolysis. It is impossible to destroy hair-growth tissue without generating sensation, because each hair follicle is surrounded by its own network of nerves. The recent approval of a new topical-anesthetic cream by the U.S. Food and Drug Administration (FDA) can now assure reduced pain to apprehensive patients.

Even the most skilled electrologists report that the rate of hair regrowth is 40 to 60 percent. This regrowth occurs because some follicles are crooked or angled, making it impossible to tell at the time of treatment whether the root has really been destroyed. Furthermore, follicles that are dormant at the time of treatment may produce hairs later. And electrolysis can destroy only existing hairs; it has no effect on the physical causes of excessive growth, some of which may require medical treatment (see sidebar below).

## More Than Skin-deep?

While people with excessive body hair are single-mindedly interested in its removal, doctors tend to want reasons for the abnormal growth. "Sometimes hirsutism has a perfectly logical explanation," says Richard F. Wagner, Jr., M.D., professor of dermatology at the University of Texas Medical Branch in Galveston. "On the other hand, the condition could signal a medical problem—even a serious one. What's more, correcting the underlying medical cause might well stop further growth of superfluous hair, although it won't remove what is already there."

All individuals inherit a genetic blueprint that determines the amount, location, and timing of hair growth. Hirsute parents generally produce offspring who grow up to be similarly hirsute. Ethnic and geographic influences matter, too: Caucasians tend to be hairier than blacks; Mediterranean and Semitic people tend to be hairier than Scandinavians and Anglo-Saxons; the least hairy peoples are Asians and American Indians.

Hormonal imbalances also bring about excessive hair growth. Normal changes in the hormonal system during puberty, pregnancy, and menopause may increase the level of the male hormones called androgens or decrease the level of the female hormone, estrogen, resulting in sudden new hair growth on the body or face. Abnormal changes in the hormonal system—due to underlying medical conditions—may also be to blame. These include polycystic ovarian disease (PCOD), in which the ovaries develop numerous cysts; tumors on the ovaries or adrenal glands; and cancers elsewhere in the body. These conditions are frequently accompanied by other masculine characteristics, such as voice changes, increased muscularity, and even balding.

Obviously, professional electrolysis does not come cheap, especially when superfluous hair growth is extensive. A one-hour session may cost $30 to $60 (some insurance policies cover the costs). But consider this, advises Trudy Brown: "When you tally up a lifetime's bills for razors, creams, waxing, and the hours of time spent pursuing temporary results, electrolysis may turn out to save money."

### Skill Equals Safety
In skilled hands the equipment and technique of modern electrolysis minimize any permanent skin damage. However, it is not unusual for redness and/or swelling to appear immediately following treatment, although this disappears within a few hours. The small whiteheads or scabs that occasionally occur are a normal part of the healing process, and they should not be picked off; scarring and even infection may result if the scabs are removed. Cosmetics, frequent touching of the area, and exposure to sunlight or tanning devices are all discouraged for several days after an electrolysis session to minimize the risk of infection or other problems.

Clients with rheumatic heart disease or mitral-valve prolapse should have prophylactic treatment with antibiotics to prevent serious heart infections from bacteria that can enter the bloodstream during the procedure. Pregnant women can undergo electrolysis, although treatment of hairs on the breasts and abdomen should be discontinued during the last three months of pregnancy.

### Safety Standards
Public fears about infectious diseases such as hepatitis and AIDS have prompted electrolysis professionals to take aggressive steps to ensure public health, safety, and welfare. "There has never been a reported case of AIDS connected with electrolysis," says Teresa E. Petricca, CPE, president of the American Electrology Association (AEA), a professional-membership organization based in Trumbull, Connecticut.

Petricca notes that only 28 states require licensure.* The organization is actively lobbying for strict regulation—first on a state-by-state basis, and ultimately on a national level. "It is unfathomable that a state would demand licensure of the cosmetology field and, at the same time, ignore the need to regulate the electrology profession," says Petricca.

The AEA sponsors the International Board of Electrologist Certification, which, with the assistance of the Educational Testing Service of Princeton, New Jersey, conducts certification examinations of electrologists to match knowledge and skills against national norms. A CPE must complete 75 contact hours of approved continuing education over a five-year period to be recertified. "Unfortunately, many electrologists are advertising 'certified' simply because they have a certificate of completion for a course of study of electrology. This certificate does *not* mean the electrologist is certified by the AEA," warns Petricca.

In 1992 the AEA updated standards developed in 1988 for sterilization, safety, and hygiene with the assistance of the Centers for Disease Control and Prevention (CDC) in Atlanta, Georgia. Even though AEA members voluntarily adhere to the standards, only state licensing laws can enforce compliance.

Professional electrologists stress that electrolysis is *not* a do-it-yourself endeavor. Electrified tweezers have been reviewed by the FDA and found to be no more effective than the ordinary hand-operated variety. And while it is possible to buy home electrolysis instruments, these may cause unnecessary damage in inexperienced hands. ◇

**Resources**
For information on electrolysis and details on how to find a Certified Professional Electrologist in your area, contact:

The International Guild of Professional Electrologists Executive Offices Professional Building 202 Boulevard, Suite C High Point, NC 27262 (910) 841-6631

American Electrology Association Public Information Committee 106 Oak Ridge Road Trumbull, CT 06611 (203) 374-6667

---

* Alabama, Arkansas, California, Connecticut, Delaware, Florida, Hawaii, Idaho, Indiana, Iowa, Kansas, Louisiana, Maryland, Massachusetts, Michigan, Montana, Nevada, New Hampshire, New Mexico, North Carolina, North Dakota, Ohio, Oklahoma, Oregon, Rhode Island, Tennessee, Utah, and Wisconsin.

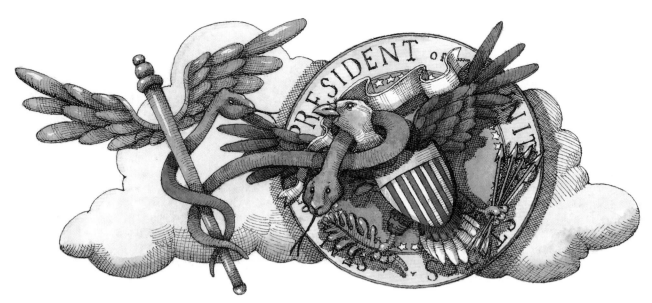

# AIL TO THE CHIEF?

*by Christopher King*

At his inauguration in 1841, newly sworn-in President William Henry Harrison took it upon himself to deliver a longer inaugural speech than any chief executive before him had attempted. Despite his advanced age, Harrison also saw fit to defy the January weather and deliver the speech without wearing his overcoat. The new president subsequently came down with pneumonia. Unfortunately for Harrison, he received the finest, state-of-the-art medical care of his day. As Robert H. Ferrell records in his book *Ill-Advised* (University of Missouri, 1992), Harrison's treatment included suction cups, stinging ointments, rhubarb—and even an Indian concoction of crude petroleum and Virginia snakeweed. He died within a month.

Less than a decade later, during a sun-baked outdoor ceremony to dedicate construction of the Washington Monument, President Zachary Taylor enjoyed a drink of cherries and ice that contained contaminated water. He fell ill with typhoid fever, and died a few days later, after only a year in office.

### Press Preoccupation

The cases of Harrison and Taylor provide particularly harsh reminders that U.S. presidents, despite the lofty stature and far-reaching powers conferred by their office, are no less prone to illness and infirmity than are the rest of us. In fact, illness has played a significant role in many presidencies, and may indeed have influenced presidential performance at critical points in American history. In some instances the public has been well-informed about a presidential ailment (and perhaps even too well-informed, as when Lyndon Johnson, president from 1963 to 1969, lifted his shirt to show reporters the stomach scars from his gallbladder surgery). More often, however, and usually with the willing participation of the president's own doctors, illness has been concealed. Despite such cover-ups—or perhaps because of them—presidential health has been an enduring preoccupation of the American press.

As early as 1813, newspapers speculated on the health of President James Madison, who suffered through a three-week episode of "bilious fever." The newspaper the *Federal Republican* whipped up public anxieties

> *The president of the United States is no less prone to illness than the rest of us.*

by publishing reports that visitors to the sick president came away with doubts about the possible "derangement of his mind." As it turned out, Madison recovered. However, nearly 200 years later, the panic-prone fascination with presidential health is stronger than ever. "Everyone, for good reasons and bad, is interested in the president's health," write political scientist Robert S. Robins and medical historian Henry Rothschild. "It can affect the stock market, an arms conference, a major appointment, and it is the biggest human interest story around." President Grover Cleveland was certainly aware of this fact in 1893, when he suddenly decided to embark on a private "pleasure cruise" aboard a friend's yacht.

### ★★★ Cleveland

In 1893 Washington, D.C., was in the midst of a financial crisis concerning the nation's currency. President Cleveland wanted Congress to repeal the Sherman Silver Act of 1890, a piece of legislation that he viewed as inflationary and a threat to the nation's financial future. Cleveland also knew that his vice president, Adlai Stevenson, saw the matter differently; Stevenson supported the Sherman Act. In the spring of that year, Cleveland noticed a rough spot on the roof of his mouth. When the spot failed to go away, the president consulted with an Army physician, who told him that the growth was likely cancerous and should be removed. Because of the financial crisis, Cleveland insisted that any operation be kept absolutely secret.

On July 1, the president boarded the large yacht *Oneida* at a pier on New York City's East River. Cleveland had spent much time sailing aboard the yacht, so the cover story of a pleasure cruise seemed perfectly believable. However, also on board was a small team of doctors. As in the earlier case of President Harrison, the finest medical knowledge of the time was brought to bear: The doctors propped Cleveland back in a chair, knocked him out with ether, and set to work. Finding what appeared to be a cancerous growth, they removed part of the president's palate and most of his left upper jaw. No external incision was made. Suspicious reporters following the president's trip were given

the official story that "no operation has been performed, except that a bad tooth has been removed." The Sherman Act was defeated, and Cleveland went on to complete his second term (he served two, nonconsecutive stints in the White House, between 1885 and 1889, and between 1893 and 1897).

As Robert Ferrell notes in *Ill-Advised,* later medical analysis of Cleveland's tumor suggests that such a hurried and hazardous operation might not have been necessary. In 1975 an investigative panel concluded that the growth was likely a "verrucous carcinoma," a relatively slow-growing tumor. But a significant pattern—involving frail presidential health and an accompanying flurry of official denials and cover-ups—had begun. The story of Cleveland's secret operation did not emerge until 1917.

### ★★★ Wilson

Woodrow Wilson served two terms as president, from 1913 to 1921. Assessing Wilson's medical history, scholars now wonder if he ever should have been nominated for the office in the first place. There is evidence that years before his election, Wilson had suffered a series of strokes—sudden attacks of paralysis or loss of sensation that are typically

*President Wilson was incapacitated by strokes during his second term in office. At the time, the severity of the president's condition was well-hidden from the public.*

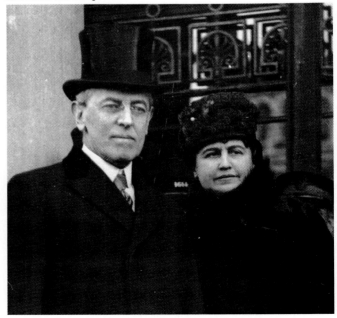

caused by blockages or ruptures in the arteries supplying the brain. In their book *Hidden Illness in the White House* (Duke, 1988), Kenneth R. Crispell and Carlos F. Gomez consider the evidence that Wilson's health problems were closely related to his driven, unyielding, workaholic personality. Wilson apparently suffered from hypertension (high blood pressure) and atherosclerosis (hardening of the arteries)—both of which underlie heart attack and stroke. Nevertheless, he refused to cut back on his work schedule, even after strokes and other neurological impairments had significantly affected the muscle strength and movement in his arms and hands. His eyesight had also been impaired. In publicly explaining the president's long periods of seclusion in the White House during medical crises, his physician and friend Cary T. Grayson cited slightly less serious ailments, blaming "colds."

In 1919, shortly after the end of World War I, Wilson went on a grueling national tour to drum up support for America's proposed entry into the League of Nations, the forerunner of today's United Nations. During the tour, he suffered two severe strokes within days of one another. These left him completely paralyzed on his left side, further damaged his vision, and impaired his speech. From then until the end of his second term, Wilson remained largely out of reach in the White House while his presidency was effectively carried out by Dr. Grayson and Mrs. Wilson, the president's wife. Some 28 acts of Congress became law without any review by the president. Without Wilson's leadership for the League of Nations initiative, America remained isolationist and did not join the organization. Wilson died in 1924.

Wilson's successor, Warren G. Harding, also suffered from heart disease, and chose as a physician Charles E. Sawyer, a man whose friendship and good intentions seemed to outweigh his medical skills. One of the weapons in Dr. Sawyer's medical arsenal was apparently a belief in prescribing pills on the basis of their color. He also consistently misdiagnosed unmistakable signs of Harding's advanced heart failure during 1923, citing such causes as food poisoning and other digestive disturbances. By the time that Harding was seen by specialists, it was too late. He died in August of that year. The cause of death, as Ferrell notes in *Ill-Advised,* was clear: "Actually, the cause was Dr. Sawyer, who allowed his charge, the president of the United States, suffering from high blood pressure and, by 1923, heart failure, to carry on daily activities as if nothing were wrong. The four other attending physicians knew of Sawyer's incompetence and covered it up."

*In 1923, President Harding died suddenly of a thrombosis, or blood clot, a condition that could have been avoided with appropriate medical care available at the time. Thousands turned out to see the funeral train that transported the president's body back to Washington from the West Coast.*

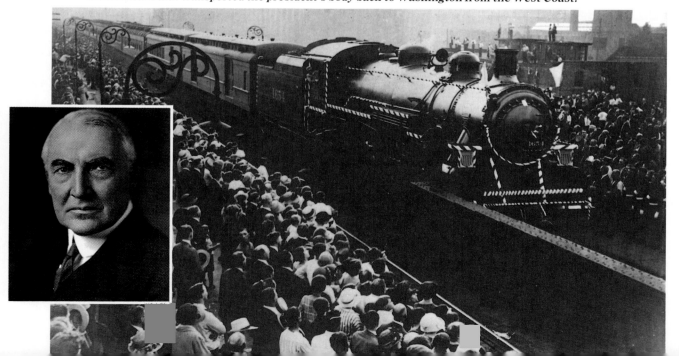

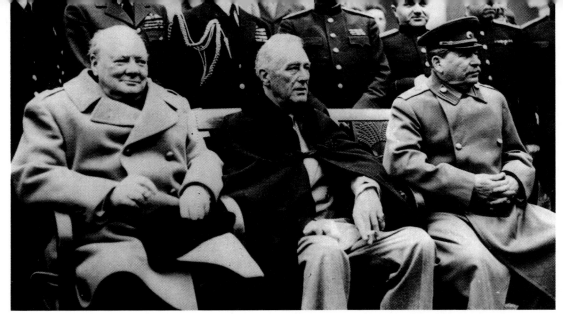

*Many historians think that Franklin Roosevelt's declining physical condition played a role in the decisions made at Yalta in February 1945. Two months after the conference, the president died.*

### ★★★ FDR

Between 1932 and 1944, Franklin Delano Roosevelt was elected to four consecutive terms, more than any other U.S. president. Roosevelt's primary physical ailment was widely known, even as it was rather cleverly concealed. In 1921, while in his late 30s, Roosevelt was stricken by poliomyelitis, more widely known as polio. This viral infection damages motor neurons—the nerve cells controlling muscles—and produces paralysis. Although now virtually eliminated by infant immunization in the United States and other developed nations, polio remains a huge health problem in Asia, Africa, and parts of Europe, as it was in this country earlier in this century.

Polio left Roosevelt without the use of his legs. This handicap, however, did not slow his political career. This fact is all the more impressive considering how differently physical disabilities were viewed in Roosevelt's time compared to today. Back then the disabled—or "cripples," as they were usually called—were expected to remain shut-ins; their mere appearance in public was considered bad taste. The concept of "mainstreaming" did not yet exist. Nevertheless, people accepted Roosevelt. As Hugh G. Gallagher notes in *FDR's Splendid Deception,* Roosevelt's condition may have struck a sympathetic chord with the American people, who had been financially "disabled" by the economic hard times of the Great Depression. "An agreement was struck," writes Gallagher. "The existence of FDR's handicap would simply be denied by all. The people

would pretend that their leader was not crippled, and their leader would do all that he could not to let them see that he was."

Whenever Roosevelt appeared in public, special arrangements were made to have him lifted from his car while out of public view. With the use of leg braces and the aid of his son James, he learned to walk with great difficulty but apparent casualness over short distances—as far as a podium, for example. And, although it may seem hard to believe given the relentless intrusiveness of today's reporters and photographers, the press assisted Roosevelt in playing down his disability. Of the 35,000 photographs collected in Roosevelt's presidential library, exactly two show him in a wheelchair. Political cartoons never depicted him as handicapped. With this artful concealment of his disability, Roosevelt was president of the United States through a critical period: up from the economic ruin of the Depression, and through the nation's involvement in World War II, from 1941 to 1945.

During the war a less visible but far more serious illness began to take its toll on Roosevelt's health. This illness, however, was entirely concealed from the public. As early as 1932, medical examinations showed that Roosevelt was suffering from hypertension. Unfortunately, the president's personal physician, Ross T. McIntire, shared the incompetence of many of his predecessors. By 1944, when the president was examined by a competent cardiologist, the outlook was grim: the left side of the president's heart was enlarged. In all, he was suffering from hypertensive heart disease, congestive heart failure, and acute bronchitis. His illness had kept him from his duties for weeks at a time.

But the business of the country—and the war in particular—continued to press. If Roosevelt was aware of the seriousness of his condition, he did not let it keep him from seeking a fourth term in 1944. His doctors did not stand in his way. His son James would later remark, "I never have been reconciled to the fact that father's physicians did not flatly forbid him to run." Yet run he did, and, in January 1945, FDR began his fourth term —a term he would never finish.

In February 1945, though gravely ill, Roosevelt journeyed to Yalta, on the Crimean Peninsula, for a meeting with British Prime Minister Winston Churchill and Russian Premier Joseph Stalin. The three leaders were to decide the postwar fate of Europe after the expected Allied victory over Germany (which would come within two months). Matters were particularly tense with the Russians, who had laid claim to Poland and other Eastern European territory. Churchill, who had met with the president previously, recorded his shock at Roosevelt's appearance: "The president looked old and thin and drawn. He intervened very little in discussions, sitting with his mouth open. I doubt, from what I have seen, whether he is fit for his job here." Historians have also wondered what part Roosevelt's ill health may have played in his dealings with Stalin and in the subsequent development of U.S.-Soviet tensions. Was he too weakened to hold a firm line against Stalin's demands? Or did his illness make no difference? Scholars can only speculate. Roosevelt would not live to see the end of the war. He returned to the United States and, in April 1945, at his retreat in Warm Springs, Georgia, died of a massive cerebral hemorrhage. Vice President Harry Truman assumed the chief executive's office for the duration of Roosevelt's fourth term. Truman then won the 1948 general election, serving as president until 1953, when the White House was taken over by the Army general known affectionately as "Ike."

### ★★★ Eisenhower

A war hero who had successfully served as supreme commander of the Allied forces in World War II, Dwight D. Eisenhower brought his accomplished leadership skills to the White House in 1953. Unfortunately, he also brought what cardiologists refer to as the classic "Type A" personality: relentlessly driven to work long hours, overexcited by stress, quick to anger, unconcerned by matters of personal health. For Eisenhower the price would be heart attacks. In 1949, even before his election, Eisenhower suffered what historians surmise was a relatively mild heart attack, with another, still milder incident in 1953. In September 1955, while visiting Denver, Colorado, Eisenhower suffered a major heart attack. And once more, in keeping with the inglorious historical pattern, there was a personal physician on hand to throw up a smoke screen. Eisenhower's doctor, Major General Howard M. Snyder, initially described the attack as a "digestive upset." The president's heart troubles were too serious to conceal, however, and he

*During his first term, President Eisenhower spent a substantial amount of time hospitalized for a heart attack and for Crohn's disease. He nonetheless ran for and won a second term.*

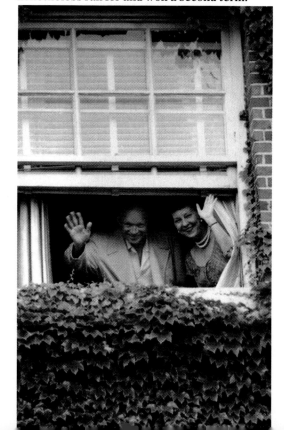

spent weeks recuperating in a Denver hospital. It was three months before he returned to his full schedule at the White House.

The next year would bring more troubles for Eisenhower. In June, he developed an intestinal obstruction due to an inflammatory-bowel disorder known as Crohn's disease. Doctors performed an operation to bypass the blocked portion of the intestines. This meant another 22 days in the hospital.

That year, Eisenhower also faced a crucial decision: whether or not to run for a second term. Back then the survival rate for patients who had suffered a major heart attack was not particularly promising—only about 50 percent lived five years. Furthermore, one of Eisenhower's doctors believed that the president had suffered an aneurysm—a swelling in the left ventricle of his heart. This made the outlook for his long-term health even bleaker. However, Paul Dudley White, M.D., a world-famous cardiologist who had taken on the care of the president in Denver, chose to gloss over the real risks when he endorsed Eisenhower's health during a press conference. As Ferrell puts it in *Ill-Advised,* "Paul Dudley White chose the next president of the United States." The neglect of Eisenhower's health appears to have played a role in his next medical crisis, a stroke suffered in 1957, which left him with impaired speech. Eisenhower's ventricular aneurysm may have been the cause of the stroke, giving off a blood clot that lodged in a brain artery. Nevertheless, Eisenhower finished his second term and lived until 1969.

### ★★★ JFK

If any president has been associated with health and vitality, it is John F. Kennedy. Images of touch-football games, sailing trips, and romps with his children all portrayed to the public a picture of a vigorous man in his prime. In truth, Kennedy spent much of his life in ruinous health. Two afflictions were particularly threatening: a congenitally weak and painful back, and another, far more serious ailment: a deficiency of the adrenal glands known as Addison's disease. In this disorder the adrenal glands fail to produce normal quantities of the hormones called steroids, leaving the victim weakened and prone to in-

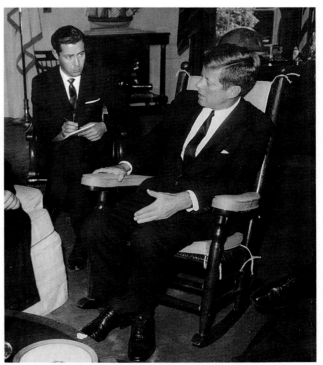

*Owing to back problems, President Kennedy used a special rocking chair in the White House. Most of his other health problems were unknown to the public until years after his death.*

fection. Previously fatal, the disease was just beginning to be treated successfully when Kennedy was diagnosed in the 1940s. Regular, lifelong doses of cortisone emerged as a successful therapy, and Kennedy was apparently one of the first Addison's patients to receive the drug.

When Kennedy's disease threatened to become an issue during the 1960 presidential campaign, the candidate and his aides simply lied to reporters about the illness. His subsequent bouts of ill health could be readily explained away: Kennedy had served in the Navy in World War II (apparently using his family connections to get around the physical examination, which the perennially sickly young man surely would have failed). His experiences in the Pacific served as a plausible basis for stories about health difficulties caused by his malaria (a tropical disease that he had supposedly contracted during the war). And a wartime incident in which his torpedo boat was rammed by a Japanese destroyer provided a suitably heroic cover story for his back troubles. In terms of medical misinformation in the Kennedy administration, the only notable difference from previous presidents was that much of the covering up was carried out by a woman, Janet Travell, M.D.

However, Dr. Travell was a model of Hippocratic decorum compared to another of Kennedy's medical attendants, Max Jacobsen, M.D. Known as "Dr. Feelgood," Jacobsen was famous for treating several Hollywood stars, and was noted for the "energizing" substances with which he injected his patients. These injections apparently included illegal drugs known as amphetamines. And although details remain sparse, it appears that Jacobsen indeed carried out his own brand of medicine on the president of the United States. Jacobsen was stripped of his medical license in 1975.

"I'm the healthiest candidate for president in the country," Kennedy had said while discussing possible running mates in the 1960 campaign, "and I'm not going to die in office." In November 1963, of course, Kennedy would travel to Dallas and be proved wrong.

### ★★★ Reagan and Bush

More recently the shooting of Ronald Reagan caused a presidential medical crisis in March 1981. His lung pierced by a bullet that ricocheted off his limousine, Reagan's condition in the days after the shooting was grave indeed. But the doctors and the president's staff did not disclose the seriousness of the wound and the accompanying trauma and infection. "There was kind of an unspoken agreement that none of us would let the public know how serious it was and how close we came to losing him," his wife Nancy would later say.

Reagan survived, of course, only to suffer still more medical difficulties. In July 1985, after a colonoscopy revealed a growth in Reagan's colon, the president underwent surgery for a precancerous lesion known as a "villous adenoma." Although medically successful, the operation may have played a part in the Iran-contra affair, one of the biggest scandals of Reagan's presidency. Subsequent

## May the Least Unhealthy Candidate Win

Sometimes health becomes an issue for politicians before they even get near the White House. In 1972 George McGovern, the Democratic candidate for president running against incumbent Richard Nixon, selected Missouri Senator Thomas Eagleton as his vice presidential running mate. The Democratic ticket looked solid—until Eagleton told reporters that he had been hospitalized for "fatigue and nervous exhaustion" three times during the previous 12 years. His treatments for depression had included psychotherapy, chemotherapy, and electroconvulsive treatments. Predictably, the press went into overdrive with speculation about the mental stability of the man who might find himself, to use the cliché, a "heartbeat away from the presidency." McGovern initially stood by his vice-presidential choice, even as the cries for Eagleton's resignation grew louder. Within days, Eagleton voluntarily withdrew from the ticket.

In 1976 presidential hopeful Hubert Humphrey's admission that he was suffering from bladder cancer likely eliminated any chance that he would be considered. And during the 1992 presidential campaign, Massachusetts Senator Paul Tsongas, who had been treated for cancer, was forced to defend his health.

Some observers have argued that all presidential candidates should be screened. Political scientists Robert S. Robins and Henry Rothschild propose that a panel of three physicians be appointed by a bipartisan congressional committee to review the health of each nominee. "A full public disclosure would be made only if the panel deems that the candidate has a hidden medical disability that might jeopardize his decision-making ability," they note in a 1981 report. Unfortunately, a dozen years later, their proposal has not exactly caused a stampede of candidates presenting themselves for examination.

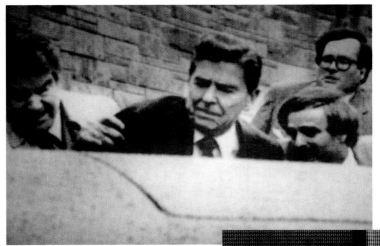

*The severity of President Reagan's condition following the 1981 assassination attempt (left) was not disclosed to the public at the time, although his cancer surgery four years later was well-publicized. Even in this atmosphere of greater candidness, most everyone found the lurid coverage of President Bush's nausea in Japan somewhat distasteful.*

inquiry into his administration's illegal arms sales to Iran suggests that the president, meeting with aides while still hospitalized, may have O.K.'d the arms-in-exchange-for-hostages deal while still suffering from lingering mental impairment caused by the anesthesia from his surgery.

There was one significant difference between Reagan's 1981 wounding and his 1985 cancer surgery: in the confusion after the shooting, the president's top aides refused to consider turning presidential power over to Vice President George Bush. Consequently, although Reagan's advisers were improvising behind the scenes, there was a period when essentially no one was in charge of the federal government. In 1985 Reagan formally signed over presidential power to Bush for the duration of the president's surgery. This act was carried out in accordance with the 25th Amendment to the U.S. Constitution, an amendment passed in 1967 in an attempt to solve thorny questions of succession following presidential death and disability. Bush was acting president for eight hours.

Bush himself would ascend to the White House in 1989, and would suffer his own health problems. In 1991 he was diagnosed with an irregular heartbeat know as arrhythmia, due to Graves' disease, a controllable disorder of the thyroid gland. During a presidential visit to Japan in 1992, an attack of gastroenteritis, an inflammation of the lining of the stomach and intestine, caused headlines, particularly as it involved Bush throwing up on Japanese Prime Minister Kiichi Miyazawa during a state dinner. There was also speculation about the president's intake of Halcion, a sleeping pill that has been known to cause adverse side effects.

In earlier times, such events may not even have become known to the public. Wilson and Roosevelt, for example, were able to conceal serious illness during crucial periods in history. Modern presidents, however, in this era of inexhaustible, 24-hour-a-day, scandal-hungry electronic news media, have no such luxury. As long as presidents are human, they will fall ill. As citizens, we can only look on, hoping for the president's good health, and the nation's.   ◇

# Housecalls

by Al Ciccone, M.D.

**Q** *My friend claims that she contracted a nail fungus while having a manicure. Is this possible? How is such a fungus treated?*

**A** Contracting a nail fungus in this way is not uncommon. It happens when manicurists don't properly sterilize their tools between clients.

The nail becomes discolored, and a crustiness forms around it. Although the infection is usually not painful, the nail can become disfigured.

Treatment for the infection can include vinegar soaks and over-the-counter antifungal creams. When those steps don't work, the individual may need an antifungal medication that actually enters the nail tissue bit by bit as it grows. The medication takes six to nine months to have its full effect on the fungus; unfortunately, such medications can also have side effects.

You should always inquire about the cleaning procedures your manicurist uses with manicure instruments. Placing the instruments in a sterile solution should prevent them from transmitting the fungus from one person to another. As a further preventive, you can soak your fingernails in vinegar a few times after the manicure. This should kill any residual fungus.

---

**Q** *I heard about the doctor on the talk show who mistakenly used the same needle to give flu vaccines to the two hosts. The first host injected was then tested for HIV, and the results were processed within hours. Do the results of an AIDS test really come back so soon?*

**A** Yes, they can, depending on which of two current tests the laboratory uses. These tests use different methods of detecting HIV (the human immunodeficiency virus, which causes AIDS).

The body's immune system produces antibodies to fight HIV. The ELISA test detects these antibodies. Doctors consider it a fairly specific and sensitive test. They use it as a quick screening step, and can easily get results within hours. If this test proves negative, then doctor and patient usually do not pursue further testing.

It is very important to bear in mind that three to six months can elapse between the time HIV infects a person and the time the ELISA test can detect antibodies to it in the blood.

If the ELISA is positive, then the test is repeated. If it is positive again, then the individual's blood is tested with a much more specific test called the Western Blot. This test detects proteins that actually make up the virus. The Western Blot takes longer, but if it is positive, doctors consider it a confirmation for their diagnosis.

---

**Q** *Is there any relationship between the sex of a baby and the point during the mother's menstrual cycle at which the child is conceived?*

**A** There does appear to be a slight relationship. Roughly equal numbers of sperm carry either a Y chromosome (which would result in a male child) or an X chromosome (which would result in a female child). But "male sperm" tend to swim a little faster than "female sperm," and they also die a little sooner. Thus, it is

*When a fungal infection is acquired through a manicure, the culprit is invariably instruments that have not been sterilized properly.*

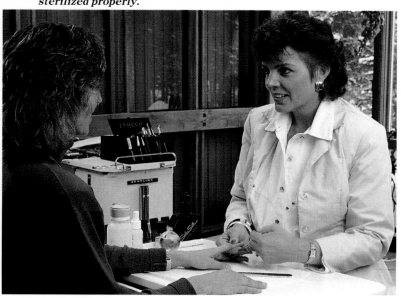

thought that if a couple has intercourse right around the time of ovulation, as the egg travels along the fallopian tube to the uterus, the woman's egg will be slightly more likely to encounter male sperm first. Conversely, if the couple has intercourse the day before ovulation, the egg is more likely to encounter a higher abundance of remaining "female sperm." Rough estimates conclude that a couple can be as much as 5 percent more likely to have a boy or a girl depending on when in the cycle conception occurs.

Consequently, some fertility specialists recommend to patients that, by carefully tracking the woman's menstrual cycle (through body temperature and other rhythm indicators) and having intercourse accordingly, they can *slightly* increase their chances of conceiving a boy or girl.

Fertility labs can take even greater advantage of this difference in sperm to offer "sex selection." By processing the man's sperm sample—using very specific steps that involve centrifuging and allowing the sperm to swim across a medium—they can artificially inseminate a woman with sperm that has an enhanced percentage of being either male or female sperm. The procedure is expensive, however, and only increases the couple's chances of having a baby of a chosen sex to about 60 to 70 percent.

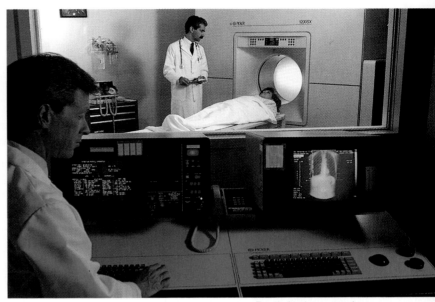

*Radiologists are physicians who specialize in the use of X rays, magnetic fields, sound waves, and radioactive compounds to produce diagnostic images and to treat various disorders.*

manipulate an organ or other structure. For instance, using percutaneous catheterization (threading tiny tubes through the skin and into the body) and X rays, interventional radiologists can open narrowed arteries in such areas as the kidneys and legs, remove gallstones, or deliver chemotherapy directly to tumors. Percutaneous techniques are less invasive, and therefore less traumatic, than surgery.

Q *Do radiologists actually see patients, or are they mostly concerned with interpreting X rays, ultrasounds, and other types of images?*

A With its many new technologies, radiology has become subdivided into a variety of areas. Some diagnostic radiologists do still primarily read X rays, and so rarely see a patient. Procedural radiologists, however, are with patients for various radiological steps of their care. For example, a radiologist subspecializing in computed tomography (CT) or magnetic resonance imaging (MRI) may assist in performing these studies on patients.

An even better example, with more direct patient care, is a growing area called interventional radiology. A new breed of radiologists in this field perform a host of different treatments, most of which require them to simultaneously image and

Q *What's the difference between registered nurses and licensed practical nurses? Why have nurses apparently abandoned their white uniforms? I was very confused about who was who when I was hospitalized recently.*

A Registered nurses (RNs) have either a four-year baccalaureate or two-year associate degree from a university or college, or a diploma from three years of training at a hospital. They have also passed their national nursing boards. They can provide complex care, direct others in providing care to patients, and make independent judgments and decisions for these duties. Most hospital nurses are RNs.

Licensed practical nurses (LPNs) have a high school diploma and one year of training, with an exam. They can provide care to patients with basic problems, give medication, and carry out treatments.

In the nursing field, there are nurses with more training than RNs or LPNs, such as nurses with master's and doctoral degrees who are administrators, supervisors, teachers, nurse-practitioners, or researchers. There are also those with less training, such as nursing assistants.

Hospitals have different dress codes for nurses, as do doctor's offices. There is no standard for uniforms, which in general came to be seen as old-fashioned in recent decades, especially since there was no requirement that doctors and many other types of health-care workers wear them. Wanting to seem current with the times, many universities, hospitals, and medical practices have eliminated the requirements for all or part of the uniforms.

Uniforms, do, however, help assure a presentable, clean appearance by nurses, enhance a sense of authority (like a doctor's white coat), and distinguish nurses from other types of medical-care workers. Eliminating them perhaps gives nurses a more relaxed work environment, disarms patients (especially pediatric and psychiatric patients), and takes emphasis away from the hierarchy of a hospital unit.

---

Q *Is testicular cancer common? Is there a recommended method of self-examination? How is someone with testicular cancer treated?*

A Testicular cancer is, unfortunately, a cancer of younger men. It is most often discovered in, and is the most common cancer among, males under the age of 30.

The primary sign is a lump or mass on the testicle that can range from the size of a pea to larger. There may also be fluid accumulation or enlargements in or around the testicle and scrotum, although such swelling may not necessarily occur until the cancer is advanced.

Any male under 30 should examine himself once a month. Hold the testicle between the thumb and first and second fingers and gently roll and manipulate it to feel around its entire surface. Bear in mind that the epididymis forms a natural protrusion at the back of the testicle. A testicular-cancer mass will feel distinct from the otherwise smooth testicle.

If you feel a lump, have it examined by a doctor, and don't jump to conclusions until you do. Benign cysts and small calcifica-

tions on and around testicles are not uncommon occurrences.

Medical teams can usually treat testicular cancer quite effectively. Except in cases of advanced disease, the cancer almost always affects just one of the testicles, which the surgeon must remove. The patient then undergoes several months of chemotherapy or radiation therapy or both.

Men who have undergone this treatment can have children and can otherwise lead normal lives.

---

Q *How do over-the-counter eyedrops that "remove the red" work? Is it dangerous to use them for extended periods of time?*

A The eyedrops treat irritation of the lining of the eyeball (the conjunctiva) caused by dust, smoke, chemicals, and fatigue. The conjunctiva can become inflamed and congested, and, as a result, blood vessels show through.

The eyedrops constrict and shrink the vessels, decreasing the redness. In most cases the active ingredient is tetrahydrozoline. The eyedrops are O.K. to use once in a while, or for two or three days, but if used every day, they will actually exacerbate the problem and increase redness.

---

Q *Whenever I get a cold, it seems to settle into my chest. Long after the other symptoms are gone, I find myself still coughing. Why is this?*

A A chest cold is caused by a viral infection, usually contracted through nasal tissue, that often works its way down to the bronchial tubes as well. Inflammation in the affected tissues helps the body fight off the infection, but brings on congestion from fluid secretion. When the infection is gone, the inside surface of the bronchial tubes is left with something much like an abrasion, which takes longer to heal and which continues the fluid secretion. The cough moves mucus out of the area as healing takes place and clears the airway.

---

*Do you have a practical question?*
Send it to Editor, Health and Medicine Annual, P.O. Box 90, Hawleyville, CT 06440-9990.

# Health and
# Medicine:
# Reports '94

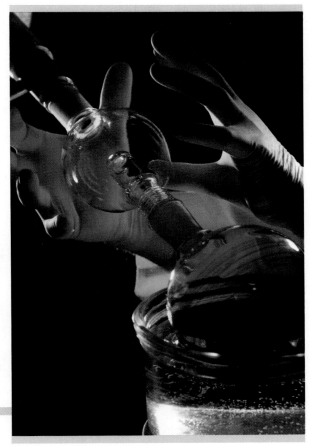

# Aging

## ▶ Alzheimer's Disease

In 1993 scientists made headway in discovering the cause of Alzheimer's disease, with several researchers proposing new theories. Approximately 4 million Americans have Alzheimer's, a degenerative neurological disease in which memory, judgment, and the ability to reason deteriorate progressively. There is no cure for the disease, and it is always fatal.

At Duke University Medical Center in Durham, North Carolina, researchers suggested that Alzheimer's may be caused by a defect in a gene responsible for the production of a cholesterol-carrying protein. In research presented at a symposium by the National Institute on Aging, Allen D. Roses, M.D., and Warren Strittmatter, M.D., explained that there are three forms of the apolipoprotein E gene: Apo-E2, Apo-E3, and Apo-E4. People who inherit the Apo-E4 gene from one or both parents have a two- to five-times greater risk of contracting Alzheimer's disease.

Roses and Strittmatter theorize that proteins produced in people with the Apo-E3 and Apo-E2 genes bind with *tau,* a protein in neurons. This prevents tau from damaging tiny channels in the axons and dendrites of brain cells, and ultimately prevents the collapse of these cells. Proteins produced by people with the Apo-E4 gene, however, do not bind with tau, so the brain cells gradually collapse. The scientists caution that their research is in preliminary stages, and that a genetic test for Alzheimer's is not yet feasible.

Another theory about the origin of Alzheimer's recently led to the development of a drug to treat the symptoms of the disease. In September 1993, the U.S. Food and Drug Administration (FDA) approved tacrine hydrochloride (Cognex), the first drug ever designed to specifically treat Alzheimer's disease.

"Tacrine is the first drug shown to have some effect on the disease's devastating symptoms," said David A. Kessler, M.D., the FDA commissioner. "It is not a cure, but it provides some relief. Tacrine briefly slows the progress of Alzheimer's in mild to moderate cases. Studies show that it will work for only about 40 percent of all patients."

Tacrine works by increasing levels of the neurotransmitter acetylcholine in the brain. Some researchers believe that low levels of acetylcholine lead to a buildup of a protein called beta amyloid. Beta amyloid, in turn, may allow too much calcium through the membranes of brain cells, which has the effect of killing the cells.

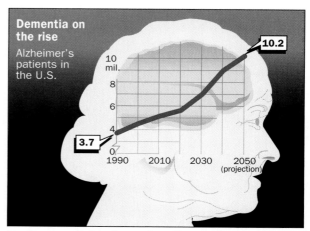

**Dementia on the rise**
Alzheimer's patients in the U.S.

*Much research has focused on discovering the cause of—and a cure for—Alzheimer's disease. Without a cure, the incidence of Alzheimer's is likely to rise dramatically over the next 50 years.*

Interestingly, Dr. Roses of Duke University disagrees with this theory. He believes that the buildup of beta amyloid is a side effect of Alzheimer's, rather than the cause of the disease.

Finally, scientists at the National Institute of Neurological Disorders and Stroke took the first step toward developing an Alzheimer's skin test that investigates ion channels, which are involved in the process of forming memories. In preliminary results reported in the *Proceedings of the National Academy of Sciences,* Daniel L. Alkon, M.D., and colleagues described a test that searched for closed potassium channels in skin cells.

Research shows that in people with Alzheimer's, "gates" in cell membranes that regulate the flow of potassium ions close up. When Alkon tested cells from the skin and nose of Alzheimer's patients, he found that potassium channels in those cells were also closed.

Currently there is no specific test for Alzheimer's. Generally the disease is diagnosed only after all other causes of dementia—such as stroke—are eliminated. Sometimes Alzheimer's is diagnosed only through an autopsy.

## ▶ Health of the Elderly Improving

As America heads toward an unprecedented increase in the number of elderly in society, researchers have come up with good news: More older Americans are in good health today than ever before in our history.

There are currently 31 million people in this country over age 65, according to the U.S. Census Bureau. Three million of those senior citizens are age 80 or older. But as the baby boomers—those people born between the years 1945 and 1965—continue to age, that number is expected to skyrocket.

By the year 2000, 4.6 million Americans will be over age 80; by 2040, 12.3 million; and by 2050, 15.3 million—five times the number of octogenarians currently alive.

As reported in *Gerontologist* and *Journal of Gerontology,* the researchers found that the number of older Americans classified as "nondisabled" increased 16.3 percent between 1989 and 1992. This trend toward better health occurred even though the population of elderly increased 14.7 percent during those same years.

Kenneth Manton, Ph.D., Larry Corder, Ph.D., and Eric Stallard based their findings on data gathered three times over seven years by the National Long-Term Survey of the Health and Human Services Department. They estimated the disability rate by counting the number of daily activities subjects could complete independently. Activities included such relatively routine things as bathing, dressing, eating, cooking, and shopping, as well as managing finances. "For just about every activity, there was a decline in disability rates," the study concludes.

The researchers also found that fewer elderly people are relying on personal assistance to cope with the daily tasks of living. Instead, people are turning more toward mechanical aids such as tub stools and special seats in the shower.

Two possible explanations for the decreasing disability rate are medical advances such as cataract surgery and joint replacement, and increasing education levels. Studies show that higher levels of education lead to higher incomes and, in turn, better nutrition and health.

## ▶ Breast Cancer and Aging

A study from the University of California, San Francisco (UCSF), suggests that women over age 50 stand to benefit the most from mammography. The study supports this year's controversial decision by the National Cancer Institute (NCI) to recommend routine mammograms only for women over 50.

As reported in the *Journal of the American Medical Association,* Karla Kerlikowske, M.D., Deborah Grade, M.D., M.P.H., and Virginia Ernster, Ph.D., studied the results of 31,814 women age 30 and up who were referred to UCSF's Mobile Mammography Screening Program from April 1985 to November 1992. The screening program offers low-cost mammograms to women of all ethnic backgrounds in six counties in northern California. Women with a history of breast cancer, those who had had a mastectomy, or those who had had a lump in their breasts were excluded from the study.

The researchers found that mammography had a positive predictive value for women age 50 and up. That is, mammograms were more likely to detect cancer among this group of women. "Although

women aged 50 years or older constituted only 38.3 percent of all women who received first-screening mammography, 74 percent of breast cancers were detected in this group," the study notes.

In fact, for every 1,000 women in the study, five times as many cancers were diagnosed in the 50- and-older group than in the younger subjects. Mammograms also had a positive predictive value in women age 40 and up with a family history of breast cancer.

The study backs up the recommendation by almost all experts that women age 50 and older should undergo regular mammograms. Among women in this age group, the researchers note, mammography "has been shown to reduce mortality from breast cancer by 20 percent to 30 percent."

Finally, the study notes that mammography was not as clearly beneficial for women younger than 50 who do not have a family history of breast cancer. For these women the results of 50 out of every 1,000 mammograms will require further additional diagnostic procedures. One in 50 of those further evaluations will reveal breast cancer, and another 1 in 50 will reveal a generally noninvasive tumor. Among women older than 50, 70 out of 1,000 mammograms will require follow-up; of those, 10 cancers will be detected.

## ▶ Vitamin Deficiencies

Deficiencies of vitamins $B_{12}$, $B_6$, and folate may be common among the elderly, according to a study in the *American Journal of Clinical Nutrition.*

Scientists from Belgium, Germany, New York City, and Denver collaborated on a study that measured blood levels of metabolites of these vitamins in 99 healthy subjects, 64 healthy elderly subjects, and 286 hospitalized elderly subjects. Metabolites of the vitamins appear in the blood when the enzyme reaction that allows the body to use the vitamins is not functioning correctly.

Although previous studies have found low blood levels of $B_{12}$, $B_6$, and folate in older people, those studies did not determine whether the low blood levels actually represented a vitamin deficiency. The researchers found that both the healthy and the hospitalized elderly subjects had low serum levels of the vitamins as well as elevated levels of the metabolites.

"These results strongly suggest that there is a higher prevalence of vitamin deficiency than could have been estimated by measuring serum concentrations of the vitamins," the study concludes. Moreover, the researchers note, elevated metabolite concentrations may play a role in both atherosclerosis and neuropsychiatric disorders. As a result the researchers urge that elderly people be screened for $B_{12}$, $B_6$, and folate deficiencies.

*Devera Pine*

# AIDS

There were few new or startling developments in AIDS research during 1993. Ever increasing numbers of people around the world have become infected with the causative retrovirus, human immunodeficiency virus-Type 1 (HIV-1). The disease, acquired immune deficiency syndrome (AIDS), continues to grind the life out of victim after victim on every continent of the world. Central Africa has been particularly hard hit, but the disease is also spreading rapidly in India, Southeast Asia, and South America.

## ▶ The International Situation

**The International AIDS Conference in Berlin.** Those who attended the annual international AIDS conference in 1993 were discouraged by the general lack of success in developing drugs for the treatment of AIDS or in developing vaccines for its prevention. In fact, the general atmosphere at the conference was one of pessimism among the world experts regarding control of the AIDS pandemic. The World Health Organization (WHO) has predicted that there will be approximately 30 million HIV-infected persons in the world by the year 2000, and few expect there to be an effective vaccine or therapy by then. Furthermore, new research shows that people can be infected with strains of HIV that have already gained resistance to the only FDA-approved AIDS drug, azidothymidine (AZT), and other drugs.

The tragedy of this pessimism is that we do know how to prevent the disease: avoid promiscuous sexual behavior, both heterosexual and homosexual; avoid sharing intravenous needles; and use condoms for all sexual activities outside of a stable relationship in which both partners are known to be HIV-negative. People seem unwilling to follow these guidelines, even when they are quite aware of the dangers. The pessimism, therefore, is as much due to the failures of human nature as it is due to the failures of laboratory science.

**AIDS in Central Africa.** Of the estimated 14 million people infected with HIV worldwide, approximately 8 million are in Africa; of those 8 million, one-quarter have developed AIDS. Unlike in the industrialized nations, most of the HIV transmission in Africa is through heterosexual sex, and there are approximately equal numbers of men and women infected.

In Uganda, the hardest-hit African country, approximately 10 percent or more of the population is already infected, and the spread of the virus there continues to be rapid. (By comparison, in the United States, about one-third of 1 percent of the population is HIV-positive, making the Ugandan rate more than 20 times as high as that in the United States.) Many observers claim that Uganda may ultimately lose most of its population to AIDS, despite considerable efforts by the government to control the

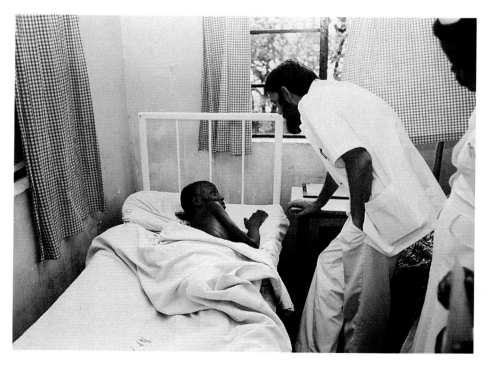

*The Central African countries have been particularly hard hit by the AIDS epidemic. In Tanzania (right), Uganda, and elsewhere in Africa, the AIDS virus is transmitted primarily through heterosexual contact, and an approximately equal number of men and women are infected.*

spread of the disease. In many families, both parents have now died from AIDS and its opportunistic infections, and older children are trying to keep the family together and earn a living.

**HIV-infected Blood in Germany.** At least six cases of HIV infection in Europe since 1989 are suspected to have been caused by contaminated blood from two German companies. The culprits, UB Plasma of Koblenz and the Haemoplas Company of Osterode, apparently sold HIV-contaminated blood or blood products. Both companies were accused of failing to test all their units of blood for antibodies to HIV, as required by law. UB Plasma, for example, was said to have tested only about one-fourth of its blood; Haemoplas apparently tested only the first unit of blood from a commercial donor (one who gets paid for donating blood), but not subsequent units from the same donor, despite the fact that a donor may have become infected with HIV subsequent to his or her first donation. All existing units of blood and blood products from these companies have been banned from use. People worried about possible exposure are eligible for free blood tests to check for HIV antibodies.

This situation has caused a public-health and political crisis in Germany, given the fact that an estimated 15 million units of blood or blood products were distributed by these two companies. In Germany the responsibility to check blood for HIV and other infections belongs to the private companies that collect and distribute blood. There is some evidence, however, that the government health ministry did not follow up on earlier reports that these companies were distributing HIV-positive blood. The political ramifications of the blood scandal are serious, and the German government has launched a full-scale investigation. There is growing pressure to put blood collection and distribution into public hands, but such a move might not be the solution. France, which has a public system, had a similar blood scandal in 1992, indicating that government control does not always guarantee safety.

**Central and Eastern Europe.** Many nations have claimed that they had little homosexuality and intravenous drug use, and therefore are safe from AIDS. Such countries have apparently ignored the fact that the most serious AIDS outbreaks in the world are due to heterosexual sex with an infected person, especially prostitution and other forms of heterosexual promiscuity. As the economies of Central and Eastern Europe struggle, more and more young women have turned to prostitution as a way to earn a living. With prostitution comes a vehicle for the rapid spread of HIV infection. AIDS experts at WHO fear that these sexual practices, and the widespread attitudes of nonchalance, will guarantee a rapid spread of HIV in these countries over the next few years.

**Brazil.** Public-health officials in Brazil are convinced that Latin America's AIDS epidemic is well on its way to becoming more serious than that in the United States. It is also likely to be different from the U.S. outbreak, because most cases are due to heterosexual activity without protection, rather than to intravenous drug use or male homosexual practices. Therefore, as in central Africa, approximately as many women as men are infected. (It should be noted that in the more prosperous areas of Latin America, such as Buenos Aires, the majority of the cases, as in the United States, are transmitted by homosexual sex or intravenous drug use.)

It is a sad commentary that the only Latin American nation that apparently has been able to stem the tide of HIV infection has been the totalitarian state of Cuba. Religious groups in Latin America have opposed programs that promote condom use, which has interfered with some of the planned educational efforts there. On the other hand, condom use has not been shown to be very effective on a population basis, although it has been effective within isolated groups with good discipline, such as some prostitution organizations.

Brazil, with only 60 percent of the population of the United States, is estimated to have as many HIV-infected individuals (about 1 million) as the United States. In some areas of Brazil, as many as 1 pregnant woman in 40 is HIV-positive. HIV infection rates are high elsewhere in Latin America, especially in Argentina, Mexico, Colombia, and Haiti.

**China.** The world's most-populous nation, with one-fifth of Earth's people, China also has had a world-class scandal centered on hypodermic needles and syringes that were washed and resold as new without being sterilized. Apparently, some people acquired dangerous infections from these needles and syringes when the equipment was not sterilized by the buyers. The infections reported so far were not due to HIV, and it is not known if any persons were infected with HIV by this means. China claims to have fewer than 1,000 HIV-infected people altogether, which, if true, would be a very low rate. Not much is known about this outbreak, however, because the leaders have not been very forthcoming about the extent of the investigation or the findings to date.

## ▶ The U.S. Situation

**AIDS Deaths Reach New High.** It was announced late in 1993 that in 1992 AIDS was the leading killer of young men (ages 25 to 44 years old)

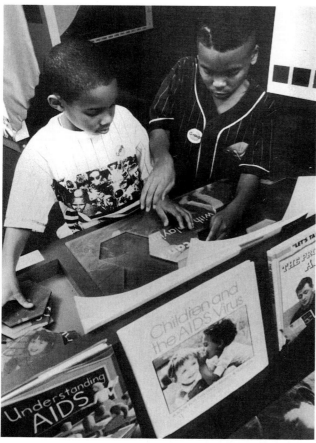

*A hands-on traveling exhibit called "What About AIDS?" is intended to educate children about the disease and the ways in which it can be avoided.*

In 1992 AIDS was the second-leading cause of death in black women 25 to 44 years old (16.5 percent of deaths), and was sixth for white women in this age range (3.8 percent of deaths). Although the proportion of all deaths due to AIDS is lower in women than in men, the AIDS death rate for black women was 12 times as high as that for white women. For Hispanics, data were available only from 1991, when AIDS was the leading cause of death for Hispanic men in the 25-to-44 age range (24.1 percent of deaths), and the third leading cause of death among Hispanic women (12.4 percent of deaths.) Therefore, AIDS is very serious for all racial groups, and is especially worrisome for some minorities in the United States. (See also the article beginning on page 50.)

**How Many Are Infected in the United States?**
The first nationwide survey to determine the level of HIV infection in a scientifically valid sample found that about one-third of 1 percent of the population in the survey was infected, or about 550,000 people in the United States. The survey did not include prisoners, those in hospitals or nursing homes, or the homeless, so this statistic is probably somewhat low. For years the Centers for Disease Control and Prevention (CDC) has estimated that about 1 million persons were infected with HIV. This survey suggests that, if the original estimate is correct, more people are dying of AIDS than are becoming infected. Taking into account the statistical margin of error, the number of HIV-infected Americans may range anywhere from 300,000 to about 1 million. Thus, the original CDC estimate may be in the realm of possibility, but many now believe it was high. Approximately 400,000 AIDS cases have developed so far in the United States, and about half of the victims have died.

**New Approach to AIDS Prevention: Spermicides.** WHO, discouraged by the general lack of success of its strategy of promoting the prevention of HIV infection through the use of condoms, and by the lack of progress toward a vaccine or a cure for AIDS, has decided to move in a different direction. The organization is now supporting and encouraging the development of a foam or gel that a woman could use before sexual intercourse. This would give women more ability to protect themselves and control their lives, even when their partners are not inclined to cooperate by using condoms. There is no ideal vaginal microbicide available yet, but WHO is shifting some research money toward developing one, and it is encouraging other organizations to do the same. The main substance now being tested is nonoxynol-9, which has been demonstrated to be effective against gonorrhea and chlamydia. In some studies of prostitutes in Africa, use of the spermi-

in the United States. This was due both to a rise in deaths due to AIDS and to a fall in the deaths due to unintentional injuries, although the biggest change occurred in AIDS. Looking at these data in another way, 73 percent of all AIDS deaths in males occurred in the 25-to-44 age range, with 2 percent of AIDS deaths occurring in those younger than that range and 25 percent of the AIDS fatalities occurring in males older than 44.

Considering these data by race, AIDS was the leading cause of death for blacks in this age range in 1991 and 1992, causing 25.3 percent of deaths; in the same age group, AIDS was the second-leading cause for whites in 1992 (18.5 percent of deaths); for all men considered together, AIDS emerged as the leading cause of death in 1992. The actual AIDS death rate was more than three times as high for black men as for white men, although it may not be obvious from the above statistics on the proportions of all deaths, because the overall death rate for blacks in this age range is much higher than it is for whites.

cide produced mixed results in terms of reducing the spread of HIV.

**Child-to-Child Transfer of HIV.** Two cases of the spread of HIV-1 infection from child to child (without needles) have frightened many people, who now fear that living together with someone with HIV infection is dangerous. However, in these cases the basic principles of AIDS prevention, as recommended by the CDC, were violated. The evidence is still strong that noninfected persons can live safely in the same household with an HIV-infected individual without danger, if due care is taken.

One of the cases involved an HIV-positive toddler with a tendency to bleed from the nose and elsewhere. In the same household lived a noninfected toddler who was suffering from dermatitis. The two toddlers apparently sometimes bit each other, and they also shared a toothbrush.

The other case involved two hemophiliac brothers, one of whom was HIV-positive. An exchange of blood apparently occurred while the infected brother was showing the other boy how to shave. Presumably, small cuts occurred when the infected boy shaved, causing blood to get on the razor. The blood was then introduced into the other's bloodstream when he cut himself with the same razor.

Both stories demonstrate violation of federal guidelines on preventing the transmission of HIV. The razor episode clearly violates the guidelines because of the significant potential for transmission. In the other episode, allowing one toddler such close contact with an HIV-positive child who bled and had open sores also should have been avoided. But what about households in which someone is HIV-positive, but no one knows? The basic rules include: avoiding blood contact; cleaning up any blood spills in the approved way; and covering any open sores. These commonsense guidelines should be practiced as a matter of course in every household, whether or not HIV infection is known.

These cases do not indicate that casual exposure has become dangerous. They do show that when blood is spilled, even though the amount is small, danger is present, at least to some degree. Neither of the above contacts is considered "casual," because blood was spilled from an HIV-positive individual. To date, almost 5,000 AIDS cases have been reported among children, and, in all but five, the infection was traced to an infected mother or to exposure to infected blood at the time of birth.

**More HIV-infected Patients from the Florida Dentist.** David Acer, D.D.S., a Florida dentist who died of AIDS, apparently transmitted the virus to at least six of his patients. The sixth of these, a young woman, was diagnosed in 1993 from a blood test performed as part of the military-enlistment process. (Although previously urged to have a blood test, the young woman had decided not to do so prior to her efforts to join the military.) Especially puzzling is the fact that this patient had not had any invasive procedures that would have caused bleeding. One of the six patients Dr. Acer apparently infected, Kimberly Bergalis, died of AIDS in 1991; in early 1994, another one of Dr. Acer's patients died of AIDS.

Dr. Acer is the only health-care professional known to have transmitted the virus to patients, despite the fact that an unknown number of health professionals are HIV-positive. Even so, the six infected people whose only HIV contact was Dr. Acer should be compared to the approximately 1,100 of his patients who have tested negative. Why, of all health-care professionals, only Dr. Acer should have transmitted the virus to his patients is simply unknown.

**Debate on AZT.** A major European study compared two similar groups of HIV-infected persons and the effectiveness of AZT in delaying the onset of AIDS symptoms. One group of subjects was given the anti-AIDS drug AZT while they were still symptom-free. In the other group, physicians waited for symptoms of AIDS to develop before the subjects were given AZT. In a surprising twist, the time from entry into the study to death was similar in both groups. However, a new study by a European-Australian collaboration found that the use of AZT in the asymptomatic period reduced the probability of developing symptoms during the study period by 50 percent; these findings are similar to those of previous U.S. trials. These contradictory studies make it difficult to know whom to

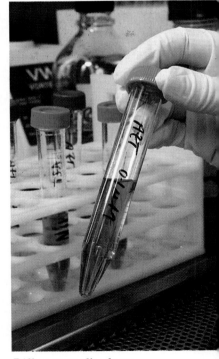

*Different studies have produced different results regarding the effectiveness of AZT in fighting the symptoms of AIDS.*

believe in AIDS research at the present time. The usual answer—which is true, but not very satisfying —is what's been heard many times over with regard to the AIDS epidemic: more research is needed.

*James F. Jekel, M.D., M.P.H.*

# Anesthesiology

With more than 25 million surgical procedures performed each year in the United States alone, anesthesia has taken on growing importance in modern medical care. In fact, anesthesia often plays a significant role in defining surgical procedures.

## ▶ Cancer Pain

The traditional focus of anesthesiology has been the control of pain and vital-organ functions during surgery. Now principles of anesthesia are increasingly being applied to chronic-pain management. In 1993 significant progress was made in controlling neuropathic pain, an especially painful syndrome associated with cancer. Morphine, the standard medication for cancer pain, can produce severe side effects, and sometimes is ineffective even at high doses. The only recourse in such cases may be to sever nerves to stop the pain, but this drastic measure can lead to the loss of sensation, and even paralysis.

Promising new research involves clonidine, a drug originally developed to treat high blood pressure. Early findings indicate that clonidine and other members of a class of drugs called alpha 2 agonists can reduce pain by stimulating the brain to release serotonin. Serotonin, a type of substance called a neurotransmitter, is naturally produced by the body to control pain and to perform other functions.

## ▶ New Use for Morphine

Despite promising research in other directions, morphine will nonetheless likely remain one of the mainstays of pain management. In 1993 researchers identified another positive use for morphine—as an effective local anesthetic for a debilitative condition called frozen shoulder. This condition is characterized by the development of small adhesions in the shoulder that curtail and eventually prevent movement. The only treatment is the manipulation of the shoulder, an enormously painful therapy. Studies have shown that locally administered morphine, an application called peripheral analgesia, can contain the pain of frozen shoulder during manipulation. The treatment is another example of the recent discovery that morphine can control pain outside the brain, suggesting that the undesirable effects associated with narcotics can be avoided for other conditions involving the joints.

## ▶ Anesthesia and Surgery

Other important developments in anesthesiology during the past year are related to its effectiveness as an adjunct to surgery, particularly in terms of patient safety and comfort.

The fear of awakening during an operation is one of the most common anxieties suffered by pre-surgery patients. While physicians are well equipped to monitor the heart, blood-circulation, and breathing functions, they have long been limited in their capacity to determine the level of awareness of patients under anesthesia. To avoid the trauma that can be associated with awakening during surgery, researchers led by G. N. C. Kenny, M.D., from the Glasgow Royal Infirmary in Scotland have focused on the auditory-evoked response, a process of measuring the brain's response to sound. Experiments have been conducted by placing earphones on patients during anesthesia and playing a recorded clicking sound. By comparing brain activity in response to the sound during unanesthetized and anesthetized states, a measurement reference point of the patient's awareness can be established. Methods for automatically administering anesthetics based on the monitoring are being tested.

By the same token, awakening from anesthesia at the appropriate time is also desirable. A timely return to consciousness helps permit patients to return home and begin the recovery process as early as possible. During the past year, Leonard Firestone, M.D., from the Department of Anesthesiology at the University of Pittsburgh has discovered a new class of drugs that can almost instantly reverse the effects of an anesthetic. Such drugs, known as anti-anesthetic monoclonal antibodies, can be tailored to reverse specific anesthetics. Thus far the research has been limited to animal subjects.

*Robert Laufer*

## A Theory of Pain Control

New government guidelines on pain relief after surgery say that it is not sufficient to give medication "as needed," or only after the patient complains. Researchers say that when doses are scheduled to prevent the onset of pain, both the time spent in pain and the levels of side effects decrease.

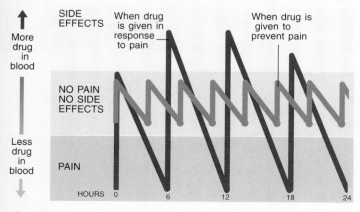

Source: *Scientific American*

# Arthritis and Rheumatism

Rheumatoid arthritis (RA) is a reaction by the body's immune or defense system triggered by an unknown stimulus. RA results in inflammation and thickening of the joint lining or synovial membrane. The inflamed joint lining invades and damages bone and cartilage. The joint loses its shape and alignment, causing pain, loss of mobility, and eventually complete destruction of the joint. The relationship of RA to the human lymphocyte antigen system (HLA), a group of genes regulating the immune response, has been recognized since 1978. This association is now recognized to actually be with a specific HLA antigen that is inherited by most patients with RA. HLA antigens are proteins on the surface of cells that are highly individualized from person to person. Scientists thus have a clearer understanding than ever before of the contribution of genetic factors to the development and severity of rheumatoid arthritis.

A paper published in the *Annals of Internal Medicine* by Cornelia M. Weyand and associates from the Mayo Clinic, Rochester, Minnesota, shows that the presence of this inherited antigen determines both the likelihood of developing rheumatoid arthritis and its degree of severity. Individuals inherit two HLA genes, one from each parent. When both of those genes specify the antigen associated with rheumatoid arthritis, severe disease is likely to develop. Those individuals with only one gene possessing this antigen are susceptible to rheumatoid arthritis, but have a lesser risk of developing severe disease. Some of the genes that specify the antigen may be associated with still-milder disease. An editorial accompanying this report suggests that analysis of HLA genes can be used to identify patients at high risk for the development of severe RA. This might permit early recognition of patients who warrant more-aggressive treatment. Further studies are needed to test this hypothesis.

## ▶ RA and Pregnancy

The HLA antigen may also be the key to why symptoms of RA abate during pregnancy. A study published in the August 12, 1993, issue of the *New England Journal of Medicine* analyzed 46 pregnancies in 38 women with RA. The researchers compared women whose arthritis improved during pregnancy with women whose arthritis remained active. The study found that in 76 percent of the women whose arthritis went away or improved, the change for the better resulted from genetic differences between the fetus and the mother—differences that triggered maternal immune responses that ameliorate arthritic symptoms. While the exact nature of the process is unknown, researchers hypothesize that some element of the mother's immune response is affected by the presence of a different HLA antigen in the fetus. The mother's body may view this HLA material as foreign matter and implement a modified antibody response. Or certain molecules from the fetus may compete or displace the mother's molecules at a specific stage in the immune response that had previously produced RA symptoms, causing a different reaction that no longer induces RA disease. Whatever the reason, these findings will help researchers explore new drug therapies for RA, including immunization.

## ▶ Implants and Rheumatic Disease

Since 1964 more than 100 patients have been reported with either a specific rheumatic disease or an undifferentiated immune-system disorder thought to be related to a cosmetic implant. In 1992 the Food and Drug Administration (FDA) restricted the use of silicone implants because of inadequate safety data, although the risk of implant-induced rheumatic disease has never been proven. To date, there have been no epidemiological studies employing an accurate database for the population at risk and an appropriate control group that accurately determines whether the incidence of specific rheumatic disorders is greater in patients who have received implants. Small controlled studies have failed to establish an association.

Two articles and a case report in the June 15, 1993, issue of the *Annals of Internal Medicine* add to the growing controversy over the safety of implants. A study by Alan J. Bridges and colleagues evaluated the findings in 156 women with silicone implants who were referred to rheumatologists because of rheumatic-disease symptoms. These women were compared to 174 women with fibromyalgia (muscle pain) without implants, and 12 women with silicone implants and no rheumatic disease. Most of the 156 referred patients were found to have no evidence of a significant rheumatic disease; none had rheumatoid arthritis. However, two unusual disease patterns were noted. Fourteen patients had a sclerodermalike illness with some distinctive features including a lower-than-usual incidence of Raynaud's phenomenon. Another group of patients had an asymmetrical, nonerosive arthritis without systemic signs of inflammation. These unusual patterns of disease suggest that they may be rare immunologic reactions to silicone implants.

Another study by Jean Cukier and associates reports that during an eight-year period in which 345,000 patients received injectable-collagen implants, eight of them developed polymyositis, a rare disease in which the muscles become inflamed and weak. This represents an increase in incidence compared to that expected in the general population. The authors suggest that an immunologic response to bovine collagen may be the cause of these cases of polymyositis.

An editorial accompanying these two papers notes that neither study establishes an association between implants and rheumatic disease. However, these reports suggest that there may be an increased incidence of atypical or uncommon rheumatic syndromes that small studies like the ones noted here lack the breadth to detect. Data from carefully designed epidemiological studies are essential for appropriate evaluation of the risk associated with implants.

## ▶ Stress and Rheumatic Disease

Anecdotal reports have often associated the onset or flare-ups of rheumatoid arthritis and other rheumatic diseases with various forms of stress. Until recently there was no strong scientific basis for such an association. Several recent papers and reviews have highlighted the growing knowledge linking stress and the immune system. The proceedings of a National Institutes of Health (NIH) conference published in the *Annals of Internal Medicine* this past year reviewed some features of this delicate relationship.

Corticotropin-releasing hormone (CRH), a hormone that increases corticosteroid secretion, and the beta-adrenergic hormones, epinephrine and norepinephrine, are released in response to stress. These hormones have mutually reinforcing effects that prepare the body for dealing with stress. CRH has recently been identified as a cause of inflammation. A counterbalancing cycle works through CRH stimulation of ACTH (adrenocorticotropic hormone), which stimulates adrenal corticosteroid release. Corticosteroids, in turn, are anti-inflammatory and suppress CRH secretion. Inflammatory mediators and cytokines released from inflammatory cells can activate this system by stimulating production of CRH.

Imbalances in this hormonal cycle could contribute to susceptibility to rheumatic disease and alter clinical response to corticosteroids. Corticosteroid release may be decreased in rheumatoid arthritis relative to the continued stress from the inflammatory disease. This could explain the clinical benefit from small doses of corticosteroids in rheumatoid arthritis. Furthermore, there is recent evidence that corticosteroid breakdown is accelerated in systemic lupus erythematosus (SLE). Large doses of corticosteroids are typically required to suppress the immune reaction in SLE.

*Herbert S. Diamond, M.D.*

# Blood and Lymphatic System

## ▶ Hemophilia

Progress was made by researchers at the University of North Carolina in Chapel Hill and at Baylor College of Medicine in Houston, Texas, toward correcting a deficiency in a blood-clotting factor that affects about 15 percent of hemophiliacs. Advances in this arena may point the way to treatments for the remaining majority of persons afflicted with this hereditary bleeding disease. Currently, treatment is extremely expensive and has the potential—however small—for contagion with blood-borne infections like AIDS or hepatitis, since hemophiliacs are transfused with human-blood products. Moreover, the treatment is not a cure.

The promising research involves genetic production of a substance called factor IX, one of the critical proteins necessary for blood clotting. Experiments

## Silicone and Rejection: A Theory

**Over time, an implant leaks tiny droplets of silicone, which travel to distant tissues.**

Blood tests that seek to determine whether a breast implant is leaking silicone are based on the immune system's escalating warfare on foreign proteins. Some researchers say silicone collects proteins that sets off the rejection process.

**FIRST STAGE**

Proteins coat the sticky, oily droplets, which are soon sought out by macrophages, immune system scavenger cells designed to devour intruders.

**SECOND STAGE**

After the macrophage attack has gone on for some time, immune system reserves are called in, causing fever, inflammation, and scarring.

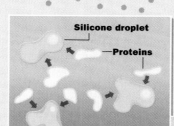

**THIRD AND FOURTH STAGES**

Deformed proteins invite a more vigorous attack, including antibody formation. In some people, the attack becomes chronic, and is directed at the body's normal proteins, too.

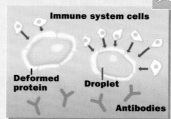

Source: Dr. Nir Kossovsky

so far have been restricted to animal subjects, but the ability of genetically engineered factor IX to halve clotting time in tests on dogs is encouraging. Many concerns will have to be resolved before gene therapy can be used for hemophiliacs. For example, the clotting factor would have to be introduced into the livers of hemophiliacs at a very young age, thereby subjecting them to the risks of a serious surgical procedure.

## ▶ Lymphoma

In developments involving the lymphatic system, advances were recorded in combating lymphomas, which are malignancies of the lymph glands. Encouraging research involved both types of lymphomas, Hodgkin's disease and non-Hodgkin's type.

Continuing research by the British National Lymphoma Investigation suggests positive outcomes when high-dose chemotherapy and autologous bone-marrow transplantation are combined for individuals with relapsed and resistant Hodgkin's disease. One study involved 40 patients, half of whom were treated with the combination therapy, and the other half with low drug doses and no transplantation. Survival rates among the former group were significantly higher than among the latter.

In non-Hodgkin's lymphoma, recent research has focused on, among other things, the bcl-2 gene. A protein produced by this gene appears to be closely associated with a form of cell destruction known as apoptosis. Not only does the bcl-2 gene prolong cell life, it is also involved in the interaction of chemotherapy drugs and their effect on tumor cells.

Other research on leukemia disorders, of which lymphoma is one type, includes the positive effects of all-trans-retinoic acid. This substance appears to convert leukemia cells into ones that age and die normally. Scientists are also examining umbilical and placental blood as a potential medium for transplanting healthy cells into a patient's system.

## ▶ Rheumatoid Arthritis

A theory further developed in 1993 focused on the role of colony-stimulating factors in rheumatoid arthritis. Produced by monocytes (one of the five types of white blood cells in the blood), colony-stimulating factors act to promote maturation of cells in the immune system. In victims of rheumatoid arthritis, a chronic inflammatory disease of the joints, the ability of colony-stimulating factors to accurately recognize cells may be impaired.

Individuals with rheumatoid arthritis may have excessive interaction of colony-stimulating factors, causing inflammation of the joints. Blocking this sequence of activity in the body's blood-making network may be possible with anti-rheumatoid medication that purposely acts slowly.

*Robert Laufer*

# Bones, Muscles, and Joints

## ▶ Osteoporosis

A new study suggests that the most important risk factors for osteoporosis are age, weight, muscle strength, and estrogen use.

Most bone fractures in elderly women are associated with low bone mass in the forearms and heels, according to the study, which was published in *Annals of Internal Medicine* in 1993. However, despite the strong association between the bone mass of the arms and legs and the risk of a fracture, there is "little consensus about the many proposed risk factors for decreased bone mass."

The study, conducted by the Osteoporotic Fractures Research Group, followed 9,704 women age 65 and older around the country. For each woman the researchers collected detailed information about smoking, alcohol use, caffeine intake, medication use, diet, exercise, weight, and other factors thought to put a woman at risk for the development of osteoporosis.

Age has a negative effect on bone mass, the researchers found, with every five years of age after 65 resulting in a 5 percent loss of bone mass among the subjects. On the other hand, as both weight and muscle strength increase, so does bone mass. Moreover, every five years of estrogen use is associated with an increase in bone mass.

To date, this is the largest and most comprehensive cross-sectional study of the factors involved in bone mass in older women, the researchers note. As a result, some of the findings are surprising. For instance, weight loss after age 50 is associated with a decrease in bone mass.

Furthermore, the correlation between dietary calcium intake and bone mass is inconsistent. However, the researchers did find that women between ages 18 and 50 who had milk with every meal had a bone mass 3.1 percent higher than women who had not had milk regularly during those years.

Pregnancy, breast-feeding, calcium supplements, alcohol use, and physical activity do not have a statistically significant association with the bone mass of the limbs, according to the study. And, contrary to popular belief, fair-haired women and women with a northern European background do not have lower bone mass, the study says.

"Our findings indicate that, with the exception of a few factors strongly associated with bone mass, most of the individual risk factors we examined do not significantly alter the overall risk for fracture," the study concludes.

In the meantime, other researchers continue to search for treatments for osteoporosis. At Israel's Tel Aviv University Sackler School of Medicine, for instance, researchers are preventing, and sometimes reversing, bone loss with magnesium supplements.

Among 31 women who took 250 to 750 milligrams (mg) of magnesium daily for two years, 75 percent increased the density of their bones anywhere from 1 to 8 percent, according to Gustawa Stendig-Lindberg, M.D. Dr. Stendig-Lindberg speculates that magnesium helps transport calcium to cells, but adds that further research is needed.

## ▶ Muscle Soreness

The over-the-counter (OTC) pain reliever ibuprofen can significantly reduce muscle soreness associated with working out, a study from the University of Texas in Galveston shows.

Researchers at the university put 20 subjects through a bench-stepping-with-weights workout that was specifically designed to induce delayed-onset muscle soreness—soreness that develops 10 to 12 hours after exercising. One group of exercis-

*Hip implants used to wear out after about 10 years. But advanced technology has added years to these implants, making them suitable for younger patients like baseball great Bo Jackson.*

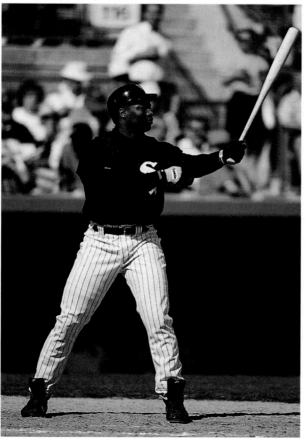

ers took three 400-mg doses of ibuprofen (equivalent to two OTC tablets), starting four hours before they worked out and continuing for the next 24 hours. A second group took a placebo before they worked out and ibuprofen afterward. Another group took placebos before and after exercising, and a fourth, control, group took nothing.

Twenty-four hours later, the exercisers who had taken ibuprofen before and after exercising were only about half as sore as all the other subjects. In addition, their leg strength decreased less than did that of the subjects in the other groups. Subjects who had taken ibuprofen only after working out reached the decreased soreness and muscle-strength levels of the first group in 48 hours.

According to researcher Scott Hasson, Ed.D., ibuprofen taken before a workout may help limit inflammation by blocking the production of prostaglandin, which is released when muscles are damaged. After a workout, ibuprofen also helps cut down on any inflammation that has occurred. However, the researchers say, ibuprofen probably does not actually reduce muscle damage.

Since long-term use of ibuprofen can cause kidney, stomach, and liver damage, the researchers warn against using the drug every day. Instead, they suggest using ibuprofen only occasionally, and then only for workouts that are brand-new or that are expected to be more strenuous than usual.

Although delayed-onset muscle soreness is extremely common and widely studied, scientists still know relatively little about it. They do know that eccentric exercises—those that stretch muscles—are more likely to cause soreness than concentric exercises, which contract muscles. Moreover, the faster, more intensely, and longer an exercise is done, the worse the resulting soreness will be. Soreness peaks 48 hours after exercising.

Indomethacin, another anti-inflammatory, has no effect on muscle soreness caused by eccentric exercises of the chest muscles, according to a study at East Carolina University in Greenville, North Carolina. Furthermore, the standard prescription for sports injuries—RICE (rest, ice, compression, elevation)—does not seem to ease soreness, according to a study from Brigham Young University in Provo, Utah.

For now, the most effective way to ease sore muscles is plain common sense: Exercise regularly, increase the difficulty of your workouts gradually, and try not to overdo it.

## ▶ Hip Replacements and Knee Surgery

It used to be that the treatment for torn cartilage in the knee was surgery to remove it. Orthopedists saw the medial meniscus, two small pieces of cartilage in the knee, as serving little or no function. If it was torn, they simply took it out.

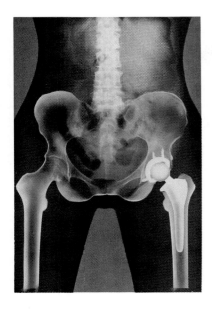

*In an artificial hip, a metal shaft with a ball on its upper end is wedged into the thighbone, and a cup-shaped socket with a plastic lining is fitted into the pelvic bone. The socket encases the metal ball, which swivels within it when the leg moves.*

Today we know that the meniscus acts as a shock absorber, cushioning the joint. Indeed, removing it can cause crippling arthritis years later. So now surgeons are experimenting with a variety of options for repairing the cartilage.

In cases where the cartilage is torn in the outer third, surgeons sew the tear together. Roughly 80 to 90 percent of these repairs are successful. For severe cases, doctors are now experimenting with transplants of cartilage taken from cadavers. Although the operations have been successful so far, the procedure is still somewhat experimental, and the long-term success of the transplants is not known.

In another area, experts are continuing to develop better hip implants. About 90 percent of hip implants installed in the past 10 years still work. The main problems with implants developed in the 1970s and 80s, however, is that the glue between the implant and the bone breaks down.

Today's implants generally do not use glue to fit the implant to the femur. Instead, some implants are custom-fitted with the help of X rays and CT scans. Others have porous surfaces to allow the bone to grow into the implant itself. A new coating that is chemically similar to bone may aid this growth. Studies show that bone quickly bonds to a coating of hydroxylapatite.

Finally, efforts are under way to prevent the polyethylene particles in the sockets of implants from rubbing off. In an implant the socket faces the constant stress of the cobalt-chromium head of the implant (the "ball" of the joint) moving in it, causing particles to flake off. These particles can trigger an immune reaction because the body sees them as a foreign invader. To counter this problem, the heads of some implants are now made of ceramics such as alumina; other implants have sockets made of ceramics or metal.

*Devera Pine*

# Brain and Nervous System

## ▶ Alzheimer's Disease

Alzheimer's disease is the most common form of dementia-causing illness. Dementia is characterized by the loss of higher cortical functioning; its symptoms include the impairment of recent memory, limitations of abstract thinking, and alterations of judgment, among other features. There are a variety of different causes of dementia in addition to Alzheimer's disease. But in all cases, no matter what the cause, affected individuals vary in their exact pattern of symptoms at the onset. Symptoms may range from getting lost on a familiar route to having problems with calculations. With progression of Alzheimer's disease, however, all victims eventually lose the ability to care for themselves.

Estimates indicate that Alzheimer's disease affects about 4 million Americans, and that it leads to the deaths of 10,000 individuals each year. Ten percent of those affected are over the age of 65, while 47 percent of those affected are over the age of 85, indicating that the disease is more common with increasing age. The cost of providing care for victims of Alzheimer's disease was calculated to be $90 billion per year in 1990, a tremendous drain on both family and public resources.

The diagnosis of Alzheimer's disease is made clinically through a process by which other possible causes of dementia are eliminated. A magnetic resonance imaging (MRI) examination is helpful to rule out strokes, especially those that are due to bleeding into a region of the brain (hemorrhagic stroke), or to a blockage of the blood supply to a region of the brain (cerebral infarct). It also helps to rule out blood clots under the skull, massive infections of the brain (brain abscesses), or tumors.

Currently there are no specific laboratory tests that yield a definitive diagnosis of Alzheimer's disease. In a patient suspected of having Alzheimer's, however, an MRI often indicates signs of atrophy of the brain. This atrophy can lead to a diagnosis of *hydrocephalus ex vacuo*. Hydrocephalus—literally "water brain"—refers to a condition in which the large ventricles where the cerebrospinal fluid (the waterlike fluid that bathes the central nervous system) is made have enlarged. Normally, about 25 teaspoons of cerebrospinal fluid are made and absorbed each day. When there is a loss of nerve cells, as occurs in Alzheimer's disease, there is more room for cerebrospinal fluid to accumulate, room that exists because of the loss of brain tissue. This condition is referred to as hydrocephalus ex vacuo.

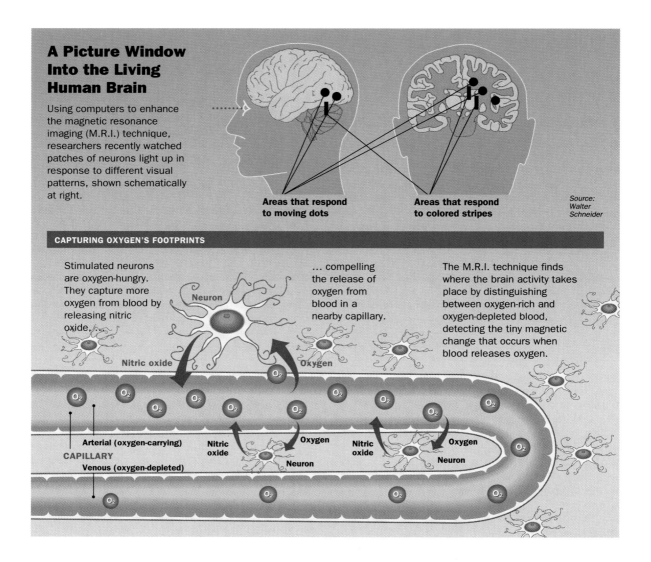

## A Picture Window Into the Living Human Brain

Using computers to enhance the magnetic resonance imaging (M.R.I.) technique, researchers recently watched patches of neurons light up in response to different visual patterns, shown schematically at right.

**Areas that respond to moving dots**

**Areas that respond to colored stripes**

*Source: Walter Schneider*

### CAPTURING OXYGEN'S FOOTPRINTS

Stimulated neurons are oxygen-hungry. They capture more oxygen from blood by releasing nitric oxide,

**Neuron**

Nitric oxide

… compelling the release of oxygen from blood in a nearby capillary.

Oxygen

The M.R.I. technique finds where the brain activity takes place by distinguishing between oxygen-rich and oxygen-depleted blood, detecting the tiny magnetic change that occurs when blood releases oxygen.

Arterial (oxygen-carrying)
**CAPILLARY**
Venous (oxygen-depleted)

Nitric oxide    Oxygen    Nitric oxide    Oxygen

**Neuron**    **Neuron**

Researchers have yet to determine a pattern that would indicate whether a person is predisposed to developing Alzheimer's. However, there do seem to be some forms of Alzheimer's that run in families; some of these familial cases manifest themselves at a relatively young age (compared to the age of most Alzheimer's patients), while others occur later. All forms of Alzheimer's are characterized by the development or presence of what are described as *neuritic plaques* and *neurofibrillary tangles*; these are believed to interfere with the function of the nerve cells that are affected by this disease. Through genetic studies, at least three genetic loci have been identified that are associated with an increased risk of developing Alzheimer's disease. A locus on chromosome 14 has been associated with the early onset of familial Alzheimer's disease, while another locus on chromosome 19 has been associated with the late onset of familial Alzheimer's disease. Finally, because of the occurrence of Alzheimer's disease in adults with Down syndrome (in which there are three copies of chromosome

21), linkage to a gene on that chromosome for the protein *beta amyloid four* has also been recognized.

Of these different candidate genetic loci, a gene for a protein known as *apolipoprotein E* (ApoE), located on chromosome 19, has received a great deal of attention this year. Allen Roses, M.D., a neurologist at Duke University in Durham, North Carolina, has found that there is an increased incidence of Alzheimer's disease in individuals who have the gene for a specific form of ApoE. This finding may lead to a blood test for at least this form of late-onset familial Alzheimer's disease.

Efforts are being made to better understand the mechanisms by which Alzheimer's disease arises and to develop new strategies for the development of treatments. Recently, a new drug has been approved by the Food and Drug Administration (FDA) for use in the symptomatic treatment of the disease. The drug, tacrine (Cognex), enhances the duration of action of the neurotransmitter *acetylcholine* in the central nervous system by interfering with its breakdown by the enzyme *acetylcholinesterase*. Alzheimer's patients have a deficiency of acetylcholine in the cortex of the brain; this deficiency is believed to result in some of the clinical manifestations of mild to moderate dementia. Although not believed to alter the course of the underlying dementing process, tacrine has been shown to improve cognitive functions in these patients. This represents an important first step in the development of additional treatment strategies for dealing with the consequences of Alzheimer's disease.

## ► Epilepsy

Epilepsy is a neurological disorder that produces recurring seizures over time. Seizures, like headaches, are a symptom of dysfunction of groups of brain cells in the cerebral hemispheres; they represent an abnormal electrical discharge by damaged cells. Although current treatments for epilepsy focus on the control of seizures, there are currently no drugs available to prevent the occurrence of seizures after damage to certain regions of the brain.

Seizures may be partial, or *focal,* involving discharge by a limited number of brain cells. They may also be *generalized,* spreading to involve the whole brain. When focal seizures spread to involve the whole brain, they are referred to as *secondarily generalized seizures.* The impact of either major type of seizure on the individual can be quite severe.

The method of treating seizures has essentially remained unchanged over the past 15 years. It has involved the use of several medications.

Surgery to remove the areas of the brain that contribute to focal seizures is sometimes recommended for individuals who do not respond to drug therapy. However, surgery is only viable for individuals in whom the affected areas do not control a vital neurologic function, such as vision or speech.

Medical treatment of seizure disorders must be individualized to control the seizure type. Doctors must monitor the drug level throughout the day, and remain alert for any side effects. A goal of therapy is to maintain a drug dose that is high enough to control seizure activity, but low enough to allow the affected individual to remain functional in his or her daily activities or employment.

This past year there have been at least three new drugs recommended for approval by the FDA for the treatment of seizure disorders—felbamate (Felbatol), gabapentin (Neurontin), and lamotrigine (Lamictal). Although the precise mechanism of action for all these drugs remains unknown at present, they do seem to be more specific in their actions, and therefore produce fewer side effects.

The strategy for epilepsy treatment in the coming years will be to continue efforts toward developing specific anticonvulsant medications, with a focus on controlling seizures while limiting side effects.

*Robert L. Knobler, M.D., Ph.D.*

# Cancer

## ► Mammography

In 1989, the National Cancer Institute (NCI) and the American Cancer Society (ACS) unified their guidelines on mammography for the screening of breast cancer in women. In mammography, X rays are used to obtain a detailed picture of the internal characteristics of the breast. Mammography can detect breast cancer at its earliest stage, before it is large enough to be felt by either the patient or the doctor in a manual examination. Mammography isn't as useful in women under the age of 35, due both to the relative rarity of the disease in these women and to the density of their breasts, which can obscure the earliest signs of cancer on the X-ray film. Nevertheless, widespread adoption of these guidelines, coupled with the consent of most insurance companies to cover the cost of routine screening mammograms, has resulted in more women obtaining screening mammograms. This, in turn, has led to a significant rise in the detection of breast cancer at its earliest, and most curable, stages.

Last year, an International Workshop on Screening of Breast Cancer was held at the National Institutes of Health (NIH) to review data from several large studies conducted to assess the impact of screening mammography on diagnosis of and survival of breast cancer. By analyzing the combined data from six different studies (a so-called "meta-analysis"), a panel of experts concluded that, with five to seven years of follow-up, screening mammography reduced breast-cancer deaths by 35 percent in women 50 to 69 years old. But in an interesting reversal, the study found no detectable effect in reducing deaths from breast cancer in women 40 to 49 years old.

These findings generated strong response from a number of groups. Since this analysis could find no benefit for women under the age of 50, the NCI revised its recommendations for screening mammography. According to these revised guidelines, women under 50 should continue to perform monthly breast self-examination and discuss their personal concerns and risk factors for breast cancer with their doctor before deciding if they should obtain screening mammograms before age 50. Critics of this recommendation contend that the studies included in the meta-analysis were not designed to detect the impact of mammography in specific age groups and, therefore, conclusions based on age were inappropriate.

Because the incidence of breast cancer rises with age, it would take a trial involving more than 500,000 women 40 to 49 years old followed for at

## Breast Cancer, by the Numbers

The estimated number of cases of breast cancer in women in 1993, by age of patient.

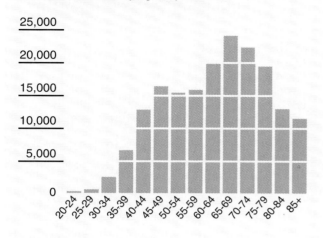

Source: American Cancer Society

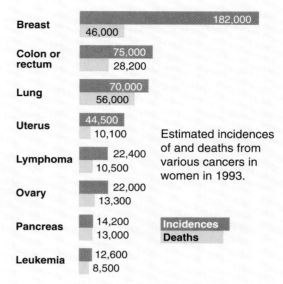

Estimated incidences of and deaths from various cancers in women in 1993.

least five years to detect a 25 percent decrease in breast-cancer death rate. Reflecting these sentiments, the American Cancer Society feels that there was insufficient information to warrant changing its stance on mammography, and it has therefore retained the 1989 guidelines.

A number of issues remain to be resolved:

1) Is longer follow-up needed in order to detect the benefit of screening mammography in younger women? Although no survival benefit was seen for women aged 40 to 49 with five to seven years of follow-up, an "uncertain" marginal benefit was detected after 10 to 12 years. Unfortunately, too few women in this age group had been followed long enough to draw a firmer conclusion than this.

2) Is there a critical age at which a woman should begin getting screening mammograms? Most of the studies included in the meta-analysis used arbitrary 10-year age groupings. Some have argued that the 10-year span is too large, and that future studies should use smaller age groupings. Certainly, the dramatic effect seen for women over age 50 contrasts sharply with the lack of benefit for women under age 50, suggesting that there is some age between 40 and 50 at which screening mammography begins to be beneficial. At the present time, however, no one knows what that age is.

3) Will this controversy deter women from obtaining appropriate screening mammograms? The new inconsistency in screening-mammography guidelines between the NCI and the ACS may confuse women and obscure the fact that this procedure remains a cornerstone of early detection of breast cancer. Ironically, older women, who stand to gain the most from annual screening mammograms, un-

derutilize the procedure, perhaps due to a misperception that they have a decreased risk of breast cancer. In fact, breast-cancer risk rises steadily with age, and this meta-analysis demonstrates a significant benefit in terms of a decrease in breast-cancer deaths for women aged 50 to 69. Unfortunately, only one-third of all women over the age of 50 obtained annual screening mammograms in the United States last year, and a quarter have never had a mammogram. Increased efforts must be focused on increasing the utilization of this lifesaving procedure by this group of women.

4) Is there any benefit to annual screening mammography for women over the age of 70? There was an insufficient number of women in this age group included in the meta-analysis to address this question. Since the 65 and older age group represents the fastest-growing segment of our society, this question will become even more important.

5) Why wasn't any benefit detected for women under the age of 50? Decreased sensitivity of mammography is the most commonly cited reason, but other explanations are possible. Could the breast-cancer growth rate in younger women be more rapid than in older women? In this case, annual mammograms would have demonstrated no benefit because the cancer occurred during the time between screenings. Following this argument, more frequent mammograms should be obtained in this group of women. Once breast cancer is diagnosed, is therapy less effective in younger women than it is in older women? This possibility could also account for the lack of perceived survival benefit from mammography, and yet have nothing to do with the sensitivity of the mammogram to detect cancer.

6) Are there any more sensitive ways to detect early-stage breast cancer? Ultrasound, magnetic resonance imaging (MRI), and injection of X-ray contrast material into the breast ducts are all being evaluated as tools to detect breast cancer. At the present time, however, none of these techniques can replace X-ray mammography as the standard imaging method for breast-cancer screening. Refinements in each of these techniques may one day make them cost-effective and accurate enough to be used in this capacity. It should be noted that technical advances have significantly improved the sensitivity of X-ray mammography over the past 10 years, and are likely to keep this method in the forefront of breast-cancer screening for the foreseeable future.

## ▶ AIDS-related Cancers

It is estimated that more than 2 million Americans are currently infected with the human immunodeficiency virus (HIV) that causes acquired immune deficiency syndrome (AIDS). Over the past decade, survival of people with AIDS has improved as a result of better therapies directed against the virus itself, as well as more effective prevention and treatment of the infections that commonly plague such patients. Now, a new problem has emerged in those individuals who are living with AIDS: cancer.

From the earliest days of the epidemic, Kaposi's sarcoma has been associated with AIDS and has served as one of the AIDS-defining criteria. In fact, suppression of the immune system from any cause (such as through immunosuppressive therapy for recipients of kidney transplants) increases the risk of Kaposi's sarcoma to 500 times that of the general population. However, its connection to immunosuppressed states, as occur in AIDS, still remains unclear. It is not a direct result of HIV infection: laboratory animals infected with the virus never develop Kaposi's sarcoma. Certain groups are more likely to get Kaposi's sarcoma in conjunction with AIDS than others: homosexual or bisexual men are five to six times more likely to develop Kaposi's sarcoma than are other groups at risk for AIDS. It appears that for Kaposi's sarcoma to occur, there must be sexual transmission of an as-yet-unidentified agent in an immunosuppressed host. It is also believed that certain HIV-related proteins act in concert with another factor to transform cells and cause the development of Kaposi's sarcoma.

More recently, it has been recognized that long-term survivors of AIDS are 50 to 100 times more likely to develop non-Hodgkin's lymphoma than is the general population. Here, too, the etiologic relationship is not known, but it appears that immunosuppression plays a key role, since individuals who are immunosuppressed for other reasons (congenital immune deficiency disorders, autoimmune diseases, or immunosuppressive therapy following organ transplantation) are also at increased risk for the development of non-Hodgkin's lymphoma. These lymphomas are typically of B-lymphocytes present in areas beyond the lymph nodes, and carry a worse prognosis compared to lymphomas that occur in nonimmunosuppressed individuals.

Cancer of the cervix also occurs more commonly in HIV-positive individuals and, as of January 1993, is included as one of the diagnostic criteria for AIDS in an HIV-infected woman. Women with AIDS-related cervical cancer frequently are coinfected with human papillomavirus, which has also been implicated in the development of this cancer. It is not known how much each virus contributes to the development of cervical cancer, but it is known that women who are infected with both viruses have a worse prognosis than those with evidence of papillomavirus infection alone.

Much remains to be learned about the relationship between AIDS and cancer, but it is likely that this interaction is quite complex and involves stimulation of tumor growth factors, chromosomal rearrangements, and impairment of the body's normal recognition and immune response against abnormal cells that can degenerate into cancer cells. In 1993, the NCI earmarked funding to create an AIDS-cancer registry to study the frequency, behavior, and biological properties of these cancers.

## ▶ Genetic Defects Associated with Colorectal Cancer

Over the last five years, researchers have uncovered a number of genetic abnormalities that are linked to the development of cancer of the colon and rectum. These genetic defects tend to fall into two categories: activation of a dormant gene that can then transform a normal cell into a cancer cell (so-called "dominant oncogenes"); or inactivation of a gene responsible for maintaining growth regulation in a normal cell ("tumor suppressor" genes). More recently, a new type of genetic abnormality has been recognized in families in which multiple members are stricken with colorectal cancer. Although the specific gene has not been identified, it has been localized to the short arm of chromosome 2 and termed the familial colon cancer (FCC) gene. When present, this gene confers a 95 percent chance of developing colorectal cancer, and may account for up to 10 to 15 percent of all colorectal cancers. If this estimate is accurate, it would make colorectal cancer one of the most common genetic diseases.

Cells possessing the FCC gene show an increase in the size of the short, repetitive sequences of DNA that are normally found throughout each chromosome. These sequences, known as microsatellite DNA, have an unknown function, but appear to be important to the normal function of cells since

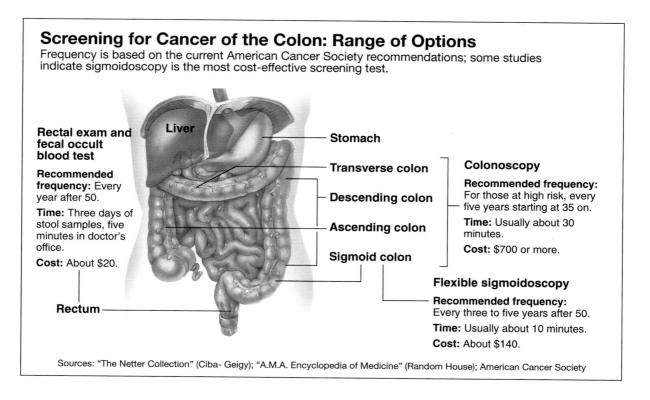

## Screening for Cancer of the Colon: Range of Options

Frequency is based on the current American Cancer Society recommendations; some studies indicate sigmoidoscopy is the most cost-effective screening test.

**Rectal exam and fecal occult blood test**

**Recommended frequency:** Every year after 50.

**Time:** Three days of stool samples, five minutes in doctor's office.

**Cost:** About $20.

Liver

Stomach

Transverse colon

Descending colon

Ascending colon

Sigmoid colon

Rectum

**Colonoscopy**

**Recommended frequency:** For those at high risk, every five years starting at 35 on.

**Time:** Usually about 30 minutes.

**Cost:** $700 or more.

**Flexible sigmoidoscopy**

**Recommended frequency:** Every three to five years after 50.

**Time:** Usually about 10 minutes.

**Cost:** About $140.

Sources: "The Netter Collection" (Ciba-Geigy); "A.M.A. Encyclopedia of Medicine" (Random House); American Cancer Society

---

they are found in all eukaryotic (multicompartment) cells. Cells that carry the FCC gene have significantly more genetic mistakes than do normal cells. It appears that the FCC gene prevents DNA from being copied accurately and prevents these mistakes from being repaired. Further research is being directed at identifying, isolating, and sequencing the gene. Additional work will be needed to identify the protein product encoded by the gene and to define how this protein exerts its effect on microsatellite DNA. It is hoped that within the next few years, tests will be developed that are capable of identifying individuals who carry the FCC gene so that they can be monitored closely to allow detection of any colon cancers at an early, and curable, stage. Ultimately, therapies may be developed to repair or replace the FCC gene with its normal counterpart, preventing the development of this form of colorectal cancer altogether.

### ▶ Cancer Vaccines

Vaccines are designed to produce a highly specific immune response against a specific disease. We are most accustomed to thinking about vaccines used for the prevention of diseases; the success of this approach against polio, smallpox, and diphtheria has virtually eradicated these diseases in the developed world. Other diseases, such as malaria and AIDS, are the focus of intensive vaccine research with a potential to save millions of lives each year.

With some cancers, such as renal-cell cancer (kidney cancer) and malignant melanoma (a form of skin cancer), the immune system is not strong enough to shrink the tumor or prevent tumor recur-

rence in patients who have had all their cancerous tissue surgically removed. Cancer vaccines are designed to activate the immune system so that a specific tumor can be recognized and "rejected" in much the same way that the body mounts an immune response against a bacterial or viral infection. But in order to do this, the T and B lymphocytes that coordinate the immune response must be stimulated in a very precise way. Early work conducted in this area during the 1970s and 1980s used crude tumor-cell preparations and nonspecific immune-stimulating drugs. Because the preparations contained so many other, unrelated molecules, the immune response was often too weak or nonspecific to have much of an antitumor effect.

Technological advances now allow researchers to isolate and reproduce specific molecules on the tumor-cell surface (known as antigens) that elicit the immune response; the researchers can thus prepare a vaccine containing only those specific components. Such vaccines may be prepared from the patient's own tumor (an autologous vaccine) or from the antigens most commonly found in cell lines or individuals with that type of tumor (an allogeneic vaccine). A third vaccine utilizes genetically engineered molecules that can mimic tumor antigens, thereby eliminating the need to obtain tumor samples.

Bearing in mind that the immune response can be impaired in people with large tumors or with widespread cancer, much recent cancer-vaccine research has focused on patients with microscopic tumors remaining after surgery who are at high risk for relapse, such as those with melanoma; chronic lymphocytic leukemia; or cancer of the colon, stomach, pancreas, breast, lung, or ovary. Within a few years, we should know whether vaccinating a patient against a specific tumor is a useful approach to preventing tumor recurrence.

## ▶ Shark Cartilage

Methods used to treat cancer that have not undergone careful evaluation through clinical trial are referred to as "unproven," "questionable," or "alternative" treatments. Discussion of these therapies tends to highlight basic philosophical differences. Proponents of alternative therapies, on the one hand, feel that the benefit of the therapy is clearly demonstrated by the experience of individual cancer patients; opponents of alternative therapies, on the other hand, contend that information obtained in this fashion is subject to so many extraneous factors that it is impossible to attribute the antitumor effect to the treatment.

Shark cartilage is one such therapy that has garnered a great deal of attention. Sharks are known to have a very low incidence of cancer and an extremely potent immune system. In addition, a component of shark cartilage called cartilage-derived inhibitor (CDI) interferes with the formation of new blood vessels (angiogenesis), a process vital to the growth and development of cancers. Laboratory tests are under way to gain a better understanding of the mechanism by which CDI inhibits angiogenesis, and how this mechanism can inhibit tumor growth. Meanwhile, powdered shark cartilage has found its way into health food stores, where it is sold as a "food supplement." By avoiding any direct reference to its potential role as an anticancer drug, it is not covered by the 1962 Food, Drug, and Cosmetics Act and is not required to abide by the Investigational New Drug guidelines enforced by the Food and Drug Administration (FDA). Opponents contend that shark cartilage is being used as an alternative cancer treatment and, therefore, should be monitored by the FDA.

The Office of Alternative Medicine (OAM) was created by a mandate from Congress in 1991 to help shed light on the value of alternative therapies. OAM received an appropriation of $2 million to support research on alternative therapies in 1993. Evaluation of the antitumor activity of shark cartilage was identified as one of the top priorities for OAM. As a result, in conjunction with the NCI, OAM has begun preliminary discussions with investigators at NCI-designated cancer centers and cooperative groups to determine whether a clinical trial with shark cartilage is feasible. It is hoped that this type of collaboration will lead to the objective evaluation of shark cartilage to determine what role, if any, it has in the treatment of people with cancer.

*Mace L. Rothenberg, M.D.*

# Child Development and Psychology

## ▶ Children of Alcoholics

Although children of alcoholics have long been thought to be at risk for many problems, few researchers have systematically examined what problems were prevalent in such children or if problems indeed exist. A study published in *Child Development* was designed to identify behavior problems in three-year-old boys whose fathers are alcoholics. Fifty-eight alcoholic fathers and 16 nonalcoholic fathers were originally recruited for the study. The groups were matched on socioeconomic status, education, years married, family size, and intelligence-test results. The families of alcoholics were recruited through probation officers after the alcoholics had given their permission to be contacted; they were paid for their participation. Nonalcoholic families were found through a door-to-door search one block away from the alcoholic families. The parent measures implemented included a demographic questionnaire, an occupation-based socioeconomic index, an intelligence test, an alcohol-problem evaluation, an antisocial-behavior checklist, and a depression inventory.

Child measures included a behavior-problem checklist (completed by the parent), a developmental evaluation, and a test designed to look at the child's ability to delay gratification. Results showed that alcoholic parents demonstrate more antisocial behavior and depression than do nonalcoholic parents. Children of alcoholics were more impulsive than children of nonalcoholics. Both groups of children were found to have a normal range of reported behavior problems. The authors' expectation of an increased number of behavior problems in sons of alcoholics was not found in this study. There were no differences in developmental level or intelligence level. The only difference between the two groups was in the ability to delay gratification, indicating an impulsivity consistent with previous findings. The authors expressed concern over the high levels of antisocial behavior found in the families of alcoholics, and the possible effects this behavior may have on children over time. It has been reported that such behavior includes spousal violence and abuse.

Although the expected behavior differences between the two groups of children did not materialize, the study's results should be interpreted cautiously. There is a tendency for the families of alcoholics to demonstrate higher degrees of adult psychopathology, which directly impacts on the adult's ability to parent. Children model their parents' behavior, problem-solving techniques, and coping abilities. If children are constantly exposed to inappropriate behavior, one would assume that over time, these styles would be emulated.

### ▶ Infant Behavior

Infant temperament has been associated with feeding, sleeping, regularity of body function, flexibility, and other behaviors. Clinicians in the pediatric setting believe there is a relationship between infant temperament and common developmental behavioral problems. The Revised Infant Temperament Questionnaire is frequently used to assess whether an infant is an easy, difficult, or slow-to-warm-up baby. It has been reported that infants with a difficult temperament demonstrate higher levels of colic, sleep, and feeding problems, and an inability to adjust quickly to change. Few studies have looked at how well infant temperament predicts problems in later childhood. A January 1993 Australian study published in *Pediatrics* measured behavior problems in four- and five-year-olds and correlated those with early temperament. The Australian Temperament Project initially engaged 2,443 infants between the ages of 4 and 8 months who came from families representative of the Australian population. The subsample used for the study was similar to the entire initial sample on the variables of sex, birth order, gestational age, and parental sociodemographic characteristics. Initial temperament measures included the Australian version of the Revised Infant Temperament Questionnaire, a global temperament scale; a questionnaire developed to assess crying, colic, and sleeping behaviors; demographic information; perinatal stress; prematurity; and nurses' ratings of infant temperament and mother-infant interaction.

The child's behavior was measured by a behavior questionnaire completed by the parent when the child was between four and five years of age. Results indicated a significant relationship between the mother's and nurses' overall perception of the infant's temperament. This is important because one can assume the infant's temperament was reliably measured. Relationships were found between infancy variables of maternal and nurses' overall perception of difficult temperament, behavior problems, prematurity, low socioeconomic status, and subsequent behavior problems. However, the study's authors felt the perception of difficult temperament in infancy was not necessarily a risk factor for behavior problems at ages 4 to 5. The authors suggest that a limitation of the study may be that the mothers who perceived a difficult infant temperament might continue to perceive their child's behavior as problematic as the child ages. Further research is necessary to determine how much past behavior contributes to present or future behavior,

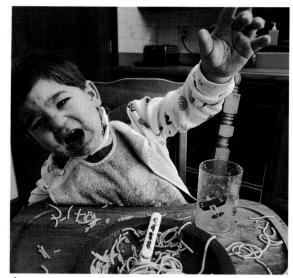
*A temperamental infant might grow into an ill-tempered child partly because parents and other adults label him or her as "difficult." That label may even follow the child into the school years.*

and what effect a parent's expectation has on a child's behavior. A child is often labeled by teachers, parents, and other adults in accordance with his or her degree of difficultness. This label may be carried with the child through adolescence.

### ▶ Maternal Depression

A study examining maternal depression and the mother's perception of her infant's behavior was published this year in *Infant Behavior and Development.* Sixty mothers and their infants participated in the study. Mothers were categorized as symptomatically depressed or nondepressed according to scores achieved on a widely used measure of depression (Beck Depression Inventory). The mothers were videotaped with their infants after having been told to pretend they were at home playing with their baby. The infant's and mother's behavior were recorded using a three-point coding scheme of behavior labeled as negative (bad/sad), neutral (O.K.), and positive (good/happy). Both the mother and a trained observer recorded behaviors. Depressed mothers were coded, both by themselves and by the independent observers, as having more negative states, an equal number of neutral states, and fewer positive states than the nondepressed mothers. The same results were found for the infants of depressed mothers. The depressed mothers coded their child's behavior as more negative and less positive when compared only with the independent observer's codes.

The authors were unclear as to why the mothers thought their babies were more negative than the observers did. It may be that symptomatically depressed mothers perceive everything as more negative. Although the results of this study, as with any study, should be carefully interpreted, they do suggest that research is needed to further explore variables that may be contributing to a mother's perception of her infant. If perceptions can be altered, then perhaps parenting skills can be influenced.

When depressed mothers of older children have been examined, overreporting of behavior problems have been observed. David M. Fergusson and his colleagues from the Christ Church School of Medicine in New Zealand hypothesized in the *Journal of Abnormal Child Psychology* that maternal depression causally influenced maternal reporting accuracy and that it is correlated with reporting accuracy. These researchers found that there is a tendency for depressed mothers to overreport problematic behaviors in their 12- to 13-year-old children. But the authors note that depressed mothers may have more parenting difficulties, and thus problems managing their child in general. It is difficult to ascertain how inaccurate their overreporting actually is; indeed, what may be problematic behavior to mothers may not be perceived by some other observers as problematic behavior.

## ▶ Dietary Intake: School Lunches

Recent attention has been focused on the food that children are served at school lunches. In previous studies, children given a choice tend to pick relatively healthy selections. A study published in *Pediatrics* by Robert C. Whitaker, M.D., and his associates from the University of Washington School of Medicine in Bellevue examined the school-lunch situation and the types of foods selected by elementary school children. The schools included in this project participate in the National School Lunch Program. Of the 6,700 students, 38 percent ate the school lunch. One-quarter of these students were eligible for free or reduced-price lunches. Two daily entrées were available to the students. For the study the number of school days in which a low-fat entrée was available was increased. The low-fat entrée was defined as deriving 30 percent or less of its total calories from fat. Observers watched to ensure that the subjects were not receiving any food from students who brought their lunch from home. The researchers were interested in analyzing how well the low-fat selections were embraced by the students over time, and in comparing the results from choices made before the low-fat selections were made available. A low-fat entrée availability was gradually increased from 23 percent to 71 percent of the days on which luncheon was served. Throughout the eight-month study, 29 percent of the students chose the low-fat item.

This study used an environmental intervention of increasing the availability of low-fat food choices to improve a child's diet. Other studies have developed programs that specifically change attitudes and beliefs in order to improve dietary habits. Most likely, the best way to improve healthy food choices is to use both strategies.

Children usually have little control over what foods are eaten in the home, except perhaps to eat only a portion (or nothing) of what is served. Problems may arise when parents do not have the knowledge or resources available to provide a nutritious assortment of foods. Children are often finicky eaters, and some parents will provide anything they know the child will eat. A child needs to be reinforced and provided with opportunities in order for a desired behavior to develop. It has been well documented that eating habits begin very early in life and are very difficult to change in adults, particularly the habits that are the least healthy.

## ▶ Adolescent Parenting

Adolescent pregnancy continues to be prevalent in our society. Children born to adolescents are at risk for developmental difficulties and psychosocial problems, to name but a few. Much literature published in 1993 focused on the adolescent parent.

In one study, Theresa Reynosa, Nancy Williams, and Ruth Sheets from the University of California, San Diego, and colleagues evaluated 50 pregnant adolescent patients at an inner-city university clinic for substance use, and reported their findings in the *Journal of Pediatric Psychology*. Self-reported substance abuse was measured using the Personal Experiences Inventory, a measure often used with adolescents to detect substance abuse. Urine tests were also conducted to detect drugs. The study observed that teenage mothers-to-be drastically reduce their substance abuse during pregnancy. The authors offer several explanations for their findings, including an adolescent's ability to make complex decisions and an awareness of the risk of substance abuse to an unborn child.

Previous studies have offered conflicting results concerning the risk of maltreatment for children born to adolescent mothers. In the journal *Pediatrics,* David M. Stier, M.D., from the Department of Pediatrics at Yale University School of Medicine in New Haven, Connecticut, and colleagues studied children born at Yale-New Haven Hospital from October 1979 through December 31, 1981, to women who were 18 years or younger (study group) and children born to women between 19 and 34 years of age (control group). Each group contained 219 children and their mothers. Data were collected from medical records over a five-year period. All medical visits with reported injuries or suspected injuries were recorded. Each episode was categorized as physical abuse, sexual abuse, neglect, or unintentional injury. Neglect was separated into three additional categories: physical, supervisional, and medical. Household violence was also included.

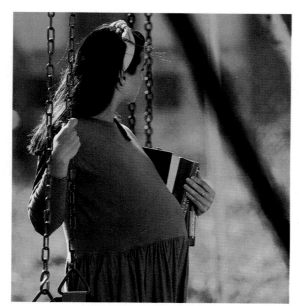

*The drastic reduction in substance abuse by pregnant adolescent girls suggests that the mothers-to-be are aware of the risks that drugs pose to their unborn children.*

Poor growth or failure to thrive was also recorded. "Parenting failure" was the third outcome variable, defined as a change in the child's primary caretaker due to the parent's inability to care for the child. Results showed that maltreatment occurred twice as often in the study group. Neglect was the only form of maltreatment that was statistically significant. Unintentional injuries with and without neglect occurred equally in both groups. Most of the abuse occurred during the first two years of life. For example, 26 of the 30 episodes of abuse occurred before age 2 in the study group, compared to 6 of the 12 episodes in the control group. Of the study children, 6.9 percent were diagnosed with poor growth (failure to thrive), usually during the first 12 months. The child's primary caretaker changed four times more frequently in the study group when compared to the control group.

By age five, 27 percent of the children born to adolescent mothers experienced some form of adverse outcome—over twice the rate experienced by the children born to older mothers. Although, in two-thirds of the physical-abuse cases, the perpetrator was not the mother, the mother's judgment was certainly questionable. The authors note several limitations, including a possible heightened sense of reporting, possible maltreatment of a child in an adolescent mother's home, poor histories of injuries reported by a young mother as opposed to more-detailed (explanatory) ones given by an older mother, and the notion that the urban environment in which this study took place may not be comparable to those experienced by adolescent mothers who live in suburban or rural communities.

*Cynthia P. Rickert, Ph.D.*

# Digestive System

## ▶ New Guidelines for Colonoscopy

Most colon cancers begin as benign polyps called adenomas. It is generally believed that the early detection and removal of colon adenomas through colonoscopy reduces the overall morbidity and mortality from colon cancer. Although cancer may be present in polyps as small as 0.2 inch, large polyps (particularly those greater than 1 inch) are more likely to be malignant. Since adenomas may recur, patients require follow-up colonoscopy at an interval that has not yet been well defined.

The general practice has been for all patients with known colon adenomas to undergo a repeat colonoscopy one year after adenoma removal. If no adenomas are detected, the next examination is performed three years later. If recurrent adenomas are present at one year, examinations are then performed yearly until no more are detected.

The results of the National Polyp Study were published in April 1993. Organized in 1978 to determine the optimal timing for postpolypectomy surveillance, this large study involved many centers across the United States, led by Sidney Winawer, M.D., and his colleagues at the Memorial Sloan-Kettering Cancer Center in New York City. The study's results confirm the hypothesis that an initial follow-up colonoscopy at three years was as effective at detecting important new adenomas as a colonoscopy performed at one year. Out of 1,418 patients with adenomas, 699 underwent repeat colonoscopy at both one and three years (group I), while 719 had colonoscopy only at three years (group II). Twenty-eight percent of patients in group I had adenomas at one year, while 32 percent of patients in group II had adenomas at their first follow-up colonoscopy at three years. This difference was not statistically significant. Furthermore, the adenomas detected at three years were no more likely to be large or to contain cancer than those found at one year.

Although new polyps may form sooner than three years, they are invariably small and have little or no malignant potential. Only those patients with a cancerous polyp, very large or multiple polyps, or incomplete removal of polyps should undergo a colonoscopy at one year, a practice that can dramatically decrease the cost of colonoscopic surveillance without compromising quality of care.

## ▶ Peptic Ulcers and Bacterial Infection

Peptic ulcer disease (PUD) refers to ulcers involving the stomach and duodenum (the first portion of the small intestine). PUD is considered a chronic disease, as 70 to 80 percent of patients will have ulcer recurrence after successful therapy with acid drugs such as ranitidine (Zantac) and cimetidine (Tagamet). Known risk factors for PUD include cigarette smoking, alcohol ingestion, and the use of aspirin and other nonsteroidal anti-inflammatory drugs (such as ibuprofen or indomethacin).

The bacterial organism *Helicobacter pylori* (see photo below) causes an inflammation of the stomach known as chronic active gastritis. At least 90 percent of patients with duodenal ulcers, and 75 percent of patients with gastric ulcers, are infected with *H. pylori*. It is not known whether *H. pylori* directly causes PUD, or simply colonizes the stomach once an ulcer has already formed.

Evidence that treatment of this organism can dramatically reduce the recurrence of PUD was published in the *New England Journal of Medicine* in February 1993 by Enno Hentschel, M.D., and his colleagues from Hanusch Hospital and the University of Vienna School of Medicine in Austria. The authors treated 52 duodenal-ulcer patients with placebo, and another 52 patients with the antibiotics amoxicillin (750 mg three times a day) and metronidazole (500 mg three times a day) for 12 days. Both groups also received standard ulcer therapy with ranitidine (Zantac) for 6 to 10 weeks. The recurrence of ulcers was followed for up to 12 months with periodic endoscopic examination of the stomach and duodenum. The recurrence rate of duodenal ulcers in the group given placebo was 86 percent (42 of 49 patients), while it was only 8 percent (4 of 50 patients) in the antibiotic group.

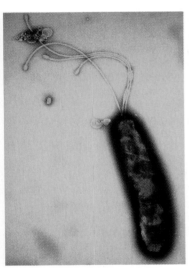

*Studies suggest that Helicobacter pylori (above) may be a primary cause of duodenal and gastric ulcers.*

These dramatic findings concur with a number of previous trials that also demonstrated a significant reduction in the recurrence rate of PUD with antibiotic treatment. These studies suggest, but still do not prove, that infection with *H. pylori* has a causative role in peptic-ulcer disease. It is not clear whether all patients with ulcers should be treated, or only those with refractory or recurrent disease. Eradication of this organism with antibiotic therapy is clearly the most effective approach now available to prevent peptic-ulcer-disease recurrence.

*Arnon Lambroza, M.D.*

# Ear, Nose, and Throat

## ▶ Poisoning Wrinkles

Edmund A. Pribitkin, M.D., of Thomas Jefferson University Medical Center, Philadelphia, Pennsylvania, and Andrew Blitzer, M.D., of the Columbia-Presbyterian Medical Center in New York City have recently presented papers in which the toxin associated with botulism poisoning, *Clostridium botulinum-A* exotoxin (Botox), was used to treat facial wrinkles. In large quantities, Botox can cause botulism poisoning, which can result in respiratory-muscle paralysis and possibly death. When injected in small amounts into hyperactive wrinkling muscles, however, Botox paralyzes offending muscles and improves wrinkles such as frown lines between the eyes, and crow's-feet on the outer corners of the eyes, both of which are felt to be caused by hyperactive muscles pulling on skin that has lost its elasticity.

Botox blocks neuromuscular conduction by binding to receptor sites on motor-nerve terminals, entering the nerve terminals, and inhibiting the release of acetylcholine. The toxin has been used extensively over the past 10 years in the treatment of patients afflicted with uncontrollable muscle spasms that close the eyelids (blepharospasm) and contort the face (hemifacial spasm).

Improvement in the frown lines and crow's-feet of these patients prompted Dr. Blitzer to treat similar wrinkles in others. Treatment involves a simple injection into the muscles producing the wrinkles. Effects are seen in two to five days, and last for up to six months. Dr. Pribitkin reports that 75 percent of patients treated with Botox for frown lines are pleased with the results and return regularly for treatment. In his series of 100 patients, no significant side effects or complications have been seen. Dr. Blitzer has extended the treatment to patients with crow's-feet, deep nasolabial folds, and unsightly neck wrinkles, with equally promising results.

## ▶ Office Lasers Treat Snoring

New hope exists for the one out of four people who snore habitually. Yosef Krespi, M.D., of St. Luke's/Roosevelt Hospital Center in New York City and Jack A. Coleman, Jr., M.D., of Vanderbilt University, Nashville, Tennessee, have imported a new laser treatment from France, where it was pioneered by Yves-Victor Kanami, M.D. The new laser treatment reduces snoring by removing excess throat tissue.

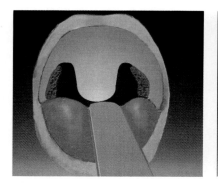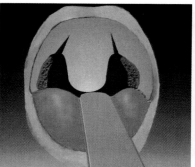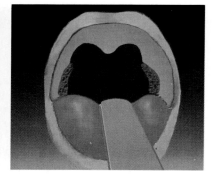

*Laser-assisted uvulopalatoplasty reduces or eliminates snoring by removing excess throat tissue. The uvula, the fleshy lobe that hangs in the back of the throat (above left), is sculpted and trimmed (middle) by a laser beam. After three to five sessions the airway at the back of the throat and nasal cavity is enlarged (right).*

Snoring usually occurs when the uvula (the fleshy lobe hanging at the back of the throat), sometimes the tonsils, and the muscles of the palate relax during sleep. These areas then act like vibrating noise-makers when inhaled air moves across them. The result is often a sleepless night—not only for the snorer's bed partner, but for the snorer as well!

Although snoring is commonly thought to be a relatively harmless and annoying condition, it can be an indicator of obstructive sleep apnea—a serious medical problem. In obstructive sleep apnea, loud snoring is interrupted by episodes during which the victim does not breathe at all. These episodes reduce the amount of oxygen reaching the brain and prevent the snorer from reaping the benefit of a good night's sleep. This can lead to morning headaches, daytime drowsiness, and accidents on the job or behind the wheel. In extreme cases, patients can develop high blood pressure and cardiovascular changes that may lead to heart attacks and strokes.

A new snoring treatment, called laser-assisted uvulopalatoplasty, is performed with the patient wide awake in the office under local anesthesia. In about 10 minutes, a carbon dioxide laser beam is used to trim the uvula and reshape the palate. The laser is fitted with a probe that carefully directs the beam to remove only one thin layer of tissue at a time, thereby minimizing pain and reducing heat damage and charring. The goal of the surgery is to enlarge the airway at the back of the throat and nasal cavity.

The full treatment is spread over three to five sessions spaced about four weeks apart. Multiple sessions keep the pain down to the level of a sore throat for a few days; there is no bleeding with the laser treatment. Patients go right back to their normal activity after each session. Preliminary results published by Dr. Kanami's group indicate a complete cure of snoring in 85 percent of patients. An additional 12 percent of patients report a significantly reduced level of snoring.

## ► Advances in Voice Medicine

Over the past two decades, a new medical specialty has developed focusing on the mechanisms of the voice. Voice medicine has benefited from scientific and technological advances in a variety of disciplines that have helped elucidate how the muscles and organs of the abdomen, chest, throat, and head act in coordination to produce vocal communication. Understanding vocal-control mechanisms, in turn, will help physicians develop better strategies for rehabilitating damaged voices.

Until the 1980s, a physician's ear was the only technique available to assess voice quality and function. Indirect laryngoscopy, in which a light source and a mirror are used to observe the vocal cords, or more precisely, vocal folds, was the only method available to observe vocal mechanisms. Both of these techniques provided only a crude and incomplete picture of vocal health.

Today, however, physicians have a variety of high-tech options at their disposal. A strobovideo-laryngoscope, or stroboscope, is the standard technique for inspecting vocal-fold vibrations. A microphone placed near the larynx triggers the stroboscope to illuminate the vocal folds. If the frequency of the stroboscope light is out of sequence with the vocal-fold vibrations, the vocal-fold vibrations appear to occur in simulated slow motion. This technique permits physicians to see abnormalities that go undetected under normal light, such as scars or early carcinomas.

Another new technique is laryngeal electromyography, which is used to evaluate neuromuscular integrity and function of the laryngeal muscles. Thin electrodes are inserted into the laryngeal muscles. Any electrical activity measured in the muscles may be used, for instance, as a predictor that a patient may be recovering from vocal-cord paralysis. In this case, surgery may then be postponed to see if a spontaneous recovery occurs.

*Edmund A. Pribitkin, M.D.*

# Emergency Medicine

Approximately 250,000 cardiac arrests occur outside the hospital each year in the United States. Published rates of successful resuscitation range from as low as 2 percent in some parts of the country to as high as 30 percent where sophisticated emergency medical systems operate. Persistent researchers are trying to improve the chances of survival from life-threatening heart attacks by studying a variety of innovative approaches to emergency treatment.

## ▶ First-Responder Defibrillation

The key to successful resuscitation of a cardiac-arrest victim is often the prompt correction of a fatal chaotic heart rhythm called fibrillation. Application of a brief electrical shock to the chest can "defibrillate" the heart, prompting resumption of a normal, regular beat. Over the past 20 years, prehospital cardiac care has been aimed at shortening the time interval from initial collapse to defibrillation.

Since paramedics have been trained to use defibrillators at the accident scene, many more lives have been saved. However, in many cases the first responder is not trained to use this special defibrillator equipment. Fortunately, firefighters and other safety personnel who often arrive first on the scene can administer this livesaving treatment. "Smart" defibrillators are now available that can electronically recognize ventricular fibrillation and advise the rescuer of the need for a defibrillatory shock.

In some areas where highly trained personnel are not readily available, these smart defibrillators may be especially valuable. However, research has shown that in cities with a fast-response urban emergency medical system served by paramedics, the impact of adding first-responder defibrillation is minimal. More important is early initiation of cardiopulmonary resuscitation (CPR). To achieve optimal rates of survival after cardiac arrest, careful attention to every link in the "chain of survival" is mandatory. The four links in this chain include: 1) 911 telephone access to emergency care; 2) widespread public training in CPR; 3) early defibrillation; and 4) prompt access to advanced cardiac life support.

## ▶ When to Call It Quits

It is common practice for emergency vehicles to transport victims of unsuccessful field resuscitation to local emergency rooms—usually at high speeds, jeopardizing both the rescue team and other motorists. Once in the emergency room, the patient usually undergoes more extensive and expensive methods of resuscitation.

Recently investigators from Memphis, Tennessee, and Houston, Texas, concluded that the survival rate of cardiac-arrest victims who are not resuscitated by a determined trial of advanced life support in the field is not improved by further emergency-room efforts. When such efforts are successful, survivors tend to suffer brain damage from prolonged periods of insufficient oxygen delivery to the brain.

Furthermore, the cost of this futile additional resuscitation is estimated at $500 million annually. Those few patients who are successfully resuscitated rarely leave the hospital alive; their health-care costs have been estimated to amount to an additional $500 million yearly.

## ▶ Clot Busters in the Field

Thrombolytic drugs, the so-called "clot busters," open clogged blood vessels in the heart muscle during a heart attack. They have been shown to be most effective when administered during the first hour after the onset of heart-attack symptoms. Unfortunately, most patients typically wait at least 30 minutes, and often longer, before seeking medical attention for their symptoms. Further delays occur in transportation to the hospital and in initial emergency-room evaluation, making it virtually impossible to meet the 60-minute goal.

Researchers at the University of Washington in Seattle tested whether outcomes would be improved if paramedics gave the clot-busting medications to patients while en route to the hospital. The researchers were unable to show an advantage of this approach. However, treatment within 70 minutes of symptom onset—whether in the hospital or in the field—was found to minimize damage from heart attack.

## ▶ New Opportunities for EMTs

An innovative use of emergency medical technicians (EMTs) may address two seemingly unrelated problems. First, there is a gross maldistribution of health-care personnel in the United States, with many rural and inner-city areas highly underserved by medical facilities. Second, the majority of calls to which EMTs respond are for nonemergencies, such as earaches in children or minor injuries requiring simple first aid.

Trained for true emergencies only, EMTs miss opportunities to provide basic health care. Now emergency medical systems across the country, including those in rural areas, are starting to redefine the roles of EMTs. EMTs are being taught new skills to allow them to treat patients who do not require transport to hospitals, to make "house calls" in nonemergency situations, and even to administer immunizations.

*James A. Blackman, M.D., M.P.H.*

# Endocrinology

## ▶ Diabetes Mellitus

Diabetes mellitus occurs when the body is unable to produce adequate amounts of insulin, a condition that causes the patient to have elevated levels of glucose in the bloodstream. Over the course of 10 years or more, diabetics may develop eye disease, kidney failure, or nerve damage. These complications have long been thought to be caused by elevated glucose levels, but no established clinical evidence existed for this theory until the past year.

At the 1993 American Diabetes Association Meeting, the results of a 10-year study called the Diabetes Care and Complications Trial were revealed. The study was designed to learn if tightly controlled glucose levels delay the onset of the eye disease called diabetic retinopathy, and if such control prevents the condition from worsening in patients with early signs of the disease.

To conduct the study, 1,141 diabetics were enrolled from 29 centers throughout the United States and Canada. One group of 726 diabetics, the primary-prevention group, had no eye disease at the start of the study. These 726 diabetics were then randomized to receive either intensive therapy, which involved three or more insulin injections daily; continuous insulin therapy by a pump; or conventional therapy, which involved one or two daily injections. Patients in the intensive-therapy treatment group monitored their level of blood glucose at least four times a day with home glucose-testing kits, and made the corresponding adjustments to their insulin doses. The intensive-therapy group also received frequent instruction about the management of their insulin, diet, and exercise.

The conventional-therapy group received standard diabetic instruction at three-month follow-up intervals, and the members home-monitored their glucose levels less frequently—sometimes only once a day.

The secondary-prevention group was comprised of 715 diabetics who had early retinopathy. This group was also randomized like the primary-prevention group into either intensive therapy or conventional therapy.

Ninety-nine percent of the patients who enrolled completed the study; the results were dramatic. The diabetics who had no eye disease and received intensive therapy reduced their risk of developing eye disease by 76 percent as compared with the conventionally treated group. Of those diabetics in the secondary-prevention group, those who received intensive therapy had slowed the worsening of their eye disease by 54 percent compared with the conventionally treated group.

The investigators also collected data on the development of albuminuria (kidney disease), and of nerve disease. Diabetics who received intensive therapy had a 56 percent reduction in the incidence of albuminuria, and a 70 percent reduction in the incidence of nerve disease.

This study showed that, with appropriate and careful instruction and follow-up by a multidisciplinary team, medical intervention can make a difference in the quality of life of diabetics who tightly control their blood-glucose levels. The risks are minimal, while the benefits are enormous.

## ▶ Women's Health

It is estimated that 3,500 women enter menopause each day, and that in the next two decades, 40 million women will enter menopause. Many of these women will live nearly one-third of their lives after menopause. These astounding numbers have helped trigger enormous interest in women's-health issues. A 1993 survey of 833 women ages 45 to 60 was conducted by the North American Menopause Society. The survey revealed that 33 percent of

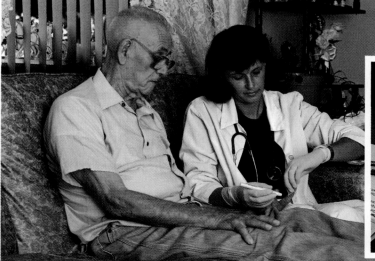

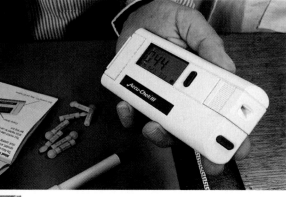

*Diabetics who monitor their glucose levels with home-testing kits (below), and who also receive instruction about diet and insulin levels, can reduce their risk for complications.*

these women were concerned about osteoporosis, 28 percent worried about their emotional well-being, and 27 percent feared the risk of heart disease as they approached or entered menopause. The survey also noted that although most physicians (84 percent) had mentioned hormone-replacement therapy to these women, few had discussed its full benefits and risks or had discussed other treatment options involving dietary changes, stress reduction, stopping smoking, and exercise. In addition, the survey found that most patients received their information about menopause from magazines, newspapers, or friends. The findings of this survey are important in order to encourage both physician and patient education and to sponsor increased research funding into women's health.

Several studies reported in 1993 addressed some of these issues. One study published in the *Archives of Internal Medicine* followed a group of 23,088 women 35 years and older who were taking noncontraceptive doses of estrogens. For six years the investigators monitored these women for the occurrence of first stroke. They discovered that the risk of first stroke was reduced by 40 percent in women taking hormone replacements. The investigators predicted 403 first-time strokes in this population over the six-year period, and yet the number of actual strokes that occurred in the women taking the estrogen compounds was only 361 cases. This study provides additional evidence of the potentially therapeutic effects of estrogens on the cardiovascular health of women.

A 1993 study reported in the *New England Journal of Medicine* examined the effect of vitamin E and the risk of coronary-artery disease. In a sample over an eight-year period of 87,245 female nurses ages 34 to 59, women who had the highest vitamin E intake were compared with those who had lower vitamin E intake. The investigators found a 40 percent lower risk for major coronary-artery disease in the group taking the higher amounts of vitamin E, particularly in those women who had taken vitamin E supplements for at least two years. Although the study could not prove a cause-and-effect relationship, the results are intriguing, especially given that the study did control for the other cardiac risk factors that would influence the results, such as smoking and age.

Many other questions are being actively studied in the area of women's health. Studies will address not only diseases such as osteoporosis, heart disease, stroke, and breast cancer, but also other issues such as psychosocial functioning, stress, diet, and exercise in menopausal and postmenopausal women. All these studies intend to provide both physician and patient with further knowledge about women's health issues.

*Alison A. Moy, M.D.*

# Environment and Health

## ▶ Secondhand-Smoke Dangers

A report released by the EPA in early 1993 warns anew of the health risks from secondhand tobacco smoke. The finding that passive smoke accounts for approximately 3,000 lung-cancer deaths per year among adult nonsmokers was among the conclusions reached in the report, titled "Respiratory Health Effects of Passive Smoking: Lung Cancer and Other Disorders."

Cigarette, pipe, or cigar smoke contains more than 4,000 substances, more than 40 of which are known to cause cancer in humans or animals. The report acknowledges that "although this environmental tobacco smoke (ETS) is dilute compared with the mainstream smoke inhaled by active smokers, it is chemically similar, containing many of the same carcinogenic and toxic agents."

By far the main groups at risk from secondhand smoke are children and infants. Children who are around smokers or whose parents smoke are at increased risk of lower-respiratory tract infections such as bronchitis and pneumonia. The report estimates that between 150,000 and 300,000 such lower-respiratory tract infections in infants and toddlers up to 18 months of age are caused by secondhand smoke. These infections result in 7,500 to 15,000 hospitalizations each year. Buildup of fluid in the middle ear (a leading cause of ear infections) and reduced lung function are also more likely to occur.

Children with asthma may take the biggest hit from passive smoke. Both the number of episodes and the severity of symptoms are increased by ETS. The report estimates that 200,000 to 1 million asthmatic children may have their condition worsened by exposure to ETS. Passive smoke may also cause thousands of nonasthmatic children to develop the condition each year.

For nonsmoking adults, besides lung cancer, secondhand smoke also causes irritation of the eyes, nose, and throat. It can irritate the lungs, leading to coughing, excess phlegm, chest discomfort, and reduced lung function.

During a hearing about secondhand smoke before the House Subcommittee on Health and the Environment held in July 1993, EPA Administrator Carol Browner said, "This is one case where individual actions make a difference." To that end, the EPA has published a brochure on secondhand smoke that tells of the dangers and gives recommendations for how adults can limit their exposure and their children's exposure to tobacco smoke.

## ▶ Pesticide-Reform Proposal

A comprehensive reform package for food- and pesticide-safety laws was presented at a joint House and Senate committee hearing on September 21, 1993, by the EPA, the U.S. Department of Agriculture (USDA), and the Food and Drug Administration (FDA). The package "represents the first significant, realistic attempt to improve and update the nation's food safety and pesticide laws in the last 20 years," wrote EPA Administrator Carol Browner. She told the committee, "Today's proposal is a giant step toward protecting all Americans —especially our children."

The coalition of government agencies feels an urgent need to change existing laws. "Nationwide, we use more than 1 billion pounds of pesticides each year. Of the 600 pesticides now in use, two-thirds have never been subjected to any health standard whatsoever. We cannot and we will not tolerate the status quo," said Browner.

The main points of the package include:
• Establishment of strong, health-based standards of reasonable certainty of no harm to consumers that would apply to all pesticide residues in food. In setting these standards, the EPA should also consider other possible routes of exposure to the same or related chemicals, such as through drinking water or nondietary exposures.
• These new tolerances must include specific findings that they are safe for infants and children. Children may be exposed to more pesticide residues than adults because they eat more food for their size than adults. The USDA would collect data specifically on children's diets, and those foods would be a top priority in pesticide monitoring.
• The EPA would require that most high-risk pesticides meet the new safety standards within three years, and that all other pesticides meet the standards within seven years.
• Allow for easier removal from the market of pesticides suspected of posing a risk to health and the environment, and give lower-risk pesticides priority review in the approval process.
• Encourage the reduction of pesticide use through greater application of Integrated Pest Management (IPM). IPM uses a variety of techniques "such as crop rotation, cultivation of predator insects, biological pesticides, and other practices, together with judicious and limited chemical pesticide use," writes the EPA. By the year 2000, the goal is that 75 percent of all farms will use IPM techniques.
• Prohibit exportation of pesticides that have been banned or voluntarily withdrawn in this country due to health concerns.
• Beef up the enforcement provisions of current laws for violations of statutes and regulations.
• Enact a "sunset" requirement that at 15-year intervals a pesticide registration is automatically canceled if it doesn't meet public-health standards. This will ensure that all pesticides are reviewed periodically. Currently pesticide registrations generally have no fixed expiration or renewal dates.

## ▶ Cleaning Up Truck and Bus Exhaust

Say good-bye to the black clouds of smoke that belch forth from buses and trucks. Two Clean Air Act rulings that took effect in 1993 will reduce the amount of particulates coming from new diesel vehicles by 90 percent, taking away almost all the black exhaust. These new rulings apply even to older diesel vehicles.

Particulates are tiny carbon particles less than 10 microns in size (1 micron equals 1 millionth of a meter). When inhaled, they can lodge in lung tissue. High levels of exposure can cause bronchitis, asthma attacks, and respiratory infections; particulates may also be carcinogenic.

The first ruling, announced on March 4, 1993, sets stricter emission standards for particulates coming from urban buses. These standards will be phased in gradually with the 1994 and 1995 bus-engine models. In 1996 new bus engines will have to meet even stricter particulate-emission levels. Manufacturers of bus engines will use catalytic converters or trap oxidizers to achieve the new goals. Particulate emissions are due to drop by 90 tons in the first full year of the program alone.

Of the new ruling, EPA Administrator Carol Browner says, "Everyone will breathe more easily from the cleaner air produced by these new standards, but the reductions will be most beneficial to those suffering from lung ailments."

*City dwellers can breathe a bit easier thanks to two Clean Air Act rulings that mandate a 90-percent reduction in the particulate emissions from buses and other diesel vehicles.*

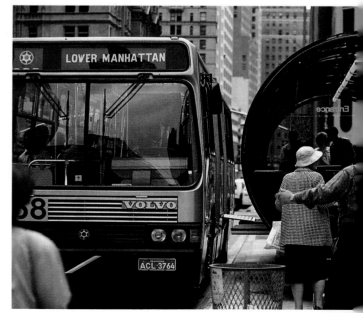

October 1, 1993, marked the date of a ruling requiring new, lower-sulfur-content diesel fuel to be used. Sulfur causes the black, sooty, particulate-filled exhaust produced by diesel vehicles. This ruling will cut sulfur in diesel fuel by 80 percent.

Since 1988 the EPA has worked with the oil and trucking industries to produce the new fuel. Browner says, "By effectively eliminating the black clouds of exhaust from diesel-powered vehicles, toward cleaning the air Americans see and breathe—especially in urban areas where particulate levels are highest—the new rule improves air quality across the board in a way that benefits us all."

### ▶ Safer Dry Cleaning

Getting your clothes dry-cleaned may seem harmless enough, but that may not be the case. Perchloroethylene (PCE, or "perc"), the chemical solvent used by most dry cleaners to clean clothes, appears on the list of 189 toxic air pollutants that Congress has told the EPA it must regulate under the Clean Air Act. The EPA writes that "with more than 34,000 commercial shops in neighborhoods and malls across the country, dry cleaners account for one of the largest groups of chemical users that come into direct contact with the public."

The agency has now started to take steps to reduce emissions of PCE at dry cleaners and to look at safer ways to clean clothes. In September 1993, the EPA announced that the total amount of PCE emissions from uncontrolled dry-cleaning machines will be cut by up to 80 percent. The rule requires pollution-control equipment called refrigerated condensers to be put on all these types of machines.

This rule affects only emissions in the air during dry cleaning, not PCE on the clean clothes picked up by customers. On that front the EPA announced the results of an EPA/industry effort that showed the viability of a "wet" cleaning process that uses biodegradable soaps, heat, steam, and pressing to clean clothes that are typically dry-cleaned.

The test project involved the collection of nearly 1,500 garments from EPA employees over a two-month period in late 1992. Half were conventionally dry-cleaned, while the other half went through this wet-cleaning method. Survey postcards were attached to 900 pieces of clothing, and about 350 surveys were returned. Consumers never knew which cleaning process their clothes underwent. The wet process was statistically preferred, particularly with regard to odor.

Total operational costs of the wet process were slightly less than standard dry cleaning as well, even though the wet process requires over three times the skilled labor in the cleaning phase. This expense is offset by the higher equipment costs, hazardous-waste disposal, electricity, and supplies used in conventional dry cleaning.

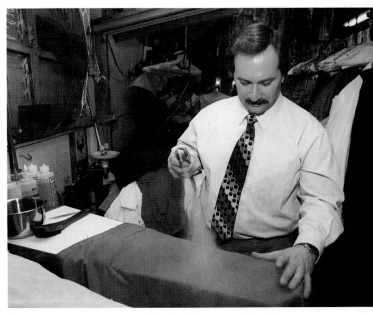

*Dry cleaners are now required to have special pollution-control equipment on their machines in order to reduce the emission of perchloroethylene, a chemical solvent used in the cleaning process.*

Overall, the cost-and-performance study "indicates that under certain situations, multiprocess wet cleaning is technically feasible and economically competitive with PCE dry cleaning," the EPA writes.

The next step, already under way, is for the EPA's Design for the Environment Program, along with the dry-cleaning industry and public-interest groups, to evaluate the health and environmental risks associated with both cleaning methods.

### ▶ Agent Orange

Decades after the Vietnam War ended, the list of recognized Agent Orange-related illnesses continues to expand. More than 19 million gallons of herbicides such as Agent Orange were sprayed over South Vietnam during the war. Some veterans have since blamed exposure to these chemicals for cancers and other health problems they have developed.

In July 1993, Secretary of Veterans Affairs Jesse Brown added Hodgkin's disease and a rare metabolic disorder called porphyria cutanea tarda to the list of diseases for which veterans can receive disability payments. Hodgkin's disease is a lymphatic cancer, while the other disorder is characterized by thinning and blistering skin. Brown added these two health disorders in response to a report by the Institute of Medicine, a branch of the National Academy of Sciences (NAS), which said there was evidence to link them to Agent Orange exposure. Before this date, Vietnam veterans were compensated only for soft-tissue sarcoma, non-Hodgkin's lymphoma, and chloracne, a severe skin disease.

In September 1993, Brown announced that, after further review, President Clinton had approved the inclusion of four more diseases. Lung, larynx, and trachea cancer as well as multiple myeloma (a cancer involving the bone marrow) will now be covered. This decision will cost the government an estimated $350 million in compensation over the next five years.

### ▶ Persian Gulf Syndrome

Confusion and frustration still surround all aspects of the mysterious "Persian Gulf syndrome" suffered by thousands of veterans of the Persian Gulf war that ended in 1991. Symptoms include nausea, diarrhea, chronic headaches, loss of breath, joint and muscle aches, and fatigue.

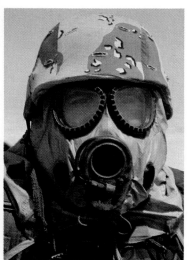

The cause of these maladies is still unknown. Speculation about chemical or biological exposure continues with no firm answers to date. At a press conference held on November 10, 1993, Defense Secretary Les Aspin said, "The upshot of all this is that a connection to the mysterious health problems that have victimized some of our veterans continues to prove elusive."

The conference was held to discuss reports from Czech forces who detected traces of nerve gas and a blister agent at one point during the war. But due to the small amounts and the location of the detection in relation to American forces, Aspin does not believe these chemicals are the cause of the health problems.

*Some Desert Storm veterans worry that their unexplained illnesses might be the result of exposure to some kind of chemical-warfare agent during the war.*

General Ronald Blanck, M.D., commander of the Walter Reed Army Medical Center near Washington, D.C., speculated at the press conference that industrial chemicals such as chlorine or ammonia may be to blame. "It is entirely possible, even plausible, that a number of these individuals . . . were exposed to multiple chemicals in small amounts that would have had a cumulative effect that might be manifesting itself now in these kinds of symptoms without objective findings," said General Blanck.

For now, the investigation continues. A panel of experts, headed by Nobel prizewinner Joshua Lederberg, has been assembled under the Defense Science Board to study the illnesses.

*Linda J. Brown*

### ▶ Alcohol Consumption and Cataracts

It has long been suggested that alcohol consumption may increase the rate of cataract formation, particularly in people who have many drinks per day. No previous reports have been able to differentiate which is the most hazardous—liquor, beer, or wine.

Beatriz Munoz, M.D., and her colleagues at Johns Hopkins University in Baltimore, Maryland, reviewed patients who developed posterior subcapsular cataracts, a particularly disabling form of cataract that forms a crystalline surface on the back of the cataract within the eye. The condition generally occurs in younger patients, and causes profound glare and a markedly increased difficulty with distance vision, disabling the patients earlier than they might be from other types of cataract. In the study the authors examined the relationship between posterior subcapsular cataract and alcohol consumption, combining the consumption data on wine, beer, and liquor for their report.

Light drinkers—those who consumed less than one drink a day—were at no additional risk for cataract formation compared to nondrinkers. Moderate drinkers—those who consumed more than one drink a day—were almost three times more likely to develop cataracts. This increased risk appeared to be independent of nutritional and socioeconomic status. (Each of these factors has also been associated with an increased risk of cataract surgery.) Future research is necessary to determine if the alcohol itself is toxic to the lens, or whether the increased rate of cataract formation is due to the nutritional abnormality typical of alcoholics.

A second study on the effect of alcohol on the rate of cataract formation, by Linda Ritter and colleagues from the University of Wisconsin Medical School in Madison, also found that heavy drinking (four or more drinks per day) is associated with an increased chance of cataract. These investigators also found a strong association between alcoholic beverages and an increased frequency of cataract.

Ritter's study separated patients into groups on the basis of the type of alcohol consumed. Perhaps unexpectedly, they found that beer was much more often associated with an increased risk of cataract than either liquor or wine. The reason for the increased risk from beer remains unknown, but there is much speculation that diet is a major factor.

### ▶ Nutrition and Macular Degeneration

The impact of nutrition on eye disease was the subject of an extensive evaluation sponsored by the National Eye Institute and the National Institutes of Health (NIH). The investigators reviewed data regarding the effect a group of micronutrients known as antioxidants have on age-related macular degeneration, the leading cause of new blindness in persons 65 or older in the United States. Macular degeneration causes the irreversible loss of central vision, while peripheral vision is preserved. The patient can readily get around, but is unable to read or drive a motor vehicle.

Much interest has been focused on the deleterious effect of oxygen on the retina. This oxygen is converted into free radicals, molecules that trigger oxidation in neighboring cells. Oxidation, the same process that causes cars to rust, has been linked to macular degeneration. Antioxidants include carotenoids, vitamin C, selenium, and vitamin E. These compounds are believed to be important in protecting the retina from damage from oxygen. The authors found a significant reduction in the rate of macular degeneration in those patients with high levels of carotenoids in their blood. High levels of vitamins C, E, and the element selenium did not appear to have any protective benefit for age-related macular degeneration. While this study does not prove the value of carotenoid dietary supplements, the results do merit additional clinical studies to evaluate the effect that a dietary vitamin and mineral supplement made with carotenoids would have on the development of age-related macular degeneration.

### ▶ Myopia Prevention

Myopia, or nearsightedness, is the most common refractive error in the United States. Myopic patients have blurred vision for distant objects, while retaining clear vision close-up. Almost 30 percent of people in this country will be myopic by age 20. Myopia is caused by inherited and environmental factors. There has been much excitement about the success of surgical treatment of myopia with radial keratotomy. However, most investigators would prefer to prevent the development of myopia.

For more than a century, physicians, optometrists, and lay personnel have attempted to prevent or slow the development of myopia. They have utilized a wide array of treatments, including bifocals, eyedrops, and avoidance of close work and reading, with the understanding that the myopic person's inherited information could not be altered, but that intervention might change the environmental influences and therefore lead to less or no myopia.

A 1993 Finnish study compared traditional treatment of myopia with full-power glasses to treatment using bifocals or distance glasses only, in which the spectacles were removed for near tasks. These two methods are the most common optical techniques currently used for the treatment of myopia. The patients were treated for three years with the selected technique. The study found that the use of bifocals or the removal of glasses for near activity does not protect the patient from myopia.

But the authors did find that certain characteristics of the patients were predictive for the development of myopia, including patient gender, age of onset, and the presence of myopia in parents. Boys had a significantly slower rate of development of myopia than girls. Both boys and girls whose parents did not wear glasses also had a marked slowing of the rate of development of myopia. The authors also substantiated the importance of environmental effects on the development of myopia. Time spent

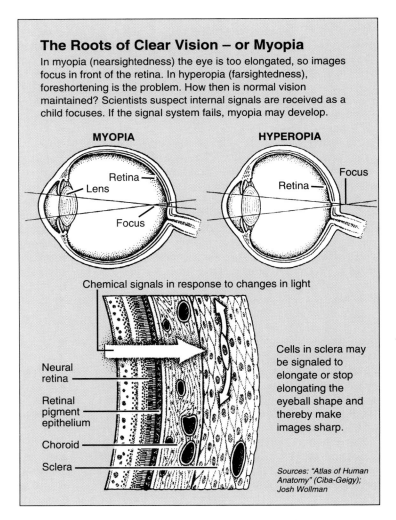

### The Roots of Clear Vision – or Myopia

In myopia (nearsightedness) the eye is too elongated, so images focus in front of the retina. In hyperopia (farsightedness), foreshortening is the problem. How then is normal vision maintained? Scientists suspect internal signals are received as a child focuses. If the signal system fails, myopia may develop.

**MYOPIA**

Retina
Lens
Focus

**HYPEROPIA**

Focus
Retina

Chemical signals in response to changes in light

Neural retina

Retinal pigment epithelium

Choroid

Sclera

Cells in sclera may be signaled to elongate or stop elongating the eyeball shape and thereby make images sharp.

*Sources: "Atlas of Human Anatomy" (Ciba-Geigy); Josh Wollman*

reading or performing other close work was closely associated with the development of myopia. Conversely, the amount of time spent outdoors was related to a delay in development of myopia. Patients who held their reading material closer to their face also had a faster rate of myopic development.

This study indicates that heredity is important in determining which patients will develop myopia and how great the myopia will be. Furthermore, patients who develop myopia at a younger age will usually develop the greatest level of myopia. Further research is needed to investigate other potential methods for the prevention of myopia.

### ▶ Diabetes and the Eye

During 1993 a successful treatment to slow the ocular complications of diabetes mellitus was reported by the Diabetes Control and Complications Trial Research Group based at the NIH in Bethesda, Maryland. Diabetes mellitus causes approximately 10 percent of the new cases of blindness in the United States each year. It is second only to macular degeneration as a cause of permanent blindness.

It has long been known that the longer a patient survives with diabetes, the more likely it is that he or she will develop abnormal-blood-vessel growth in the eye, predominantly in the retina. Such abnormal vessels leak fluid and protein, distorting the retina and reducing vision. Such abnormal blood vessels may also bleed. The blood clot will produce a scar, which will naturally contract, often causing a retinal detachment. This will likely result in permanent and uncorrectable blindness. Though there have been great advances in the surgical repair of damaged eyes, the preferred method is to prevent these complications in the first place.

Until recently medical therapy has been unable to prevent ocular disease associated with diabetes. The NIH investigators speculate that aggressive maintenance of a normal blood-sugar level could delay development of the abnormal-blood-vessel growth. Normally diabetics have blood sugars that range widely during the course of every day. The investigators evaluated the eye disease in two groups of patients. The first group followed the traditional diabetic management of two injections of insulin a day. The second group received four injections of insulin a day or used an insulin pump, which constantly supplied insulin. The more aggressive therapy used by the patients in the second group resulted in much lower blood-sugar levels than those achieved by the traditional-therapy group.

After three years the investigators found that intensive therapy reduced the risk of development of new retinopathy by 76 percent. For those patients with retinopathy, the aggressive therapy slowed progression by 54 percent.

*Michael X. Repka, M.D.*

## Genetics and Genetic Engineering

Researchers continue to make great progress in identifying the defective genes that cause many inherited diseases, as well as the healthy genes that take part in cellular metabolism. By the most recent count available, researchers have identified and determined the structure of 3,837 of the estimated 100,000 genes that serve as the blueprint for a human.

### ▶ Lou Gehrig's Disease

In March 1993, a multicenter team headed by Robert H. Brown, Jr., M.D., of Massachusetts General Hospital in Boston reported that they had discovered the defective gene that causes amyotrophic lateral sclerosis (ALS), better known as Lou Gehrig's disease. ALS is characterized by the death of nerve cells in the brain and spinal cord that control muscle activity, producing progressive muscle weakness and paralysis. Most patients die within two years after its onset, but some live much longer. It strikes about one in every 100,000 people, and afflicts an estimated 30,000 people in the United States.

Scientists were surprised by the identity of the gene, which turned out to be the blueprint for a well-known enzyme called superoxide dismutase. Superoxide dismutase normally scavenges a highly reactive form of oxygen—called a free radical—in the body before it can react with and destroy crucial tissues. Impairments of the enzyme's function have previously been associated with the deterioration of bodily functions that accompany aging. Last summer, based on the discovery of the gene, the Muscular Dystrophy Association began clinical trials of several well-known drugs, including Vitamins A and E, that scavenge free radicals in the hope that they could retard the progress of the disease. No results have been announced yet.

### ▶ Huntington's Disease

Also in March, a team of researchers from six U.S. institutions announced that they had discovered the defective gene that causes Huntington's disease, ending one of the longest and most intensive searches for the source of a genetic disorder. The disorder, which affects 30,000 Americans, generally strikes in a person's mid-30s and is invariably fatal. It begins with small involuntary movements that gradually overwhelm all parts of the body. It also interferes with thought processes, leading to dementia and other mental disturbances, particularly depression. Identification of the gene will allow researchers to identify those who will develop the disease with near-100 percent accuracy, but the team has not yet discovered the protein produced by the gene and are thus not yet able to begin working on a therapy.

## ▶ Colon Cancer

Researchers reported in December 1993 that they had identified the genetic defect that produces a strong susceptibility to colon cancer, the second-most deadly form of cancer in the United States. The research suggests that virtually every person who carries the defective gene—about one in 200—will develop the disease, making it one of the most common causes of inherited disease.

Colon cancer strikes an estimated 158,000 Americans each year, killing 60,000. Researchers had previously isolated the gene that causes an inherited form of colon cancer called familial adenomatous polyposis, but that form accounts for only about 1 percent of colon cancer. The newly discovered gene, in contrast, accounts for about 15 percent of all colon-cancer cases, or about 24,000 cases per year. Furthermore, the researchers have discovered the gene in many noninherited cases and they believe that it accounts for a significant fraction of those 134,000 cases as well.

The new gene is virtually identical to a well-known gene found in yeast and bacteria. In its healthy form, the gene corrects mistakes made in reproducing deoxyribonucleic acid (DNA) during the proliferation of cells, much like the spell-check function of a word-processing program eliminates errors in text. When the gene is defective, errors accumulate at 1,000 times the normal rate. The combination of all these errors produces cancer. The team hopes shortly to have a blood test to identify people who have the gene.

## ▶ Homosexuality

Two new studies indicate that genetics plays a strong role in the development of homosexuality in both men and women. In March 1993 researchers at Northwestern University in Chicago, Illinois, and the Boston University School of Medicine in Massachusetts reported on their study of identical female twins. Such twins have an identical genetic complement, in contrast to fraternal (non-identical twins), who share some genes but not all.

The researchers identified 71 sets of identical twins in which at least one sister was a lesbian. They found that 48 percent of the second twins were also gay. A similar study in male twins had previously shown that 52 percent of the second twins were gay. In contrast, among 37 sets of non-identical female twins in which one was lesbian, the second twin was also lesbian only 6 percent of the time. Finally, the researchers identified 35 adoptive sisters who were raised in the same households, but shared no genes. Only 6 percent of this group were lesbians. The fact that not all the identical twins were lesbian, the researchers said, indicates that environment also plays a role. It is not known what those environmental factors might be, but possibilities include birth stresses and differential treatment by parents.

In July 1993, researchers at the National Cancer Institute (NCI) reported that much male homosexuality may be caused by a gene located in a small region of the X chromosome, the sex-linked chromosome that men inherit from their mothers. They reached this conclusion by studying families in which more than one male was homosexual. In such families, they occasionally observed fathers and sons who were both gay. Far more often, however, they observed that a gay male had a maternal uncle or a maternal cousin who was also gay. The incidence of such maternal links was about four times the normal rate, sug-

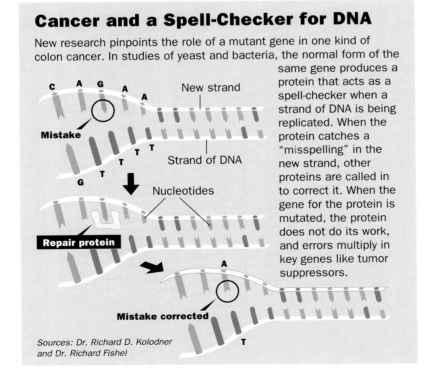

## Cancer and a Spell-Checker for DNA

New research pinpoints the role of a mutant gene in one kind of colon cancer. In studies of yeast and bacteria, the normal form of the same gene produces a protein that acts as a spell-checker when a strand of DNA is being replicated. When the protein catches a "misspelling" in the new strand, other proteins are called in to correct it. When the gene for the protein is mutated, the protein does not do its work, and errors multiply in key genes like tumor suppressors.

New strand

Mistake

Strand of DNA

Nucleotides

Repair protein

Mistake corrected

Sources: Dr. Richard D. Kolodner and Dr. Richard Fishel

gesting that the gene assumed to cause male homosexuality lies on the X chromosome.

To check this, the researchers identified 40 pairs of gay brothers and studied genetic markers on their X chromosomes, the same technique that is used for identifying gene defects in inherited illnesses. They found that 33 of the pairs shared markers in a small region of the chromosome, suggesting that the gene is in that region. The area contains an estimated 100 genes, however, so they are attempting to narrow their search down to a specific gene. The research has implications far beyond the study of homosexuality, however. Neuroscientists note that this represents the first time that a behavioral trait has been linked to a specific gene, and a study of how the gene works should provide insight into a variety of mental disorders.

## ▶ Aggression

A Dutch family with a long history of violence has enabled Dutch and American researchers to identify a gene associated with aggressive behavior. Researchers from Massachusetts General Hospital in Boston and University Hospital in Nijmegen, the Netherlands, reported in October 1993 that affected males in the family had a defect in the gene that serves as a blueprint for the well-known enzyme monoamine oxidase A. The enzyme is a brain chemical that helps break down several neurotransmitters that—if permitted to build up—might cause a person to overreact to stress.

The family traced the origin of the disorder to a couple who married in 1780. The disorder affects only men, and their "aggressive outbursts" have included a rape, two arsons, and an incident in which a man tried to run over his boss with a car after receiving a negative performance evaluation. The researchers found that none of the affected men showed the presence of the enzyme in their urine and all had a subnormal IQ, averaging about 85. The defective gene for the enzyme was then traced to the X chromosome.

## ▶ Alzheimer's Disease

North Carolina researchers have found a gene that may account for as many as two-thirds of the cases of Alzheimer's disease, a debilitating disease of aging that affects as many as 4 million Americans. It causes loss of memory and mental functions, and, eventually, death, primarily in people over the age of 65. Surprisingly, the newly identified gene is one that has previously been linked to heart disease, and its identification is leading not only to new ways of looking at the disease, but also to potential new therapies.

The gene in question serves as the blueprint for a protein called apolipoprotein E (ApoE) that ferries fats through the bloodstream. The North Carolina

team did not find that the ApoE gene is defective in Alzheimer's patients. Rather, they found that it exists in three normal variants, called ApoE 2, ApoE 3, and ApoE 4. An individual has two copies of the ApoE gene, one from each parent, and the identity of the variant determines the risk of developing Alzheimer's. An individual with two copies of ApoE 4 is as much as 15 times more likely to develop Alzheimer's as a person with no copies, while an individual with one copy is about five times as likely. About 20 percent of those with no copies of ApoE 4 develop Alzheimer's by age 75, compared to 60 percent of those with one copy and 90 percent of those with two copies. The work has subsequently been confirmed in several laboratories.

In November 1993, the researchers offered a potential explanation of how the gene works. The protein produced by ApoE 3, they said, acts to stabilize the structure of minute channels, called microtubules, that carry nutrients through nerve cells. ApoE 4 does not stabilize them nearly as well, so that the microtubules break down during the aging process, leading to the death of cells and development of the disease. They think it should be possible to design a synthetic molecule that would take the place of ApoE 3, stabilize the microtubules, and prevent the disease. Giving the drug, they say, would be like taking vitamin C to prevent scurvy.

## ▶ Genetic Engineering

In May 1993, researchers at the National Institutes of Health (NIH) declared the first approved gene therapy in humans an unqualified success. The subjects were Cynthia Cutshall, now 12, and Ashanthi De Silva, now 7. Both of the Ohio girls suffered from a rare condition called severe combined immunodeficiency disease (SCID), a complete malfunction of the immune system resulting from their bodies' inability to manufacture an enzyme called adenosine deaminase (ADA). Three years ago, the researchers removed white blood cells from each of the girls, used a virus to insert the gene for ADA, and reinfused the blood.

The cells then began making the missing enzyme, allowing their immune system to function. Both girls are now attending public schools, playing with friends, and participating in the normal activities of childhood—all of which they were unable to do before the treatment. Because the white blood cells die out after a few months, the process must be repeated periodically. To overcome that limitation, the researchers in June 1993 treated stem cells from the girls. Stem cells are the progenitor cells from which all other blood cells are made; they reside in the bone marrow permanently. The scientists hope that this treatment will result in a permanent cure for the disease, but they have not yet announced results.

Also in May 1993, researchers at Children's Hospital Los Angeles and the University of California at San Francisco performed stem cell therapy on three newborns who also suffered from SCID. In these three cases, however, the researchers isolated stem cells from the umbilical cord rather than the patients' bone marrow. The umbilical cord has proven to be a rich source of stem cells. Preliminary results disclosed in October 1993 suggest that the stem-cell therapy was effective in at least one of the infants.

The use of human gene therapy accelerated dramatically in 1993. Although there were no gene-therapy protocols approved in the United States until the end of 1990, more than 50 had begun or been approved by the NIH by the end of 1993. Although some of the projects are designed to treat genetic disorders, such as SCID, familial hypercholesterolemia, and cystic fibrosis, the majority were designed to treat AIDS and cancer, primarily by bolstering the immune system to make it better able to fight off the diseases.

Familial hypercholesterolemia is a liver disorder that results in extreme cholesterol buildup and early death. The disease results from a defect in the gene that serves as the blueprint for a protein called the LDL receptor. LDL is the so-called "bad" form of cholesterol that causes heart disease. In 1992, researchers now at the University of Pennsylvania treated a 29-year-old Canadian woman who had such severe coronary disease that bypass grafts were failing after only three years. Surgeons removed about 15 percent of her liver, separated individual cells, inserted a healthy gene for the LDL receptor into each, and infused them back into her body, where they took up residence in her liver. They reported in February 1993 that her cholesterol level, initially three times normal, had been reduced by 40 percent. They then hoped to bring it within the normal range by conventional therapy. Four other patients are being treated in the same fashion.

Researchers have also had some preliminary success in treating cystic fibrosis. These patients have a defective version of a gene called CFTR that allows thick mucus to build up in the lungs, where it impairs breathing and traps bacteria that can cause lethal infections. Three separate groups are conducting experiments in which a healthy version of the CFTR gene is inserted into a defanged form of adenovirus, one of the viruses that cause the common cold. A team from the University of Iowa reported in October 1993 that the virus is taken up by cells in the nose and throat, which then begin producing the protein. The researchers were simply studying safety of the technique, however, and the patients were not given a large enough dose to cure their disease.

## ▶ Malaria

Colombian scientists reported in March 1993 that they had made substantial progress with a genetically engineered vaccine for malaria, one of the most serious health problems of the developing world. Malaria kills 3.5 million people worldwide each year and affects 100 times that many. Researchers at the National University of Colombia in South America used a vaccine that contained three artificially produced proteins from the malaria parasite *Plasmodium falciparum*.

Over a six-month period, 152 of the 738 volunteers who received the vaccine had a total of 168 infections. In contrast, 242 of the 819 people taking a dummy vaccine had a total of 297 cases. The vaccine thus produced a 40 percent reduction in cases. The vaccine was particularly successful in children under the age of 4 (a 77 percent reduction in cases) and in those patients over the age of 45 (a 67 percent reduction).

## ▶ Sickle Cell Disease

A new way to turn genes on and off in order to facilitate the treatment of sickle cell disease and beta-thalassemia was reported in January 1993 by researcher teams at the Boston University School of Medicine in Massachusetts and the Oakland Children's Hospital in California.

In sickle cell disease, which affects an estimated 50,000 blacks in the United States, a genetic defect causes the production of a defective form of hemoglobin, the molecule inside red blood cells that transports oxygen through the bloodstream. That defect causes the cells to assume characteristic sickle shapes that clog capillaries, causing pain and organ damage. In beta-thalassemia, a serious condition which affects 10,000 Americans, the body does not produce hemoglobin at all and victims become severely anemic.

For reasons that are not entirely clear to scientists, the fetus uses a slightly different hemoglobin molecule produced by a different gene. This gene is not normally defective in either sickle cell disease or beta-thalassemia. If the gene could be activated or turned on, it would produce healthy hemoglobin that would greatly reduce the symptoms of the two diseases. The team studied a new drug called arginine butyrate, a derivative of an amino acid. In preliminary safety trials, they infused the drug into the bloodstream of six hospitalized patients, four with sickle cell disease and two with beta-thalassemia. Not only did the drug prove safe, but all of the patients had a significant improvement in their diseases and one of the beta-thalassemia patients even had a "complete reversal" of her symptoms. Trials using larger doses of arginine butyrate are now underway.

*Thomas H. Maugh II*

# Government Policies and Programs

In the fall of 1993, President Clinton unveiled his health-care-reform proposal. The plan was developed by a large task force chaired by the president's wife, Hillary Rodham Clinton, and directed by a fellow Rhodes scholar, Ira Magaziner.

### ▶ How the Clinton Plan Would Work

The key administrative elements in the plan are new organizations called Regional Health Alliances, which would contract with health plans, collect premiums from individuals and their employers, and pay health-care providers. The alliances would monitor the quality of care and provide information to help consumers make their decision on which plan to choose. These alliances would be run by boards of consumers and local employers.

All employers except the largest national corporations—those employing 5,000 workers or more —would have to be members of an alliance. A large corporation could self-insure its employees as long as its health plan is at least equal in quality to those available through the alliances.

Employed individuals would sign up for a health plan at their place of work. Information would be provided on the health plans available—prices, the participating physicians and hospitals, and information on the quality of care that each plan provided in the past. Those individuals who are self-employed or unemployed would be able to sign up for a plan through their local health alliance. Once a year, participants would be able to change plans if they were not satisfied with their current one.

*Under the Clinton health plan, a health-security card would be issued to each and every American.*

The Medicare program would remain, but those eligible for Medicare could elect to remain in health-care plans offered through their alliance.

### ▶ Principles of Clinton Health Plan

**Security.** This is a guarantee that all Americans would receive comprehensive health coverage. Re-gardless of changes in job or family status, this health coverage could not be taken away.

**Simplicity.** Clinton proposes to simplify the health-care system by creating a uniform, comprehensive package of benefits comparable to the ones that most Fortune 500 companies offer their employees. Like most current insurance plans, the Clinton benefit package would include physician and hospital care. Prescription drugs and certain other services would also be provided. Administrative procedures would be simplified by creating a standard form for all health-care claims, and standardized administrative procedures for processing claims.

**Savings.** The president predicts that this system would save money. Although there was much skepticism about the cost estimates, the Clinton administration continues to argue that the proposal would reduce the federal deficit by $58 billion through the end of the century.

The administration claims that implementation of its program would cost $331 billion, but would save the government $389 billion. These savings would derive from several sources, including: $189 billion from the Medicare and Medicaid program; $40 billion from other federal programs; tax increases of $89 billion; and additional revenue of $71 billion because employers would have lower health-care costs, and thus lower deductions in their corporate income tax. Included in the tax increases is a 75-cent-per-pack hike in the tax on cigarettes. (This tax hike presents a curious moral dilemma. On the one hand, the Clinton administration is committed to reducing smoking. On the other hand, a significant portion of the revenue to finance health-care reform is going to come from tax revenues that would decline if people stopped smoking.)

The costs of $331 billion are broken down to include $116 billion in premium discounts for business and families; a tax deduction for health-insurance costs for the self-employed, which would cost $10 billion; the new prescription-drug benefit in the Medicare program, which would cost $66 billion; a new program for long-term care, which would cost $65 billion; and increased spending for public health and administration of $29 billion. The Clinton administration's health plan also includes a $45 billion cushion in the event that these predicted costs are higher than anticipated.

One of the key issues involving cost was the extent to which cost increases could be controlled, particularly since those Americans who currently lack health insurance would be covered under the Clinton plan. The administration proposes global caps on health-care spending, and limits on allowable health-premium increases. Controversy rages over what would happen if demand for medical care causes these global caps to be breached.

The most important way that the Clinton administration thinks that its plan would save money is by increasing competition among health plans. This would be done by increasing the economic power of consumers and businesses who purchase health insurance. The proposed health alliance, in negotiating with insurers and the health-care-delivery system, would likely have more clout than small businesses or individual consumers do now.

The Clinton plan also hopes to achieve savings in drug prices. For existing drugs, the administration assumes that competition will limit price increases. For new drugs on which the manufacturer holds a patent, competition will restrain prices. At the same time, demand would increase because of the new Medicare prescription-drug program and through the inclusion of drugs in the standard medical plan proposed by the administration. To forestall unreasonable cost increases, the administration proposes to establish an advisory council to monitor the prices of new drugs. While the administration insists that there would not be price controls on drugs, there were skeptics, such as Senator Arlen Specter (R-Penn.), who argues that the administration would rely on controls rather than market forces.

**Quality.** The Clinton administration argues that its proposal will not only maintain the quality of care in the current system, but will increase the quality through several changes.

First, consumers would get information on the quality of services provided by different health plans, thus encouraging competition between plans on the basis of quality.

Second, the administration plan would emphasize preventive health measures with the objective of reducing costs by keeping people healthy. Consumers would not have to pay for a number of preventive services, including: prenatal care; well-baby care; immunizations; disease screening for adults, such as mammograms, Pap smears, and cholesterol tests; and health-promotion programs, like stop-smoking classes and nutrition counseling.

Third, the administration proposes to encourage more medical students, nurses, and other health-care professionals to enter primary care instead of specialties, with the objective of increasing the supply and quality of primary-care physicians.

**Choice.** The administration proposal contains three features designed to give consumers choice.

First, everyone would have a choice of health plans. At a minimum, each Regional Health Alliance would offer three different kinds of plans. These would include: the traditional fee-for-service, in which the consumer selects the health-care provider, and health insurance reimburses the provider for part or all of the bill; and two forms of managed care. One managed-care option would be Health Maintenance Organizations (HMOs), in which the

consumer goes to a health facility and is assigned a primary-care physician. The second option would be Preferred Provider Organizations (PPOs), a hybrid between fee-for-service and HMOs, in which the consumer chooses a primary-care physician from a list. Many health-care experts consider managed care to be less costly than fee-for-service because there is a greater ability to introduce controls to prevent unnecessary medical procedures and to limit reimbursement rates.

The second type of consumer choice that the administration emphasizes in its plan is the right to choose one's doctor. Nevertheless, to encourage participation in managed care, consumers would likely have higher out-of-pocket costs if they elected traditional fee-for-service. The maximum annual deductible for traditional fee-for-service would be up to $200 for an individual and $400 for families. The out-of-pocket limit for catastrophic expenses would be $1,500 a year for an individual and $3,000 for a family.

The third consumer choice that the administration emphasizes is a series of initiatives to give elderly and disabled Americans the option to remain at home in their communities while they receive long-term care. As an alternative to nursing homes, the administration proposes a new federal program to cover home- and community-based care. This program would be administered by the states, which would have flexibility in the approaches they adopted. Options available to the states would include homemaker and chore services, respite services, assistive technology, adult day care, rehabilitation, and supported employment.

For the disabled, the Clinton plan would provide comprehensive health-care coverage with no lifetime dollar limit on benefits that are often included in current health-insurance policies. The administration considers this the most important protection in the plan for the disabled. In addition, disabled persons who could work would be able to take jobs without fear that their government-financed health coverage would end. Disabled workers who needed personal assistance in order to continue working would be eligible for tax credits covering 50 percent of their costs up to $15,000 each year.

**Responsibility.** The final objective in the administration's plan is to make everyone responsible for paying part of the cost of health care. Small firms with low average wages would receive subsidies to keep their health-care costs down, but all employees and employers would have to pay part of the cost of health care.

Workers would have to pay about 20 percent of the cost of health insurance unless their employer elected to pay all of the premium.

Discounts would be provided to households with incomes below 150 percent of the poverty level.

In 1994 dollars, this translates to incomes below $22,200 for two-parent families with children, $18,400 for single parents with children, $14,600 for married couples without children, and $10,800 for single persons.

In addition, individuals will pay limited co-payments or deductibles to their health plans. Those who are either self-employed or unemployed, if they can afford to make payments, will have to pay part of the cost of their insurance.

Employers would have to pay 80 percent of the health-insurance premiums for their employees. No company, however, would be forced to spend more than 7.9 percent of its payroll for health coverage. For some firms, this would be a considerable savings. The Clinton administration estimates that some employers currently pay up to 20 percent of their payroll for health care.

The administration paid particular attention to the problems of small businesses, arguing that its plan would help small firms in the following ways:
• Administrative costs will fall because employees will be part of a Regional Health Alliance.
• The rates they pay would be the same that large firms pay.
• Certain insurance practices that hurt small firms will become illegal, such as price gouging and redlining entire industries by refusing to insure them.
• The workers' compensation system would be reformed. The Clinton administration notes that the current system is a particular source of problems and cost for small businesses.
• Small companies would receive special discounts. For the smallest firms that pay the lowest wages, such as restaurants, health costs could be as low as 3.5 percent of payroll.

The Clinton administration also proposes to reduce the litigation associated with medicine. Arbitration procedures would be established so that patients and physicians could attempt to settle disputes without going to court. In addition, lawyers' fees in medical-malpractice suits would be limited.

After the Clinton plan was announced, heated controversy erupted about who would benefit from the plan. The administration conceded in a hearing before the Senate Finance Committee that 40 percent of Americans would pay more for health insurance under the Clinton plan. This estimate was subsequently refined. The secretary of Health and Human Services, Donna E. Shalala, stated that only about 15 percent of the population would pay more for health insurance and not get more benefits. One of her senior staffers explained that of the currently insured, 60 percent would pay less and get more benefits, 20 percent would pay more and get more benefits, and the remaining 20 percent would pay more and get fewer benefits. The last category consisted primarily of young, healthy people.

## ▶ Other Reform Proposals

As 1993 drew to a close, health-care reform threatened to become a bazaar of competing proposals.

The most liberal approach is the single-payer concept, which would essentially nationalize the health-care industry. Only the government would provide health insurance. Former U.S. Representative Marty Russo (D-Ill.) originally introduced the legislation for a single-payer system. Senator Paul Wellstone (D-Minn.) and Congressman Jim McDermott (D-Wash.) took up the cudgels for this approach after Russo left Congress.

Another approach is called managed competition, a concept developed by a group of economists and health experts who brainstormed health-care problems at annual meetings in Jackson Hole, Wyoming. U.S. Representative Jim Cooper (D-Tenn.), yet another Rhodes scholar, introduced the managed-competition legislation. While the Clinton plan mandates that employers provide health insurance, the Cooper plan would provide subsidies to individuals who cannot afford health coverage. The subsidy would extend up to 200 percent of the poverty level. Like Clinton, Cooper would create pools for the purchase of health insurance at lower rates. Cooper's plan would not impose global-health-spending budgets as Clinton's would, however.

A third proposal, sponsored by U.S. Representatives Pete Stark (D-Calif.), the chairman of the House Ways and Means Health Subcommittee, and Richard Gephardt (D-Mo.), the majority leader in the House, would expand the Medicare and Medicaid programs, while limiting overall health spending.

Finally, Republicans offered several approaches. One is a proposal for incremental reform through regulating employment-based health insurance, providing a tax deduction for the self-employed, and reforming medical-malpractice-liability laws. This proposal, which is largely based on measures developed by the Bush administration, was introduced by House Minority Leader Bob Michel (R-Ill.).

Some moderate to liberal Senate Republicans led by John Chafee (R-R.I.) introduced legislation that many political observers feel might eventually enable a bipartisan coalition on health-care reform. Chafee proposes to require individuals to purchase health insurance, while providing subsidies to low- and moderate-income persons who could not afford it on their own. Like both the Clinton and Cooper plans, Chafee would create insurance cooperatives to reduce health-care premiums, but employer participation in these plans would be voluntary. This is a sharp contrast to the Clinton mandate that all but the largest employers participate. The Chafee plan also rejects the global-budgeting approach in the Clinton plan. Instead, the Chafee plan would control cost escalation by slowing down increased access to the health system if savings did not materialize.

## ▶ Health-Budget Costs

Even as the Clinton administration proposed health-care reform, major cuts were made in the current program to bring the federal budget deficit down. In August, Congress agreed to a package of cuts, which, over the next five years, was estimated to save $55.8 billion in Medicare and $7.1 billion in Medicaid. These cuts were an example of how difficult it will be to reform the health-care system while the federal government continues to run major deficits. The Clinton administration proposed Medicare and Medicaid cuts to help finance health-care reform. It argues that most of the savings could come from preventing health-care providers from shifting costs from non-Medicare patients to Medicare patients. The Clinton cuts would be on top of the cuts in the budget package approved in August. Their magnitude was sufficient to lead Gail Walinsky, a former senior Bush administration health official, to warn that the proposed reductions as part of health-care reform were "unwise" and "impolitic."

## ▶ Health Officials

The Clinton administration moved quickly to make its mark with key appointments. David Kessler, M.D., the highly respected commissioner of the Food and Drug Administration (FDA), who had been appointed by President Bush, was one of the only Republican appointees permitted to stay on. In September 1993, after an acrimonious debate, the Senate confirmed M. Joycelyn Elders, M.D., as surgeon general. Dr. Elders had administered the public-health program for the state of Arkansas and was an outspoken proponent of making birth-control information and devices available to teenagers. In November 1993, Harold E. Varmus, M.D., became director

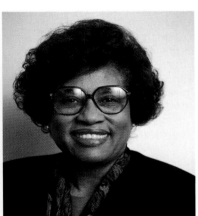

M. Joycelyn Elders, M.D.

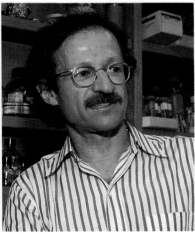

Harold E. Varmus, M.D.

of the National Institutes of Health (NIH). Dr. Varmus is the first Nobelist to achieve that position.

*James A. Rotherham, Ph.D.*

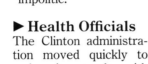

# Health-Care Costs

## ▶ Reform Afoot

From beginning to end, the prospect of reform dominated the health-cost agenda for 1993. As the nation's total health bill soared above $940 billion and flirted with the trillion-dollar mark, it was far from clear what direction reform would take. By year's end, however, the health-reform effort was officially under way: Congress had a massive, 1,342-page reform proposal from the Clinton administration, as well as several serious reform proposals from its own members to deliberate. But as policy makers prepared for what promised to be the most sweeping legislation since the New Deal—legislation that would affect every citizen and fully one-seventh of the nation's economy—the massive health-care system was already in the midst of change.

Throughout the country, employers were finding ways to hold the line on costs, and doctors and hospitals were banding together to find new ways of delivering health care. Many insurers reported single-digit premium increases—a few held at no increase—for the coming year. It seemed that reform was already well under way beyond Washington's Beltway.

Even before Bill Clinton formally assumed office in late January, a transition team was struggling to frame a program to deliver on his promise of health reform. Clinton had campaigned on a program that would provide health care to all Americans and, at the same time, control costs and maintain quality. Health economists repeatedly pointed out that the three were mutually incompatible, that any two were possible, but not the third.

Clinton had initially embraced a concept known as managed competition as a way to deal with the nation's soaring health costs, now approaching 15 percent of the gross domestic product. As the campaign progressed, Clinton added several elements —among them a global health budget—to the original concept, which relied on market forces to control costs.

The transition team's proposal was quickly rejected as too costly. The new president immediately appointed his wife, Hillary Rodham Clinton, to head a task force that would deliver a health-reform plan within 100 days that would meet all the president's objectives. With longtime Clinton friend and business consultant Ira Magaziner at the helm, the task force set up shop behind closed doors at the Old Executive Office Building next to the White House. With lobbyists, the press, and most of the experts who had been preaching health reform for the past few years shut out, the more than 500 task-force members struggled to deliver an acceptable plan in an atmosphere of secrecy.

While the task-force members were attempting to figure out how the managed-competition structure favored by the president could work, Mrs. Clinton and Tipper Gore, wife of Vice President Al Gore, traveled the country for hearings and town meetings where citizens aired their problems with the current system. More secretly, political strategists worked on techniques for selling the president's proposal once it was formed. At one point a spokesman said they were prepared to resort to demonstrations in the streets to gain public support for the program.

The effort quickly bogged down. Advocacy groups and the press complained about the secrecy; several groups went to court, accusing the administration of violating legal requirements for open meetings since neither Mrs. Clinton nor Mrs. Gore, both task-force members, were government employees. To pacify interest groups, the task force held a token public hearing at which witnesses were allowed three minutes to present their cases. Even though task-force members were sworn to silence, internal grumbling about the unwieldy process started to surface. After pirated lists of members were published, the White House finally identified most of the task-force members. Many, it turned out, were staff members of key Democratic members of Congress, a strategy would-be critics saw as an effort to win votes even before legislation was drafted.

As it became increasingly clear that the 100 days was an impossible target, the process loosened somewhat. Mrs. Clinton made repeated forays to Capitol Hill to brief key members of Congress and solicit their views, eventually reaching out to key Republicans as well as Democrats. Members of key interest groups began meeting with task-force members, offering their ideas on health care and outlining their concerns about the perceived direction the plan was moving. The press was briefed about the process, and "trial balloons" began appearing with increasing regularity on the front pages of major newspapers to test public reaction to such funding proposals as a value-added tax (VAT) or a mandate that all employers pay for the health insurance of their workers.

Throughout, the overall framework of the Clinton approach remained clear, even while the details were being worked out. Structurally the plan would create huge purchasing alliances that would negotiate with "accountable health plans"—networks of hospitals and doctors—to offer a number of competing health plans from which members of the alliance could choose. All employers with fewer than 5,000 workers would have to join the alliances; providers would compete for business on the basis of both cost and quality, and would have to offer the same basic package of specified benefits to all Americans. A new entity, a National Health Board, would oversee the process and draw up a national health budget if competition failed to control costs, although states would be granted great flexibility to design their own health systems.

▶ Alternate Approaches

Meanwhile, reform advocates and interest groups on the outside pursued their own agendas. After the administration attempted to portray both the drug industry and insurers as the villains responsible for uncontrollable increases in health costs, both groups fought back in an attempt at damage control. Pharmaceutical groups stressed that drugs were less expensive than other therapies, and pledged to hold down price increases; the insurance industry issued its own reform agenda, including proposals to guarantee a basic benefit package for all Americans and eliminate discriminatory practices that block many Americans from obtaining decent health insurance. Though Magaziner and Mrs. Clinton repeatedly assured physicians that reform would reduce red tape and paperwork, and put them back in charge of patient care, physicians on the whole remained guarded, worried by talk of budgets, price controls, and an end to traditional fee-for-service medicine, where doctors are paid for care that is given.

As the details of the Clinton plan became clearer, advocates of alternative approaches became louder. Proponents of a Canadian-style single-payer system pursued a vigorous grass-roots campaign; legislation backed by Senator Paul Wellstone (D-Minn.) and Representative James McDermott (D-Wash.) garnered more than 80 co-sponsors. Representative Jim Cooper (D-Tenn.) and Senator John Breaux (D-La.) pushed a "pure" form of managed competition that would require employers only to offer insurance, not pay for it, and would rely on the free market, not budgets or controls, to hold down costs. Led by Senators John Chafee (R-R.I.) and Robert Dole (R-Kans.), Republicans offered a reform proposal close to the Cooper approach, while conservative Republicans, led by Senator Phil Gramm (R-Tex.), urged a health savings account/voucher system that would permit Americans to purchase their own insurance.

From those proposals, the reform plans that had been urged by various coalitions and leading interest groups, and from the outlines of the Clinton plan, consensus emerged on the broad principles. All Americans should, at the very least, have access to health care and some form of insurance that assures a basic package of benefits. Though polls repeatedly show that most Americans are satisfied with their

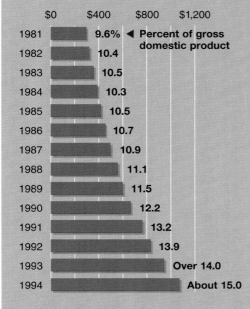

## Health Spending: Reaching $1 Trillion

Spending on health care in the United States, in billions of dollars.

| | $0 | $400 | $800 | $1,200 | |
|---|---|---|---|---|---|
| 1981 | | 9.6% | | | ◀ Percent of gross domestic product |
| 1982 | | 10.4 | | | |
| 1983 | | 10.5 | | | |
| 1984 | | 10.3 | | | |
| 1985 | | 10.5 | | | |
| 1986 | | 10.7 | | | |
| 1987 | | 10.9 | | | |
| 1988 | | 11.1 | | | |
| 1989 | | 11.5 | | | |
| 1990 | | 12.2 | | | |
| 1991 | | 13.2 | | | |
| 1992 | | 13.9 | | | |
| 1993 | | | Over 14.0 | | |
| 1994 | | | About 15.0 | | |

Figures for 1992-94 are Commerce Department estimates.

| BREAKDOWN OF ESTIMATED COSTS | | |
|---|---|---|
| | **1993** | **1994** |
| **Total** | **$942.5** | **$1,060.5** |
| **HEALTH SERVICES AND SUPPLIES** | 914.0 | 1,029.6 |
| Personal health care | 830.2 | 934.8 |
|  Hospitals | 363.4 | 408.8 |
|  Physicians' services | 175.2 | 194.9 |
|  Dentists' services | 44.2 | 47.5 |
|  Other professional services | 47.4 | 54.0 |
|  Home health | 16.5 | 22.2 |
|  Nondurable medical products | 72.6 | 80.2 |
|  Durable medical equipment | 14.2 | 15.5 |
|  Nursing home care | 76.0 | 85.5 |
|  Other personal health care | 20.7 | 26.2 |
| Administration | 54.3 | 61.9 |
| Government public health activity | 29.4 | 32.9 |
| **RESEARCH** | 14.1 | 15.0 |
| **CONSTRUCTION** | 14.4 | 15.8 |

Sources: Department of Health and Human Services, Department of Commerce

health coverage and care, reform would protect Americans from their greatest fear: loss of coverage and/or a catastrophic illness that would overwhelm existing insurance. One study calculated that as many as 2 million Americans lose insurance coverage each month, joining, at least temporarily, the pool of 37 million without coverage.

### ▶ Number Crunching

Another point of broad consensus revolved around the need to control the growth of health-care costs, which by 1991 consumed 97.5 percent of the after-tax profits for business and, as President Clinton repeatedly warned, threatened to undermine the nation's overall economy. He proposed that the enactment of his health program would slow growth in health spending to the rate of inflation within a period of two years.

After missing repeated self-imposed deadlines, then bowing to congressional pressure not to confuse the legislative agenda by pushing health reform until after the annual budget deliberations were resolved, the Clinton administration waited until late summer to revive the health-reform proposals. Though the structure of the Clinton plan had been clear since the campaign, two major stumbling

blocks persisted: the cost of reform and how to pay for it. Those were superimposed on a number of other interrelated details, such as how generous the basic benefit package would be. Though the ultimate decisions rested with the president, official task-force members and presidential advisers were split from the outset between those who advocated generous coverage and those who urged caution and a slower, more measured approach to reform until all of the cost implications of the health-care proposals were clear.

The cost and funding details remained obscure even after a 239-page draft plan was circulated in mid-September, after the president unveiled his plan for a joint session of Congress 10 days later, and after Mrs. Clinton and task-force members began testifying before congressional committees. While White House advisers maintained those details were still being changed, and "number crunchers" were still working to make sure the numbers were correct, outsiders started sniping at the "fantasy" financing. Even Senate Finance Committee Chairman Daniel Patrick Moynihan (D-N.Y.) questioned, in public statements, the Clinton administration's plan to pay for the system through sharp cutbacks in Medicare and Medicaid, a new tax on cigarettes, and anticipated savings within the system, while at the same time guaranteeing generous coverage to all Americans (even those who now have no insurance coverage), subsidizing the cost to small businesses that are threatened by the added burden of paying for health coverage for all of their employees, adding new drug and home-health benefits for Medicare recipients, and subsidizing the costs of coverage for early retirees.

When the legislation was formally introduced in late October, it contained few surprises, but it had been toned down. Deadlines were stretched, and cost estimates were revised. As it stands now, administration number crunchers figure the additional costs to the government for coverage and the benefit package to be $389 billion over the five-year period from 1995 to 2000. Avoiding the notion of new general taxes—the employee contribution was dubbed a "premium," not a "tax," though business leaders pointed out that any mandatory payment they could not control was equivalent to a tax— the administration promised this money would come largely from savings in Medicare, Medicaid, and other government health programs, and from a new tax on cigarettes. Most of this money would go to subsidies for small businesses and low-income Americans, and to new drug and long-term-care benefits for Medicare recipients, with a hefty $45 billion contingency cushion to cover any possible miscalculations.

Though political optimists predicted quick action on health reform, realists wondered if Congress could complete the immense and complex task of reform before the 1994 congressional elections are held in November. Indeed, beneath agreement on the broad goals of reform, and despite Clinton administration warnings that all the details of the health-care package were carefully interwoven, tinkering threatened the whole effort, and tinkering with the details is certainly inevitable. As Senator Dole acknowledged, "Everyone here, be they Republican or Democrat, agrees that America's health-care system can be improved. Rather, the debate will be over the prescription."

## ▶ Reform without Reform

Even as Congress began hearings and as committees jockeyed for jurisdiction on key parts of the Clinton initiative, the reform movement was already well under way outside of Washington. Blue Cross/ Blue Shield plans reported that the days of double-digit cost increases were over, with an average premium rise of 5.5 percent. In some tightly managed systems, the reports were even more encouraging: Some HMOs announced a zero inflation rate. Health analyst KPMG Peat Marwick recorded an 8 percent increase in premiums after surveying more than 1,000 employers selected at random.

The "reform-without-reform" movement began in the early 1980s, when businesses, confronted with ever-escalating costs, began to limit benefits, offer only HMOs to employees, or negotiate with preferred-provider networks for discounts in return for volume. In some parts of the country, doctors and hospitals began forming networks of their own as a means of survival. As with many health-care innovations, the new wave got its start on the West Coast and spread. "The growth has been explosive," reports Donald Fisher, head of the American Group Practice Association. "The practice of medicine is changing very rapidly even without health reform."

The Washington Business Group on Health, which represents a hefty portion of the Fortune 500, reports that more than half its members have managed-care networks, and 95 percent have some form of managed care as part of their health programs. Individual firms and business coalitions are experimenting with different approaches. Southern California Edison has set up its own system, with company doctors and in-house clinics providing routine care. In central Florida a purchasing alliance, representing 300,000 employees, began bargaining for discounted prices, analyzing outcomes of care, and creating an insurance pool for small- and medium-sized businesses; it projected eventual savings of more than $100 million. A major health-promotion program for city employees in Birmingham, Alabama, saved the city more than $10 million in health costs.

The government's efforts to hold down spending for its two programs, Medicare for the elderly and Medicaid for the poor, were not as successful. Medicare's 1992 spending reached $129 billion, and was expected, according to Congressional Budget Office (CBO) projections, to double by 1998; Medicaid's $68 billion price tag was expected to reach $146 billion by that time. At the same time, even though faced with a growing Medicare population, Congress cut $69 billion from Medicare over a five-year period, largely by reducing payments to doctors and hospitals. The Clinton plan proposes even deeper cuts.

How much of the grass-roots reform was due to the need of employers to control their own costs and how much was due to the looming inevitability of major reform remains unclear. What was clear, though, was that with the combination of ongoing change and the efforts of the administration and Congress to produce sweeping reform, health care in the United States in the years to come will be dramatically different. Whether the emerging new system will meet the goals of cost-effectiveness and quality health care for all Americans remains to be answered.

*Mary Hager*

# Health Personnel and Facilities

▶ **Health Networks**

A key portion of the Clinton administration's plan for reforming the U.S. health-care system involves the creation of integrated health networks. As envisioned by President Bill Clinton, the health-care-reform movement will create large-scale networks of physicians and hospitals. These networks will provide care to patients who are covered by purchasing cooperatives that represent all residents of a particular geographic area or all employees of a major corporation.

As it turns out, these networks are not distant pipe dreams; they are already reality in many parts of the country, and hospitals are the prime movers.

The emerging health networks take several different forms. Some are composed only of hospitals and physicians; others include any combination of outpatient clinics, nursing homes, home-health agencies, hospices, pharmacies, and mental-health programs in addition to physicians and hospitals.

Many act like massive health maintenance organizations (HMOs) to provide a full range of health services for a fixed price. A network headed by Henry Ford Health System in Detroit, Michigan, for example, includes 13 hospitals and hundreds of physicians. As a group the network contracts with local employers to provide everything from immunizations for schoolchildren to open-heart surgery for adult retirees in exchange for a designated monthly payment per employee.

The goal of the integrated health networks is to meet all or most of the health-care needs of patients in a community or company, and to do so in an economic manner. The networks consequently are working to enhance existing local health services. Butterworth Health System, a new network in Grand Rapids, Michigan, strengthens its position by sharing expertise among its 11 hospitals. The linchpin institution of the network, Butterworth Hospital, is a large tertiary-care center that specializes in cardiology, neonatology, obstetrics, oncology, and pediatrics. Butterworth has sent some of its own clinical specialists or administrators to help upgrade particular health programs, such as physical therapy, and improve the buildings and facilities in other network hospitals.

Networks also are trying to fill gaps in existing services. When it was first formed, Butterworth Health System discovered that the 13 counties in and around Grand Rapids had far too few primary-care physicians to adequately care for the area's 1.3 million residents. The network therefore established seven urgent-care centers to treat minor emergencies among the counties' 165,000 indigent patients. Butterworth formed a primary-care clinic, school-health program, and four rural family-health centers. The network at the present time is building a special-care center that will treat and rehabilitate occupational injuries, provide ambulatory surgery, and house modern diagnostic equipment.

**Streamlining operations.** New integrated health networks plan to reduce costs by improving the efficiency of health-care delivery, and they are targeting in particular costly duplicative hospital services. According to the U.S. Commerce Department, hospitals account for more than 40 percent of all health-care spending in this country—more than is spent on doctors, dentists, and drugs combined. Hospitals also have large numbers of unused beds and services. On any given night, fully 33 percent of the hospital beds in this country are not occupied.

Because health networks merge several hospitals in a particular area, the networks are able to slash the number of unused beds; reduce the amount of little-used, expensive diagnostic equipment; combine basic-support departments, such as dietary, housekeeping, and the laboratory; and cut administrative expenditures by downsizing management and decreasing paperwork.

▶ **Emergency Rooms for Emergencies**

Visits to hospital emergency rooms have grown steadily over the past 15 years. In the first three months of 1993 alone, visits to emergency departments in community hospitals jumped 8.7 percent; many of these visits were for nonemergencies. As a result, hospital emergency rooms are overcrowded with patients who often must wait for hours to see a doctor to treat a minor problem.

Several hospitals have attempted to alleviate emergency-room overcrowding by instituting so-called fast-track programs. These programs use staff members to screen patients as soon as they enter the hospital emergency department. Those who have mild infections or injuries are then directed to a designated waiting area for walk-in ambulatory patients, freeing up the emergency-department area for seriously ill patients, and shortening the length of time the walk-in patients have to wait to see a doctor. The fast-track programs also are priced differently. Instead of the standard $150 charge for a typical nonemergency visit to an emergency department, fast-track programs charge only about $75.

A number of hospitals have used home-care programs to keep patients out of the costly emergency department. Home-care nurses at some hospitals act as case managers for patients in various high-

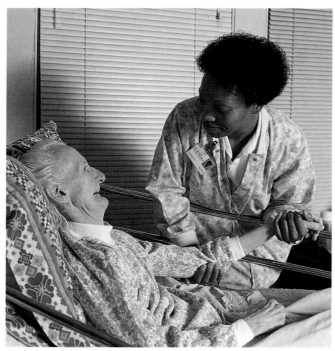

*In many hospitals and continuing-care facilities, nurses' aides have assumed many of the responsibilities traditionally held by registered nurses.*

risk groups, such as elderly individuals with heart disease or children with asthma. Patients who fall into these high-risk categories are assigned a case manager who conducts a complete medical examination and treats the immediate problem. The case managers then develop an ongoing relationship with the high-risk patients. In the future, whenever a patient experiences distress of any kind, he or she can call the case manager directly and receive medical attention before the situation deteriorates into a true medical emergency.

### ▶ The Changing Hospital Professional Staff

As hospitals become more involved in large health networks that offer wide ranges of services, they are adding more nonphysicians to their professional medical staffs. A recent report from the American Hospital Association showed that between 1989 and 1991, hospitals had increased the number of non-physician and nurse specialists in all categories. The report found that 6 percent more hospitals had doctors of osteopathy on staff in 1991 than in 1989, 8 percent more had podiatrists, 7 percent more had psychologists, 9 percent more had physician assistants, 6 percent more had nurse practitioners, and 6 percent more had nurse midwives.

**Nurses' aides.** Acute-care hospitals also are relying more on nurses' aides than they have in the past few years. As recently as five years ago, nurses'

aides were almost completely absent from the wards of American hospitals. In 1991, however, the Hospital Nursing Personnel Survey showed that hospitals increased their budgets for nurses' aides by more than 9 percent.

Hospitals have begun rehiring nurses' aides for two principal reasons. One is the long-standing overall shortage of registered nurses (RNs)—as high as 15 percent for hospitals in some parts of the country over the past few years. The other is the severity of illness of patients in the hospital. Cost-containment pressures have forced hospitals to admit only the sickest patients. Because registered nurses, the primary caregivers in hospitals, need to devote most of their on-duty time to direct clinical care of these critically ill patients, hospitals have turned to nurses' aides to perform many of the RN's nonnursing duties, such as transporting patients and changing linens.

**Patient helpers.** A new class of health worker is offering hospitals the chance to improve patients' satisfaction with their treatment and at the same time keep personnel costs to a minimum. Called patient-service associates, the staffers perform a number of personal-care activities for patients, such as serving meals, running errands, and cleaning rooms. The patient-service associates coordinate tasks that usually are handled by as many as 16 different workers during a typical hospital stay. The patient helpers reduce the need for hiring temporary nurses or requiring on-staff nurses to work overtime in order to meet basic patient needs.

Minorities have traditionally been poorly represented in health-care professions. Although minorities accounted for 22 percent of the total U.S. population in 1991, only 8 percent of physicians, 14 percent of nurses, and 10 percent of health administrators were members of minority groups. This situation will likely change as the need for educated health-care workers in the next 12 years grows dramatically, increasing between 42 and 92 percent in various job categories.

In order to provide health education and career opportunities for minorities, groups of hospitals in several cities are participating in Project Achieve, an effort funded by the Kaiser Foundation. Project Achieve provides minority students with special education in the sciences and mathematics, field trips to health-care settings, health-career mentors, and help in entering college. One of the most telling examples of Project Achieve success has occurred in North Memphis, Tennessee. Before the program began in 1989, fewer than 10 percent of the minority students in the area finished high school and went on for further schooling. In 1992 more than 50 of the 200 Project Achieve students headed for college.

*Karen M. Sandrick*

# Heart and Circulatory System

Cardiovascular disease (CVD) is the cause of 1 million deaths annually in the United States. Even though preventive strategies, early diagnosis, and improved treatment for cardiac disease have reduced CVD deaths by 50 percent in the past 30 years, CVD nonetheless remains a most important public-health problem.

Several 1993 studies have added new risk factors for coronary-artery disease (CAD) to the established list. These include: male pattern baldness; chronic infection with the respiratory bacterium *Chlamydia pneumoniae;* oxidized LDL (a particularly bad form of the "bad" cholesterol); lack of emotional support; low socioeconomic status; elevated levels of the natural clot dissolver t-PA; trans-fatty acids (found in margarine and shortening); triglycerides; women with six or more pregnancies; and physical inactivity. Other 1993 reports defined certain protective factors: phenols in red wine; the anti-breast-cancer drug tamoxifen (Nolvadex); high intake of walnuts; and the antioxidants vitamin E and beta-carotene. Other studies found that aspirin, when combined with the blood thinner warfarin (Coumadin), prevented artificial blockages in the neck and prevented death and embolism in patients with artificial heart valves; the related blood thinners picotamide and indobufen prevented myocardial infarction (MI) and other complications.

## ▶ Treating Myocardial Infarction

Three 1993 studies support the use of emergency angioplasty to open arteries blocked by blood clots. In this procedure a balloon mounted on a catheter is passed through the groin artery and into the heart's arteries. Angioplasty was found to be a more effective, safer, and cheaper means of opening arteries than are thrombolytic ("clot-busting") drugs. Another study showed that the combination of angioplasty and thrombolytic drugs was no more effective—and actually less safe—than angioplasty alone. The chief limitation of angioplasty is the fact that only 18 percent of U.S. hospitals have angioplasty facilities.

Given this situation, thrombolytic drugs continue to be a crucial weapon against the coronary-artery blood clots that cause myocardial infarction. A 1993 European study confirmed that the sooner the drugs are used, the more heart muscle—and thus lives—will be saved. The best results of all occur when the drugs are given immediately in the home or ambulance.

The results of the Global Utilization of Streptokinase and t-PA for Occluded Arteries (GUSTO) study, the largest heart study ever mounted, were released in 1993. The study found that using a rapid infusion of t-PA (Activase) saved more lives than did the thrombolytic streptokinase (Streptase, Kabikinase) or the combination of both agents, despite having the effect of causing more brain hemorrhages. The study also shows that the earlier a patient is treated and the faster the artery is opened, the better the survival and the more heart muscle is saved. Because t-PA opens arteries faster than streptokinase, the use of t-PA for MI could save 2,000 extra lives annually, though at an extremely high cost compared to streptokinase (t-PA is 10 times more expensive than streptokinase).

Another study showed that aspirin given after thrombolytic medications to patients suffering myocardial infarction is as effective as the more powerful blood thinner warfarin in keeping arteries from re-clotting. Still another 1993 paper found that the leech-saliva protein hirudin is more effective in preventing reclotting than is the standard blood thinner heparin. Finally, t-PA was shown to be superior to heparin in removing dangerous pulmonary emboli (blood clots that arise in veins, break off, and lodge in the lungs).

## After a Heart Attack

A new study reported a marginal advantage of using the combination of tissue plasminogen activator (t-PA) and heparin over streptokinase in dissolving blood clots that form to cause a heart attack.

| Treatment | Number of patients | % Died | % Disabling stroke |
| --- | --- | --- | --- |
| Accelerated t-PA with intravenous heparin | 10,344 | 6.3 | 0.6 |
| Combination of t-PA and streptokinase with intravenous heparin | 10,328 | 7.0 | 0.6 |
| Streptokinase with subcutaneous heparin | 9,796 | 7.2 | 0.5 |
| Streptokinase with intravenous heparin | 10,377 | 7.4 | 0.5 |

Source: GUSTO Heart Attack Study

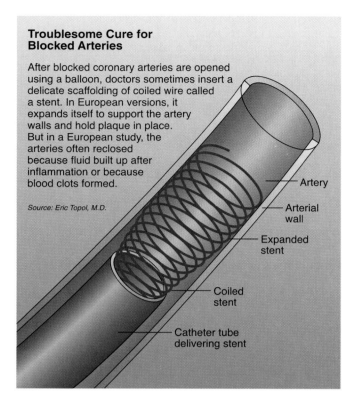

**Troublesome Cure for Blocked Arteries**

After blocked coronary arteries are opened using a balloon, doctors sometimes insert a delicate scaffolding of coiled wire called a stent. In European versions, it expands itself to support the artery walls and hold plaque in place. But in a European study, the arteries often reclosed because fluid built up after inflammation or because blood clots formed.

*Source: Eric Topol, M.D.*

Artery

Arterial wall

Expanded stent

Coiled stent

Catheter tube delivering stent

## ▶ Unblocking Coronary Arteries

In chronic coronary-artery disease, fixed blockages cause chest pains, weakening of the heart muscle, and predisposition to MIs and sudden death. Two 1993 studies compared treatment of the blockages by conventional balloon angioplasty to the newer catheter technique of atherectomy. Atherectomy is performed the same way as balloon angioplasty, but involves a motorized shaving cutter instead of a balloon; it destroys blockages by cutting away the plaque, not by flattening it against the artery wall like balloon angioplasty. The studies found that while atherectomy results in better and more reliable initial arterial dilating, with less renarrowing over time, the procedure causes more complications and is more costly than the balloon method.

In 1993 the Food and Drug Administration (FDA) approved the use of two new devices for coronary blockages: the rotational atherectomy catheter (literally, a diamond-studded drill bit that pulverizes plaque); and the coronary-artery stent, a cylindrical metal coil that is placed inside the narrowed artery (also via a catheter) to prop it open.

A 1993 interim report from one of several studies comparing angioplasty of multiple blockages with multivessel bypass surgery concludes that the procedures are equivalent in preventing MI and death, but surgery leads to fewer residual symptoms, less need for medications, and fewer repeat procedures.

Another study found that aspirin is more effective than the blood thinner warfarin or the combination of aspirin and dipyridamole (Persantine) in preventing the clotting of bypass vessels.

## ▶ Cholesterol and Hypertension

In 1993 the first update of national cholesterol guidelines in five years was released. The guidelines recommended intensified treatment of elevated LDL CAD patients, but suggested restraint in treating the young. This suggested restraint is a result of recent data indicating that lowering cholesterol, while helping to reduce CAD, actually increases non-CAD mortality. Thus, only those at high risk of death from CAD should undergo such treatment. The report also highlights the risk of low levels of HDL, or "good," cholesterol.

Last year also saw the updating of national guidelines on high blood pressure. Diuretics (water pills) and beta-blockers are recommended as first-line drugs, since only these classes of antihypertensives are proven to reduce stroke and coronary-artery disease. A 1993 study of mild hypertensive medications found that such drugs reduce blood pressure more effectively than do nondrug measures (reducing salt, alcohol, tobacco, and caloric intake, as well as increasing the frequency of exercise).

## ▶ Congestive Heart Failure

The incidence of heart failure, a syndrome marked by severe weakening of the heart's pumping function and caused by a variety of cardiac insults, continues to grow as patients with severe heart disease are kept alive with improved treatments, only to eventually manifest heart failure. Severe heart failure afflicts 2 million Americans, with a 50 percent annual mortality (worse than most cancers).

Last year saw the quick rise and fall of the drug flosequinan (Manoplax), the first new drug for heart failure in many years. Flosequinan works by a novel molecular mechanism to improve symptoms and exercise capacity. Unfortunately, soon after FDA approval, its manufacturer voluntarily withdrew the drug from the market after a major study found that at high doses the drug increases the rate of hospitalization and death due to worsened heart failure. The drug was a major disappointment, and is one of many heart-failure drugs that appeared initially promising, but paradoxically worsened survival.

Another promising drug, vesnarinone, not only improves symptoms of heart failure, but also survival rates, at low doses. Again, strangely, it worsened survival at higher doses in a 1993 trial.

In other drug studies, the 18th-century drug digoxin (Lanoxin) is very efficacious in heart failure; a study examining its effects on survival is in progress. A Swedish trial of metoprolol (Lopressor, Toprol XL), a beta-blocker, found that it was very effective in preventing death or the need for heart transplantation (the only effective treatment for "end-stage" heart failure); in the past, beta-blockers were thought to be lethal for such patients. Finally, the ACE inhibitor drug enalapril (Vasotec) was shown to prevent angina and MI in patients with heart failure.

## ▶ Treating Arrhythmias

Arrhythmias are heartbeat irregularities that cause the heart to pump less effectively. Many types of arrhythmias can occur in healthy or diseased hearts. The condition can range in severity from trivial nuisances causing palpitations (usually arising in the atria or upper chambers) to sustained, malignant disorders causing loss of consciousness or sudden death (usually arising in the ventricles or lower chambers). The death of basketball star Reggie Lewis from a lethal ventricular arrhythmia, and the diagnosis of a very benign arrhythmia by one of his doctors, has heightened public interest in these disorders.

A major 1993 study found that the new drug sotalol (Betapace) was superior to six other antiarrhythmic drugs in preventing death and recurrent arrhythmias. The study also found that the cheap technique of Holter monitoring (whereby the patient wears a tape recorder, which records 24 hours of continuous EKGs) is as useful as the invasive and costly technique of electrophysiological study (EPS) in predicting which drugs are most effective for dangerous ventricular arrhythmias. (EPS involves the insertion of several catheters through groin veins and into the heart, followed by electrical stimulation of the heart in order to provoke arrhythmias.) Another study found that the related drug amiodarone (Cordarone) reduced mortality after MI, and still another study found that in victims surviving sudden cardiac death, the routine use of amiodarone was superior to using EPS to test all other drugs to find the best one.

The type of arrhythmia called atrial fibrillation does not cause death, but can lead to stroke if blood clots form in the fibrillating atrial chambers. Recent studies show that the blood thinner warfarin prevents these strokes; a 1993 study now shows that the safer and more convenient aspirin is equally effective in preventing stroke. A study of neurocardiogenic syncope, a form of fainting caused by an overactive nerve reflex involving the heart and brain, finds that medications such as beta-blockers are a more effective treatment than pacemakers.

Finally, many types of arrhythmias are being cured by catheter ablation, whereby radio-frequency energy is delivered through catheters (passed into the heart via the groin veins) into the sources of arrhythmias, where it destroys them.

*Richard L. Mueller, M.D.*

# Immunology

## ▶ Removing Immune-Cell Blinders

The immune system is an amazingly deadly foe for most invaders of the body. Immune cells act as vigilant sentries, quickly identifying and destroying such foreign agents as viruses and bacteria. But in the case of cancer, immune cells seem to be continuously duped. Cancer cells manage to slip by these watchguards and escape destruction, only to produce widespread devastation wherever they go.

Recent advances have unveiled a more precise picture of how T cells, the scout cells of the immune system, recognize foreign agents. This emerging picture, in turn, has led to research using a novel gene-therapy approach that may overcome the immune system's blind spot for cancer cells.

Immunologists have long thought that T cells are activated by a single signal—encountering an antigen on the surface of another cell. But recent studies have shown that a second signal is also required to spur T cells into action. This "co-stimulation" occurs when B7, a surface protein on the invading cell, binds with a molecule on the surface of a T cell called CD28. Without this co-stimulation, the T cell remains inactive and does not recognize the invader. Since tumor cells do not carry the B7 protein, researchers believe that this may be one reason why tumor cells are permitted to proliferate.

This newly identified double signal has led some researchers to use innovative gene-therapy schemes with tumor cells that have been genetically enhanced with a B7 molecule. In one study, Peter Linsley and colleagues at Bristol-Myers Squibb Pharmaceutical Research Institute in Seattle,

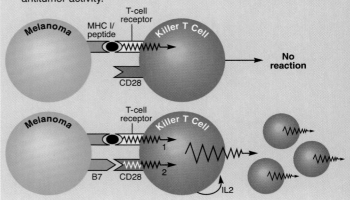

**A Stimulating New Approach to Cancer Treatment**
Cancer cells have been genetically altered to add the B7 surface molecule needed to gain the ability to stimulate killer T cells with antitumor activity.

Washington, introduced the B7 gene and a gene for a viral antigen (known to provoke an immune response) into melanoma cells. When these cells were injected into mice, tumors developed, but regressed completely within two to three weeks.

To further challenge this new immune approach, the Seattle group then injected mice with unaltered melanoma cells so that growing tumors would be present when treatment was initiated. This method more closely mimics a human clinical trial. The researchers next injected the genetically altered melanoma cells into the mice. The results: All treated mice survived longer than untreated controls, and 40 percent of the survivors appeared tumor-free. This dramatic outcome seemed to indicate that mel-

anoma cells, traditionally unable to evoke an immune response, can do so if they display B7 and a viral antigen on their surfaces.

In other studies, Sarah E. Townsend and James P. Allison from the department of molecular and cell biology at the University of California, Berkeley, found that mice injected with melanoma cells enhanced with B7 *alone* also developed tumors that slowly regressed. The researchers surmise that antigens already on the tumor surface were sufficient to provide the first signal to the T-cell receptor, and the addition of a viral antigen was unnecessary.

Townsend and Allison were also able to exploit B7-positive melanoma cells as a sort of vaccine. They first prepped the mouse immune system by introducing the altered tumor cells. After 25 days, the researchers injected the mice with unaltered tumor cells. The "vaccine" protected 89 percent of their test mice for more than three months.

Both laboratories believe that the altered melanoma cells directly co-stimulate tumor-specific "killer" T cells of the immune system. Usually killer T cells require the aid of "helper" T cells to spring into action and fight invaders. But this gene-therapy procedure apparently bypasses this step.

These preliminary results using co-stimulation therapy are promising. But researchers remain wary, recognizing that a great deal of further research will be necessary to see if co-stimulation will be effective in naturally occurring tumors in human patients.

### ▶ Signal Transduction Deciphered

Immunologists may be a step closer to defining how T cells recognize foreign invaders. Now other cell biologists have deciphered the mystery of how a T cell that has identified a foreign agent in the body signals its own DNA to initiate cell division and recruit other cells to the area to fight the intruder. Understanding this process, called *signal transduction,* may lead to new therapies for a variety of illnesses, from allergies to cancer.

Independent research results from diverse fields have converged to illuminate a complex pathway. Scientists now know that a T cell has a protein receptor poking through its cell membrane. When this T-cell receptor encounters a foreign substance, the part of the recep-

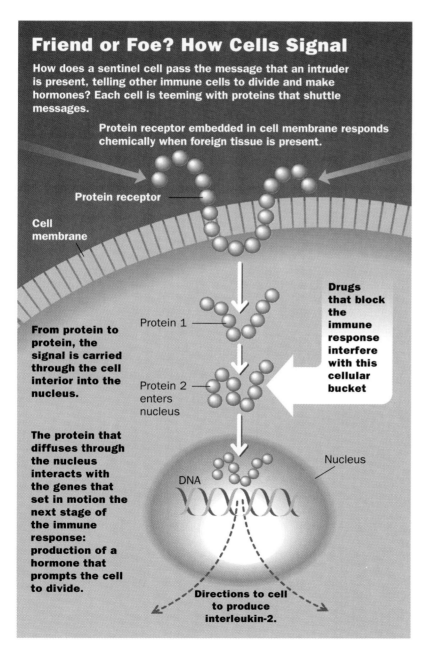

**Friend or Foe? How Cells Signal**

How does a sentinel cell pass the message that an intruder is present, telling other immune cells to divide and make hormones? Each cell is teeming with proteins that shuttle messages.

Protein receptor embedded in cell membrane responds chemically when foreign tissue is present.

Protein receptor

Cell membrane

**From protein to protein, the signal is carried through the cell interior into the nucleus.**

Protein 1

Protein 2 enters nucleus

**Drugs that block the immune response interfere with this cellular bucket**

**The protein that diffuses through the nucleus interacts with the genes that set in motion the next stage of the immune response: production of a hormone that prompts the cell to divide.**

DNA

Nucleus

Directions to cell to produce interleukin-2.

tor inside the membrane undergoes a chemical alteration that turns it into a molecular magnet, attracting proteins inside the cell. The T-cell receptor signals a protein inside the T cell to alter yet another protein. This altered protein then enters the cell's nucleus, and triggers the gene to make interleukin-2, a hormone that stimulates the cell to grow and divide, and attracts other cells to the area to fend off the invader.

Among the players in this signaling cascade is the ras protein, the quarterback of cell growth and division. This protein is so central to the process that defects in it are believed to account for one-third of all human cancers. In its inactive state, the ras protein is attached to a small nucleotide called GDP. When the T-cell receptor is stimulated by a foreign body, the resultant protein-signaling system boots the ras protein into action. The protein detaches from its GDP molecule and picks up a GTP molecule. This chemical alteration spurs the ras protein to send an excitatory message into the nucleus to direct cell division and growth.

Once transmission is finished, the ras protein switches back to an inactive state by breaking down its attached GTP to a GDP molecule. But the tiniest mutation can destroy this procedure, causing the ras protein to stay hitched to the GTP and remain in a continuously active condition. This may lead to cancerous cell growth.

Understanding the step-by-step interactions of signal transduction has raised hope among scientists that drugs can be developed that can enter the T-cell membrane and block or enhance any of these key steps. For example, Merck Research Laboratories in West Point, Pennsylvania, has devised a cancer drug that alters the ras protein. If this drug is successful in clinical trials, its mechanism of altering a specific part of the signaling pathway would be a marked improvement over standard chemotherapy, which attacks and kills any cell that is dividing.

In other therapeutic arenas, Ariad Pharmaceuticals, Inc., in Cambridge, Massachusetts, is working on drugs that block certain intracellular signals in mast cells, the immune-system cells that release histamines—substances that trigger the sneezing and itchy eyes characteristic of allergies.

The emerging picture of signal transduction may also have implications for AIDS research. In a June 1993 issue of the journal *Cell,* Stephen Goff, M.D., from the Columbia-Presbyterian Medical Center in New York City, and colleagues found that a protein made by the human immunodeficiency virus (HIV), which causes AIDS, may bind with a protein in the cell-signaling system. This alteration ultimately causes the suppression of the immune system, which makes AIDS patients subject to opportunistic diseases.

*Lisa Holland*

# Kidneys

## ▶ Limited Results for Dialysis

Some 200,000 Americans suffer from chronic kidney failure, a condition known as end-stage renal disease (ESRD). Roughly three-fourths of these people receive kidney dialysis therapy, at a total annual cost in excess of $5 billion. Despite the vast financial and scientific investment dedicated to extending dialysis treatment to all ESRD patients, researchers issued somber reports in 1993 about the success of this expensive, pervasive therapy.

A joint study conducted by the New York State Health Department and the State University of New York Medical Center at Stony Brook found that the older a patient is when beginning dialysis, the worse the chances for survival. In particular, researchers measured very low survival rates for diabetics who began dialysis therapy past the age of 55. A separate study released by the State University of New York Health Science Center at Brooklyn found that dialysis treatment did not restore kidney functions to pre-therapy levels for most older patients. Many older dialysis patients said they feel unable to go outdoors due to fatigue and weakness; some even withdraw from dialysis due to physical discomfort and emotional despair from the treatment.

*Diabetics fitted with an insulin pump (below) or who otherwise rigorously control their blood-glucose levels have less risk of developing kidney problems.*

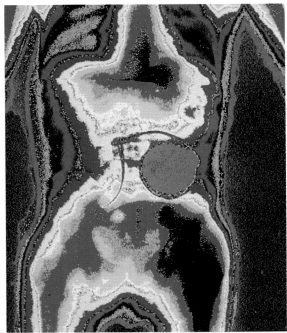

The survival rate of Americans undergoing dialysis treatment is among the worst in the world. For example, researchers found the five-year survival rate for chronic Japanese dialysis patients to be 52 percent higher than for Americans with similar conditions. Researchers suspect that the significant differences in mortality could be caused by the comparatively shorter treatment times and smaller dialyzers typically used in the United States. For more information on kidney dialysis, turn to the article beginning on page 26.

### ▶ Allocating Kidney Transplants

For most patients with ESRD, a kidney transplant offers the best odds for a successful recovery. However, the majority of these people must rely on dialysis therapy because the supply of donor organs is quite scarce. As the supply of organs remains stagnant and transplant waiting lists continue to grow longer, the scientific and medical communities have begun to study and dissect the process of allocation to determine who is getting these valuable organs.

Numerous studies have determined that sociodemographic factors appear to affect a patient's access to a kidney transplant. In particular, nonwhite patients, women, older people, and lower-income patients have a poorer chance of receiving a renal transplant than do other people.

A great deal of attention has been focused on the disparity between white and black patients. Some of this imparity may be the unintentional result of government regulations intended to decrease the incidence of organ rejection. These regulations mandate that donor organs and potential recipients be tissue-typed; organs are then distributed to patients with similar blood markers. This matching process has increased the survival rate of transplant recipients. Unfortunately, since blacks comprise one-third of those waiting for an organ and only 8 percent of the organ-donor pool, a black ESRD patient must wait much longer for a tissue-typed transplant than a white patient.

In a related study, a team headed by Daniel Gaylin and Philip Held, Ph.D., of the Urban Institute in Washington, D.C., also examined the impact of other existing conditions on access to kidney transplants in a report published in the *Journal of the American Medical Association*. The researchers found that patients with heart disease, obesity, and a history of smoking had low transplantation rates.

### ▶ Fish Oils and Renal Transplants

One of the most common immunosuppressive drugs used to improve the success of a kidney transplant is *cyclosporine*. This drug, derived from a soil fungus, chemically disables T lymphocytes, cells that can cause the immune rejection of a transplanted organ.

However, cyclosporine also has numerous side effects, including *nephrotoxicity*, a serious complication marked by decreased kidney function and increased blood pressure. This cyclosporine-induced renal dysfunction can also lead to rejection of the donated kidney.

A team of Dutch researchers found that cyclosporine-treated kidney-transplant patients who regularly ingest fish oil develop increased renal function. These patients show lower blood pressure and an improved glomerular filtration rate—an indicator of the kidney's ability to form urine. The researchers also found that fish-oil supplementation reduces the incidence of acute kidney rejection in the first year following transplantation.

### ▶ Tumor-Suppressor Gene Linked to Kidney Growth

Wilms' tumor, the most common type of kidney cancer in children, generally occurs before the age of 10. Researchers at the Whitehead Institute for Biomedical Research in Cambridge, Massachusetts, discovered a link between one gene that normally suppresses the development of Wilms' tumor and the lack of kidney growth in embryos. Scientists implanted cells containing faulty copies of this tumor-suppressor gene into mouse embryos, which later transmitted the altered genes to some of their own offspring. Researchers found that embryos that contained two copies of the faulty gene did not develop kidneys at all. This discovery, published in the journal *Cell*, leads researchers to believe that the normal suppressor gene plays an important role in kidney development in embryos.

### ▶ *E. Coli*-induced Renal Failure

Early in 1993 hundreds of Americans became sick and three children died after eating undercooked hamburgers served in restaurants in several western states. The outbreak was traced to a virulent strain of *Escherichia coli* (*E. coli*) bacteria that was present in the undercooked hamburger meat. That strain, *E. coli* 0157:H7, produces a toxin that attacks kidney tissue.

Most of the younger children that were affected by *E. coli* 0157:H7 developed *hemolytic uremic syndrome* (HUS), a condition that can cause kidney failure. HUS is an infectious disease that can persist in stool for weeks. Elderly people and children under the age of 4 are at the greatest risk of developing HUS. Researchers have also linked the incidence of HUS to fresh-pressed apple cider from mills that do not wash their apples. Fortunately, there are steps people can take to avoid getting HUS. Experts recommend that people try to avoid such cider and to properly cook beef to at least 190° F to ensure killing the causative *E. coli* strain.

*Peter A. Flax*

# Liver

Disorders of the liver are extraordinarily diverse in their underlying causes and the mechanisms by which they induce disease. Their most important common denominator, however, is their capacity to cause progressive scarring of the liver and, ultimately, cirrhosis or even liver cancer. Some liver disorders also cause acute illness that may be debilitating and, even in exceptional cases, fatal.

Clinical and basic research proceed steadily in almost all areas of hepatology. The most intensively studied liver diseases are the various forms of viral hepatitis, particularly hepatitis B and C, because of their high worldwide prevalence and ability to cause chronic, irreversible damage to the liver.

## ▶ Hepatitis B

Recombinant alpha interferon (interferon alfa-2b) remains the only approved form of treatment in the United States for chronic hepatitis B. Widespread experience with interferon has often been gratifying. Still, about 50 percent of patients do not respond to the drug, and it does produce toxic side effects. Other drugs under study to combat hepatitis B include beta interferon and thymosin, an immunomodulator.

Scientists continue to refine their knowledge about important mutant strains of the hepatitis B virus. These strains lose the capacity to synthesize an important viral protein called hepatitis B e antigen, yet they are still capable of causing disease. A growing body of data suggests that patients infected with these strains have a poor response to antiviral therapy with interferon.

One of the most dramatic developments in hepatitis B research was the tragic outcome of a study involving a previously promising new drug called Fialuridine (FIAU). This antiviral drug, which interferes with DNA replication, had shown potent inhibitory effects on the hepatitis B virus (HBV) in pilot studies. In a larger National Institutes of Health (NIH) study that followed, several deaths related to liver and/or pancreas failure occurred after months of treatment. These deaths appeared to be due to a toxic effect of FIAU on mitochondria, the energy-producing units of the cell. This very unfortunate development resulted in the cancellation of a large multicenter study of FIAU.

Meanwhile, another drug in the same class as FIAU called lamivudine, has shown promise against HBV in an early trial. The lessons learned with FIAU underscore the need for continuous close surveillance of patients using this class of drugs during clinical investigations.

Ultimately our best weapon against hepatitis B is prevention by universal immunization of children. Following a recommendation by the Centers for Disease Control and Prevention (CDC) to this effect, such immunization, which is safe and highly effective at inducing long-term immunity, is being widely applied in the United States.

## ▶ Hepatitis C

Perhaps the most active area of basic research on the hepatitis C virus (HCV) is the discovery of the staggering number of genetic mutations that characterize this agent. Hepatitis C is an RNA virus (in contrast to HBV, which is a DNA virus). The RNA codes for a number of proteins, both structural and nonstructural. Virtually every portion of the genome that has been evaluated shows genetic variation, though some portions are much more variable than others. A "hypervariable" portion codes for one of the envelope or surface proteins, and may be characterized by significant genetic variation even in the same patient.

The implications of this genetic variation are enormous. It may impair the ability of the host to make antibodies that can effectively neutralize the virus and confer immunity. In a similar vein, genetic variation may substantially impede the prospects for the development of a vaccine. Some genetic types (called genotypes) of the virus may have the capacity to produce more severe liver disease than others, and some may be more resistant to treatment. Patients with genetically diverse viral infections within their own liver also seem more resistant to treatment. This may help explain why patients with more advanced cases of the disease (and therefore generally long-standing disease) are more resistant to treatment.

Numerous classifications of the virus have been proposed, but they are usually based on a limited portion of the genome. There is a need for collaboration to develop a uniform classification scheme even as research on the implications of this biological feature continues.

As with hepatitis B, recombinant alpha interferon is currently the only approved therapy for hepatitis C, and, like hepatitis B, there is a response rate of about 50 percent. But the relapse rate after successful remission is much higher (over 50 percent) with hepatitis C. Physicians have refined their ability to predict which patients are more likely to respond well to interferon. Patients with more-advanced liver disease, especially those with cirrhosis, have a lower likelihood of response. In contrast, those with mild liver-biopsy findings, as well as those with lower levels of virus, have more favorable response rates.

Diagnosing hepatitis formerly relied exclusively on antibody tests, with unreliable results. Newly available tests, most notably the polymerase chain reaction (PCR), can detect tiny quantities of viral RNA in the blood of infected patients. These improved diagnostic tests should further the ability of doctors to diagnose hepatitis C virus infection accurately and, potentially, to base treatment decisions on the level of virus in infected blood. New drugs under study for hepatitis C include beta interferon, ribavirin, and thymosin, as well as combinations of the latter two with interferon.

Hepatitis C is one of the most common indications for liver transplantation. Using PCR testing, it has become clear that virtually all patients with hepatitis C who undergo transplantation will develop infection with HCV in the new liver. Although the outcome of this recurrent infection is frequently favorable (at least in the short-term studies reported thus far), significant liver disease may occasionally result. Therefore, studies on antiviral therapy for these transplant patients will be important in the next several years.

## ▶ Liver Failure

Acute viral hepatitis or toxic injury to the liver, such as that resulting from overdoses of acetaminophen, can lead to overwhelming disease in which the liver is destroyed within a short period of time. Liver failure develops so quickly that donor livers for transplantation, the only hope for these patients, may not become available in time.

Liver specialists have long hoped that an artificial means of support may be developed for patients with acute liver failure, something akin to kidney-dialysis machines for patients with kidney failure. That dream might soon be fulfilled. Scientists have developed a bioartificial liver device that uses millions of pig-liver cells through which the patient's blood is filtered. Promising early results have recently been reported.

## ▶ Cirrhosis Causes

Contrary to the general perception, cirrhosis of the liver is not a disease that exclusively afflicts alcoholics. Indeed, according to Mark Zern, M.D., director of the division of gastroenterology at Thomas Jefferson University in Philadelphia, Pennsylvania, fully half the cases of cirrhosis diagnosed each year are not related to alcohol consumption. Probably one-third of the cases are caused by the liver damage wrought by hepatitis B or C. Another 15 percent arise from hemochromatosis (abnormal handling of iron by the body), Wilson's disease (abnormal handling of copper), inherited conditions, prolonged exposure to toxins, and other conditions. Despite these facts, cirrhosis carries the stigma of an alcoholic's disease, making it all the more difficult for victims to deal with this illness.

*Ira M. Jacobson, M.D.*

# Medical Ethics

## ▶ National Health-Care Reform

President Clinton submitted to Congress a plan to completely overhaul the current health-care-insurance system, replacing it with a new system that would guarantee health insurance for all American citizens and legal aliens, regardless of their prior medical history or employment situation.

Titled the "Health Security Act," the proposed plan would utilize a concept called "managed competition" to open up access to the currently uninsured, while at the same time controlling the escalating costs of our health-care-delivery system. Under the act, each state would set up health-care "alliances," into which all state residents would be grouped. Such alliances would bargain with the various insurers in the state, using their leverage to structure a range of health-care-insurance options to provide quality care at reasonable prices. Each alliance would offer individuals essentially three options from which to choose: a health maintenance organization (HMO) option; a costlier fee-for-service option; or a combination of the two. Cost savings are expected, as it is anticipated that most individuals would choose the least-expensive option, an HMO. Employers would be obligated to pay for approximately 80 percent of the standard package, while individuals would be responsible for the remaining costs, plus any additional costs associated with more-expensive options.

Self-employed individuals would be required to purchase insurance, and government subsidies would be available to assist those unemployed individuals who are not in the Medicaid system. As insurers would be competing for patients, the act anticipates that costs would be kept low while quality would be maintained. Data would be collected to monitor the costs and quality of various plans, and patients could choose new plans if they were unhappy with their original choice.

Under the new plan, individuals receiving Medicaid would receive the standard package through an alliance. The act anticipates that for the next several years, the Medicare system would remain intact, although the ultimate plan is to fold Medicare into the alliance system. The intent of the plan is to allow market forces and insurer competition to regulate prices and costs, although there would be government oversight and intervention if such cost savings failed to materialize. A new National Health Board would oversee the system, set the national health-care budget, and regulate the private insurers.

The Health Security Act attempts to incorporate several basic principles considered essential to frame a new system of health insurance. It guarantees health insurance for individuals and families regardless of their income level, employment status, or health condition. Under the act, all individuals would have a legally enforceable right to a standard package of health-care benefits. The plan is expected to simplify the current system by developing uniform insurance-claim forms and standardized packages of insurance options. Every individual would have several options from which to select, and the cost to the individual would be directly related to the choice selected by the patient. The administration asserts that significant cost savings would occur if, as expected, most individuals enroll in HMOs, which would compete with each other for patients. The quality of care would likely be maintained by insurers, or they would risk losing patients to other, more-desirable plans. The act intends that individuals bear the responsibility of recognizing the costs of their health care and incorporating such considerations into their health-care choices.

Numerous practical and philosophical criticisms of the plan have surfaced that question the fundamental premise of the entire act. From a practical perspective, many critics doubt the claims that significant cost savings or a more simplified, streamlined system will result. Moreover, the plan rests on the notion that individuals will purchase health care as they do other "commodities," with price foremost in their minds, a premise that has yet to be tested in the health-care arena. Furthermore, there has been significant concern raised that in the attempt to control costs, HMOs may scrimp on the quality and quantity of treatment available, a charge made against many already-existing HMOs. The plan does permit individuals with sufficient financial means to buy additional treatment on their own, raising the specter that a rigid, two-tier system of care will ultimately develop. Finally, and perhaps most critical, the plan fails to address the fundamental question concerning what health care *ought* to be provided in an era of an aging population and continued quests for new technological innovations. Many critics have faulted the plan for not addressing the politically contentious and ethically troubling issue of health-care rationing, and such critics have argued that cost will never be controlled unless explicit decisions are made concerning prioritization of expenditures and limitations of access to new and expensive technology.

The plan has yet to be formally taken up by Congress, and it is expected to be significantly revised prior to passage and enactment.

### ▶ Oregon's Health-Care-Rationing Plan
Moving ahead with its own individual plan, the state of Oregon received federal approval to enact a five-year experimental program to dramatically expand the number of people eligible for Medicaid, while at the same time explicitly limiting treatment options available to those on Medicaid, based upon a list of 688 ranked medical procedures. The plan is intended to add 120,000 more Oregonians to the Medicaid roll, and will also require all employers to provide insurance to employees.

The plan was developed over several years, through many public forums, to directly address the question of what the state can, and cannot, afford to pay for medical care. A list of 688 medical procedures was developed, and the procedures were ranked according to their cost and the number of individuals whom they benefited. Once the list was developed and a budget was established, the state determined that it could afford to pay for the first 568 services on the list. Any services above that number—which tend to relate to self-limiting conditions, cosmetic procedures, or therapy of unproven value—would not be paid for by Medicaid. For example, the Medicaid system will not pay for liver transplants for individuals with liver cancer, but it will pay for such costly procedures as organ transplants in cases where there is proven benefit.

A previous draft was denied federal approval, as there was concern that its evaluation of the quality of a patient's life might discriminate against disabled individuals. The new plan does not consider such factors, and is ultimately considered more of a cost-containment system than an overt method of rationing. The system is expected to save approximately 3 percent of Medicaid costs over time.

### ▶ Separation of Siamese Twins
Angela and Amy Lakeberg were born in Lakewood, Illinois in June 1993, co-joined at the chest with one abnormal heart shared between them. Their par-

*Despite overwhelming odds, one of the two Lakeberg Siamese twins surgically separated in 1993 has recovered well since the operation; the other twin died.*

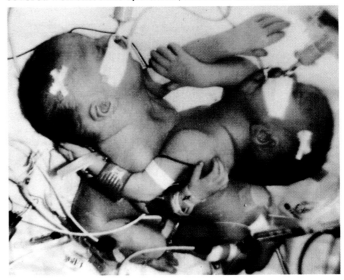

ents were aware of their condition prior to birth, but chose not to abort the fetuses. Upon the birth of the children, doctors estimated that there was a less than 1 percent chance that even one of the girls would survive the surgical separation, and a 100 percent certainty that one would die in surgery, as the single heart was apportioned to one of the two. Despite the overwhelming likelihood of failure, the parents wished to pursue the option of surgery, and the twins were transferred to Children's Hospital in Philadelphia for the complex procedure. The surgery took place seven weeks after the twins were born, and, as anticipated, Amy died during the surgical separation. However, despite massive complications and physical abnormalities, Angela not only survived the surgery, but has continued to make slow and steady progress toward recovery. She will nonetheless face considerable physical challenges in the future, as numerous additional surgeries will have to occur to correct other congenital abnormalities. In previous cases of this sort, it has been very rare for the surviving twin to live longer than six months after the initial surgical separation.

Despite the apparent success of the surgery, many have argued that it was wrong to even offer to the parents something so likely to fail, and that the twins should have been allowed to die, as would have been the natural outcome had the surgery not been performed. Arthur Caplan, M.D., a renowned bioethicist from the University of Minnesota, publicly declared it to be a violation of medical ethics to attempt such an operation, given the near impossibility of its success, no matter what the parents desired. Other commentators suggest that while the choice of the parents was extreme, nonetheless, it was not the job of individual physicians to withhold potential therapy, despite its unlikely success and extraordinary expense. If such treatment decisions are to be based on cost considerations, that would have to be a public-policy decision, rather than at the discretion of individual clinicians.

## ▶ Genetic Cloning of Human Embryos

Researchers at George Washington University Medical Center in Washington, D.C., reported in the journal *Science* that, for the first time, single human embryos had been cloned into identical twins and triplets through a process of splitting the embryos. Using techniques common to the cloning of animal embryos (which has taken place for quite some time), Jerry Hall, M.D., reported his success with procedures that were performed as part of an in-vitro-fertilization program, where sperm and eggs were brought together in a laboratory setting for later implantation into a previously infertile woman.

The intent of the researchers was to create more embryos for implantation, enhancing the probability that the woman would subsequently become pregnant. Since it would be unethical to experiment on viable embryos, Hall used abnormal ones—eggs accidentally fertilized by more than one sperm. The cloned embryos in this case were ultimately discarded, as they were unsuitable for implantation for technical reasons.

The news of the expansion of this technique into the arena of human embryos caused considerable uproar, and raised significant concerns regarding the ethical propriety of such research and the guidelines in place to monitor it. The procedure of cloning involves the creation of organisms with identical gene structures, as occurs with the birth of identical

## How the Cloning Process Works

Researchers at the George Washington University Medical Center in Washington have possibly extended a cloning process, known to work on amphibians and some mammals, to humans.

1. In vitro fertilization occurs.

2. Fertilized egg develops into young embryo.

3. Egg is taken apart into separate cells or nuclei.

4. An egg is obtained from another woman and the material containing genetic information is removed through a surgical procedure. Proteins and fats necessary to egg development remain.

5. A nucleus from the first fertilized egg is then implanted into the second unfertilized egg. This process, called nuclear transplantation, imbues the second egg with the genetic characteristics of the first.

This process can generate one or more clones with the same characteristics.

*Source: "Cloning of Frogs, Mice and other Animals," McKinnell, Robert G.; University of Minnesota Press*

twins or triplets who naturally break off from a single embryo. While this technique is not new, its application to human life has arisen without any public discussion or monitoring of such procedures. In fact, many publicly questioned the propriety of expanding upon such research, or opening it up to public use, without significant public discourse on the range of ethical dilemmas that arise in its consequence. Some people have voiced fundamental concerns regarding the uniqueness usually cherished in distinct individuals.

Others support the research in the name of privacy and procreative freedom. A consensus seemed to develop, however, that no matter what the future implications and application of such a procedure, the need for public consideration and debate about its consequences was both timely and urgently necessary.

## ▶ Physician-assisted Suicide

The propriety of physician involvement in patient decisions to commit suicide remains a topic of public debate. In the United States, Jack Kevorkian, M.D., escalated his involvement in such suicides, despite a new state law outlawing such assistance. In the Netherlands the Dutch Parliament finally took public action to acknowledge the significant number of physician-assisted suicides in that country, and to decriminalize such activities, provided they take place in accord with strict government guidelines.

In February 1993, Michigan enacted new legislation making it illegal for either physicians or laymen to "knowingly and intentionally" assist in another's suicide. Such an act is now considered a felony in Michigan, punishable by up to four years in prison and a $2,000 fine. The law was specifically aimed at addressing the actions of Dr. Kevorkian, the suburban Detroit pathologist who believes physicians are obliged to assist certain terminally or chronically ill patients to commit suicide. Dr. Kevorkian has to date been involved in 20 such acts of assistance, and was charged with violating the new Michigan law in three of those cases. While the law has been declared unconstitutional by a lower county court, that case was appealed, and the matter is now being considered by the Michigan Court of Appeals, which, as of early 1994, had yet to render any decision in the case.

Dr. Kevorkian publicly acknowledged his intent to challenge the law, which he calls immoral. In fact, his increased involvement in patient suicides led to the accelerated pace of the legislation's passage, as lawmakers grew fearful of the number of individuals who were seeking out Dr. Kevorkian's assistance prior to the law's enactment. After his indictment for the third act of suicide assistance, Dr. Kevorkian refused to post the $50,000 bond, and was placed in a Michigan jail. He refused to eat while he was jailed, saying that to do so would be a form of cooperation with the "immoral" system that had put him there. Two of the three charges against Dr. Kevorkian were subsequently dismissed. After he was released from jail, Dr. Kevorkian agreed to stop his euthanasia efforts and instead devote his energies to resolving this dilemma in the political arena.

Dr. Kevorkian states that all patients he assisted sought him out, and that they each underwent an extensive series of discussions and examinations prior to his decision to assist them. He maintains that he ultimately responded to only a few of the requests he received, and then assisted such individuals with a device that allowed them to inhale carbon monoxide through their own triggering of the device. Thus, while Dr. Kevorkian provided the means to commit suicide and while he offered assistance, he did not directly activate the device, which would then implicate him directly in the deaths.

Meanwhile, the Dutch Parliament voted in 1993 to establish a public policy acknowledging that physicians may at some times wish to assist their patients in suicide, or actually directly bring about their deaths. This new policy permits such actions to occur without criminal prosecution if the involved physician follows a strict protocol, which includes providing a detailed report to the coroner following the death of the patient. In addition, the patient must be well informed about other options available, and must have the mental capacity to make such a decision; the patient's choice must be consistent and long held; the patient must be afflicted with unbearable and hopeless suffering; and the physician must seek out the consultation of another physician with experience in this matter.

While such actions technically remain criminal, this new policy recognizes that such assistance is widespread in the country, and sets out specific guidelines for doctors to follow in order to ensure that they will remain free of liability.

Critics of this plan argue that the policy fails to consider the documented cases of over 1,000 instances in the country where euthanasia was performed without the explicit request of the patient, raising the specter that approval of such a policy will lead to a slippery slope of regular, nonvoluntary killings of vulnerable patients. In fact, the Dutch Parliament, following approval of this policy, announced that it would next take up the matter of nonrequested euthanasia for extremely impaired newborns and the mentally incompetent. The Netherlands is the only country to have formally established a national dialogue on this issue and to have subsequently developed policy. Several U.S. states have placed the legalization of physician-assisted suicide on their ballots, but no state has yet to successfully pass such a measure.

*Connie Zuckerman, J.D.*

# Medical Technology

### ▶ Regulating Irregular Heartbeats

Every year, nearly 400,000 Americans die of cardiac arrest when their hearts begin to beat too fast, a condition known as *ventricular tachycardia,* or at an irregular rate, a state called *ventricular fibrillation.* During episodes of ventricular tachycardia, the heart cannot pump enough blood, causing dizziness, weakness, and nausea. Tachycardia can lead to ventricular fibrillation, when the heart quivers spasmodically and does not pump any blood. Fibrillation frequently causes sudden death.

A new medical device approved by the Food and Drug Administration (FDA) on February 11, 1993, will help prevent these serious heart conditions. Called the Pacer Cardioverter Defibrillator (PCD) Tachyarrhythmia Control System, and marketed by Medtronic Incorporated of Minneapolis, Minnesota, the implantable device can detect when the heart is not beating normally. Depending on the severity of the problem, the PCD then sends a gentle, moderate, or intense electric shock to the heart to restore its normal rhythm.

Medtronic's device was the first implantable cardiac defibrillator to provide three different levels of electric shock. (A similar three-stage defibrillator, the Cadence V-100, produced by Ventritex Incorporated of Sunnyvale, California, received FDA approval in May 1993.) The lowest level delivers several mild and rapid shocks one after another to decrease the rate of a heart beating too fast (tachycardia) or increase the rate of a heart beating too slow (brachycardia). This pacing action is similar to that provided continuously by a cardiac pacemaker. The next level of electric shock is more like a moderate jolt—it is used when mild pacing does not return the heart to a normal rhythm. The third and highest level of electric current is used to restart the heart in the event of ventricular fibrillation. The sensation it produces has been compared to a strong hiccup.

The new device will be used in patients with chronic abnormal heart rhythms caused by coronary-artery or heart-muscle disease. The defibrillator is expected to reduce the incidence of sudden death in these patients. It will also reduce the need for antiarrhythmic drugs, which can cause unpleasant side effects in some people. Gust H. Bardy, M.D., associate professor of medicine at the University of Washington in Seattle, studied 50 patients implanted with the new device, and found that 82 percent were able to stop taking antiarrhythmic drugs. The new defibrillator will also improve the quality of life for heart patients previously at risk for sudden cardiac arrest.

The PCD consists of three components: a pulse generator that monitors the heartbeat and sends electric shocks; wire leads that run from the generator to the surface of the heart; and an external programmer that stores information about the device's function, such as the number of shocks sent to the heart and the success rate of these shocks in re-

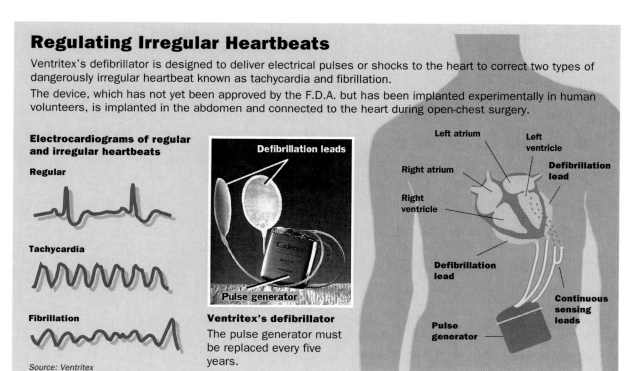

## Regulating Irregular Heartbeats

Ventritex's defibrillator is designed to deliver electrical pulses or shocks to the heart to correct two types of dangerously irregular heartbeat known as tachycardia and fibrillation.

The device, which has not yet been approved by the F.D.A. but has been implanted experimentally in human volunteers, is implanted in the abdomen and connected to the heart during open-chest surgery.

**Electrocardiograms of regular and irregular heartbeats**

Regular

Tachycardia

Fibrillation

*Source: Ventritex*

**Defibrillation leads**

*Cadence*

**Pulse generator**

**Ventritex's defibrillator**
The pulse generator must be replaced every five years.

Left atrium

Left ventricle

Right atrium

Right ventricle

Defibrillation lead

Defibrillation lead

Pulse generator

Continuous sensing leads

turning the heart's rhythm to a normal rate. The external programmer also allows a doctor to specify the intensity of the electric pulses sent to the heart. Medtronic's CEO, William W. George, says that the PCD "simply stated . . . is a computer in the heart."

The pulse generator is the size of a cassette tape, and contains a lithium battery good for five years. It also houses the computer used to program the device. This generator is implanted under the skin or muscles of the abdomen. The wire leads are connected to the heart in an open-chest procedure called a thoracotomy or in a recently approved and less risky procedure that allows the wires to be threaded through a vein to the heart.

Medtronic's new device is actually a third-generation version of the implantable cardiac defibrillator marketed by Eli Lilly's Cardiac Pacemakers Inc. (CPI) division in St. Paul, Minnesota. That device, called the Ventak, was only able to deliver an intense and often painful shock to the heart when it detected abnormalities in its rhythm, regardless of the severity of the irregularities. The Ventak-P, a later version of this defibrillator, introduced the external programmer that allows a patient's doctor to adjust the severity of the shock. Since their approval, the Ventak and Ventak-P have been implanted in 48,000 heart patients; of these people, 35,000 were still alive at the beginning of 1993.

Sales of implantable cardiac defibrillators, which cost about $20,000 each, are expected to reach $1 billion annually by the year 2000. One reason for this growth is that the new devices regulate irregular heartbeats without the painful shock associated with earlier versions, making them a more attractive option to many heart patients. The PCD and Cadence V-100 are also better at determining when an abnormality is serious and when it is harmless, and thus they reduce the number of shocks overall.

Another factor predicted to dramatically increase the use of the new device is the recent FDA approval of two new wire-lead systems that allow defibrillators to be attached to the heart without a thoracotomy. This will reduce the chance of postoperative complications, such as pneumonia and excessive bleeding. In addition, it will decrease the cost of implanting a defibrillator by $7,500, and reduce the length of hospitalization.

In mid-1993 Eli Lilly's CPI division received approval for the Endotak wire-lead system, while Medtronic was given the marketing go-ahead for its Transvene wire-lead system. In each system the wires are first attached to the defibrillator's pulse generator, and then threaded through a vein and into the heart. A patch sewn under the skin above the heart is also attached to the pulse generator; it sends electrical impulses of varying intensities to the heart when the wires detect arrhythmia.

Medtronic will use the Transvene wire system with its PCD device. Until Eli Lilly receives FDA approval for a three-stage cardiac defibrillator, it will use the Endotak system with its Ventak and Ventak-P defibrillators. Ventritex also plans to use the Endotak system with its three-stage Cadence V-100.

### ▶ A Portable Home Dialysis Machine

Medical supplier Baxter International Incorporated hopes to receive FDA approval by the end of 1993 for a portable dialysis machine that weighs less than 25 pounds and that fits under an airplane seat. The Home Choice Automated PD System is already available in Canada, Europe, and Japan.

Dialysis filters impurities from the blood of patients whose kidneys have failed. It can be administered in two forms: hemodialysis or peritoneal dialysis. In hemodialysis the patient is hooked up to a machine that filters the blood outside of the body. In peritoneal dialysis, the type administered by Baxter's new machine, the patient is also hooked up to a machine that purifies the blood, but this process is performed inside the body—in the peritoneal cavity, or abdomen. The average peritoneal-dialysis machine in use today weighs about 200 pounds. Patients can use these machines at home or at dialysis centers and hospitals.

The new machine contains a computer to run the dialysis process, and a warming tray to keep the temperature of the dialysis solution constant. In addition the three main components required to perform dialysis—pumps, valves, and measuring devices—are encased in a hard plastic, disposable cassette about the size of a videocassette. Once placed in the compartment provided for it in the machine, the cassette uses pneumatics (very low air pressure) to pump fluid in and out of the patient's abdomen. Most other peritoneal-dialysis machines rely on gravity to perform this function, which takes more time and is less efficient.

To use the machine, a patient simply places the cassette in the front of the machine and closes the lid, forming a sterile seal. He or she then attaches several bags of dialysis solution, and an empty bag to store used fluid, to the appropriate tubes that lead away from the chamber that holds the cassette. The bags of solution are laid in the warming tray on top of the machine. The patient then attaches the cassette tube to the permanent catheter implanted in his or her abdomen, presses the machine's "Go" button, and lies down. The computer, which has been programmed by the patient's doctor to administer the exact dialysis required for the patient, then takes over the process of pumping the fluid in and out of the patient's abdomen. Computer algorithms control the amount of fluid pumped in and the amount of time allowed to elapse before it is pumped back out. They also maintain the temperature of the dialysis solution. Other computer operations include checking for and correcting malfunctions and periodically purging the lines that lead in and out of the cassette.

The Home Choice Automated PD System will be ideal for home use, freeing many kidney patients from regular visits to dialysis centers and hospitals. Its portability will also allow patients to once again travel long distances from their homes. In addition, since the system makes little noise while running, patients will be able to use it while sleeping. The Home Choice Automated PD System will also be affordable: in the United States, it will cost about $10,000 a year to operate. Much of this expense will be covered by Medicare, the federal health-insurance program for the elderly and severely disabled, which has covered dialysis as part of the End-Stage Renal Disease Program since 1972. Most important of all, the new machine will be easy to use. New Hampshire inventor Dean Kamen says he developed the Home Choice Automated PD System so that someone could use it "blindfolded, wearing hockey gloves."

## ▶ New Test for Chlamydia

On June 15, 1993, the FDA approved a new, rapid test for detecting chlamydia, one of the most common sexually transmitted diseases (STDs) in the United States. Chlamydia, which infects approximately 4 million Americans every year, is caused by a parasitic bacterium. In men, the primary carriers of the bacteria, the disease causes few if any symptoms, but, if left untreated, can result in sterility. Women infected with chlamydia may have a thin white vaginal discharge and uncomfortable urination. If the infection is not treated, it can lead to pelvic inflammatory disease (and eventually infertility), ectopic pregnancy, and—in babies born to women with a chlamydia infection—pneumonia and other respiratory conditions, as well as eye infec-

tions such as conjunctivitis. In Third World countries, women with chlamydia often give birth to blind babies.

Chlamydia is easily cured with antibiotics, such as tetracycline. But until now the tests used to detect it have been slow, undependable, and, in some cases, painful enough, especially for men, to discourage them from being tested. The recently approved *Amplicor Chlamydia Trachomatis Test* (or assay) relies on the polymerase chain reaction (PCR), a relatively new method for cloning large amounts of a specific fragment of DNA from a single sample. It is performed on a specimen taken from a man's urine or a woman's cervix. If chlamydia is present in the sample, it appears in large quantities at the end of the test, which takes about four hours. The traditional chlamydia tests require samples from a man's urethra or a woman's cervix to be grown in a culture for three to seven days. (The urethral sample is taken by inserting a swab in the urethra, an uncomfortable procedure for most men.) While urine samples can also be used in these standard tests, they are only 68 percent effective, compared to the 95 percent detection rate for the Amplicor assay. David A. Kessler, M.D., the FDA commissioner, believes that the new test will overcome men's resistance to testing, since it requires only a urine sample. Infected men can then be treated before passing the disease on further.

## ▶ Long-Distance Medical Care

Physicians in urban areas across the United States are combining the telephone with a television or computer screen to treat patients in small communities as far away as Somalia—without patients or doctors ever leaving their hometowns. This new phenomenon, called telemedicine, is expected to significantly improve the quality of medical care provided to patients in rural areas and other remote locations. Patients in small towns are usually treated by general practitioners; until now, if they

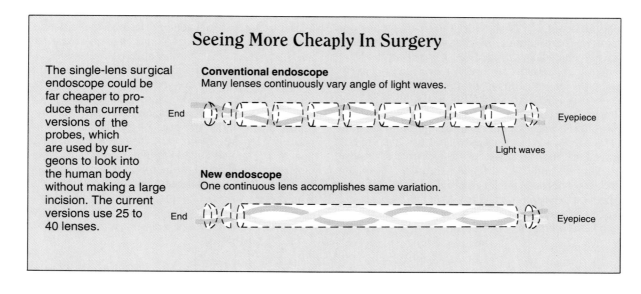

## Seeing More Cheaply In Surgery

The single-lens surgical endoscope could be far cheaper to produce than current versions of the probes, which are used by surgeons to look into the human body without making a large incision. The current versions use 25 to 40 lenses.

**Conventional endoscope**
Many lenses continuously vary angle of light waves.

End — Eyepiece

Light waves

**New endoscope**
One continuous lens accomplishes same variation.

End — Eyepiece

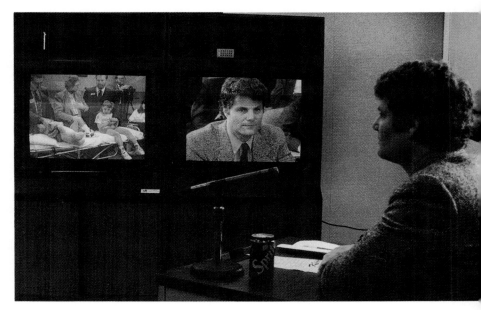

*With the advent of telemedicine technology, specialists in urban areas can diagnose the medical problems of patients in remote locations.*

required the care of a specialist, they had to travel to a university or city hospital, since many specialists work in urban areas, where their services are most needed. But for some rural residents, the trip to a specialist is too expensive or simply not feasible.

With telemedicine a patient visits his or her local family doctor, who then sets up a teleconference with a specialist at a participating medical center. Using special tools, such as a stethoscope that transmits a patient's heartbeat over fiber-optic phone lines, the local doctor conducts an examination, the results of which are analyzed by the specialist. This examination may include taking digital pictures that can be viewed on the specialist's television or computer screen. For example, a cardiologist might see a close-up of a patient's jugular veins to see if they are distended.

Of course, not every disease or medical condition can be treated long distance. Obviously, telemedicine cannot be used to set a broken bone or deliver a baby. The system is best suited for patients who do not require extensive physical examinations. The service is also not yet available on a widespread basis. Some of the areas currently using or testing it include Kansas City, Kansas; Austin, Texas; Buffalo, New York; and Augusta, Georgia. The state of Pennsylvania has just started participating in a $400,000 telemedicine pilot program designed to improve the quality of health care for rural residents. "It will also lower the cost for citizens who reside in rural areas," says Richard M. Walsh, the governor's special assistant for telecommunications. And Baylor College of Medicine in Houston, Texas, in conjunction with the National Aeronautics and Space Administration (NASA), will soon provide satellite teleconferencing to doctors and patients in Russia, Turkey, and Saudi Arabia.

The U.S. military is also using telemedicine. It recently spent $60,000 to set up a remote teleconferencing site in Mogadishu, Somalia. The system consists of off-the-shelf computers and software, portable telecommunications equipment, and a computerized digital camera. Medical personnel in Mogadishu use the system to consult with experts at Walter Reed Army Medical Center in Washington, D.C., when they encounter unfamiliar illnesses or medical problems; in some cases, this allows them to start treating a patient before he or she is airlifted to a hospital in Europe. In other cases, it completely eliminates the need to transfer a patient to a hospital. A typical teleconference between Mogadishu and Washington, D.C., relies on a written medical profile of the patient and still photographs of the injury or condition: for example, pictures of head injuries or malarial parasites. Using a suitcase-sized transceiver, these data are sent by modem to a satellite linked to a computer at Walter Reed. The expert receiving the data then responds to the remote personnel by cellular phone or computer.

Telemedicine is being used in other settings as well. For example, hospital emergency rooms are linking up with prison infirmaries to diagnose sick inmates. And some major companies are buying portable defibrillators made by the Medphone Corporation in New Jersey that can be used to restart a person's heart by remote control over a phone line. Designed for use while waiting for paramedics to arrive at a heart-attack scene, the MDphone automatically dials the nearest participating hospital, where an emergency-room doctor then instructs the person on the other end of the line to attach the MDphone's adhesive electrodes to the patient's chest. An electrocardiogram is transmitted to the doctor, who determines if and when to press a button that sends an electric shock to the defibrillator to restart the heart.

Some hospitals are using the picture-transmitting capabilities of telemedicine equipment to display magnetic resonance images (MRIs), computer-assisted tomography (CAT) scans, and X rays stored at remote sites. This eliminates the need to store vast numbers of records on-site, freeing up storage space for more-critical supplies or equipment. Yellowstone National Park is using a similar system to transmit X rays of hikers with possible fractures to a hospital in Wyoming.

*Abigail W. Polek*

# Medications and Drugs

## ▶ Advances in Cancer Therapy

Prior to the release of cladribine (Leustatin), by Ortho Biotech, patients afflicted with hairy-cell leukemia had little hope of a cure, and treatment was aimed at controlling the symptoms of the disease and preventing other complications.

Those patients with active hairy-cell leukemia treated with Leustatin have shown an 88 percent overall-response rate with a 66 percent complete-response rate. A complete response means an absence of any identifiable hairy cells in either the blood or bone marrow, a normal hemoglobin level, and normal counts of neutrophils and platelets in the blood. To date, patients who have achieved a complete response have done so for an average of more than eight months. The longest complete response recorded exceeds 25 months.

Leustatin is given as a single, seven-day continuous intravenous infusion, with the dose being based on the patient's weight. Leustatin is well tolerated; its reversible and manageable side effects include fever, fatigue, infection, rash, nausea, and headache. It has not been shown to cause hair loss or severe nausea and vomiting.

Myelosuppression, or low counts of white blood cells, red blood cells, and platelets, occurs in 70 percent of patients, usually within the first month following therapy. Cell counts usually return to normal within two months. Patients should avoid people with colds or flulike symptoms both during treatment and for a few months afterward, as their resistance to disease will be reduced at this time.

Leustatin may produce teratogenic effects on the fetus. Women of childbearing age should be advised to avoid becoming pregnant while taking the drug. Leustatin should be used during pregnancy only if the potential benefit to the patient outweighs the potential risk to the fetus.

### Refractory acute lymphoblastic leukemia.

Acute lymphoblastic leukemia (ALL), a disease that affects the blood-forming cells of the body, is most commonly seen in children and young adults. Over time the cancerous changes in the blood-forming cells interfere with the normal blood-forming cells and the ability of the body to fight infection. Symptoms include frequent bruising, bone tenderness, enlarged lymph nodes, and anemia. In the early 1950s, most children with ALL did not survive longer than three months. Today therapy for ALL is one of the few success stories in the field of cancer

treatment. Current therapy provides more than 50 percent of afflicted children with long-term remission (a disease-free state), and sometimes a cure. More than 95 percent of children treated for ALL respond well to initial treatment with a variety of antileukemia drugs.

Unfortunately, some children do not respond to this initial therapy due to a resistance to the drugs or severe infection. This condition is called refractory ALL. For such patients, Bristol-Myers Oncology has introduced teniposide (Vumon), a new anticancer drug used to treat refractory ALL. Used alone, Vumon has successfully treated advanced cases of the disease. When used in combination with other anticancer drugs, Vumon has also been successful in inducing remission, although in some cases a secondary leukemia develops. The side effects caused by Vumon are similar to other antileukemia drugs: diarrhea, nausea, vomiting, hair loss, and bone-marrow suppression. Vumon is being investigated for use in lung and breast cancer, lymphoma, and in preparation for bone-marrow transplantation. For now at least, Vumon may provide new hope for children with refractory ALL.

## ▶ Pain Management for Patients with Bone Cancer

Metastron, by Medi-Physics/Amersham Healthcare, is a new radiopharmaceutical analgesic used to relieve the debilitating pain suffered by bone-cancer patients. In most cases the pain is caused by either breast or prostate cancer that has spread (metastasized) to the bone. Although it does not cure the cancer, Metastron allows the patient a better quality of life.

The active ingredient in Metastron is strontium 89 chloride. The strontium behaves similarly to calcium in that it is taken up into areas of the bone where active osteogenesis (bone growth) is occurring, such as in primary bone tumors and metastases. Metastron is administered as a two-minute intravenous injection every 90 days on an outpatient basis.

Seven to 20 days after administration of the drug, Metastron begins to relieve the patient's pain. The pain relief lasts for as long as six months. Because of the delay in effectiveness after injection, it is not indicated for use in patients with very short life expectancies.

Side effects of the drug include a temporary lowering of the white-blood-cell and platelet counts. These blood counts reach their lowest points about 12 to 16 weeks after the injection, and then return to normal before the next dose is due. Metastron carries a Food and Drug Administration (FDA) Pregnancy Classification of Category D, and should not be administered to pregnant women or nursing mothers.

## ▶ No-Doze Allergy Relief

Schering Laboratories has introduced loratadine (Claritin) nonsedating antihistamine for use in patients over 12 years old who suffer from hay fever or other seasonal allergies. Like other nonsedating antihistamines such as terfenadine (Seldane) and astemizole (Hismanal), the new drug causes little drowsiness in most people. But Claritin has the added advantage over terfenadine in that it has to be taken only once a day. A daily 10-milligram (mg) dose has been shown to work as effectively as both sedating and nonsedating antihistamines in relieving such symptoms as sneezing, nasal itching, and runny nose.

Another advantage that Claritin may have over both terfenadine and astemizole is that it does not produce any adverse heart effects. Nor have there been any cases of interaction when the drug is taken with the antibiotics erythromycin, ketoconazole, or itraconazole. Both terfenadine and astemizole have been reported to cause irregular heartbeats when taken with these drugs.

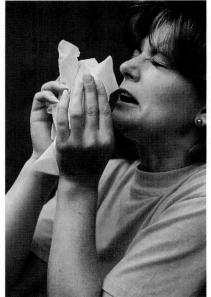

*There is new hope for allergy sufferers. A single-dose medicine is available that doesn't cause drowsiness.*

## ▶ AIDS-Related Infections

Patients infected with the AIDS virus die from opportunistic infections rather than from the virus itself. One of these infections, *Mycobacterium avium complex* (MAC), occurs in the respiratory and gastrointestinal tracts and is found in about half of AIDS patients at autopsy. Treatment of this disease is difficult and requires the use of several drugs.

Rifabutin (Mycobutin) is the first drug to be approved for the prevention of MAC disease. It is given to patients with advanced HIV infection and white-blood-cell counts of less than 200 per cubic millimeter. It should be given for the patient's lifetime unless MAC disease develops, at which time Mycobutin should be administered in conjunction with the antibiotics clarithromycin or azithromycin.

Recent studies published in the *New England Journal of Medicine* have shown that AIDS patients taking Mycobutin were half as likely to develop MAC infection as were other patients taking a placebo. Mycobutin also helped delay symptoms of infection with MAC such as fatigue, fever, night sweats, weight loss, and abdominal pain. However, the drug did not have an effect on the overall survival of these patients.

The most common side effects of Mycobutin are neutropenia (a decrease in a type of white blood cell that helps fight off other bacterial infections), stomach upset, and rash. It may also temporarily change body fluids (such as urine, saliva, perspiration, and tears), feces, and skin to a brown-orange color, and in some cases the drug may permanently stain contact lenses.

Mycobutin must not be used in people with active tuberculosis (TB), because such patients may develop resistance to both Mycobutin and to the TB drug called rifampin, making the tuberculosis harder to treat.

Another opportunistic infection that causes disability and death among AIDS patients is *Pneumocystis carinii* pneumonia (PCP). This infection has traditionally been treated with either trimethoprimsulfamethoxazole (TMP-SMX) or pentamidine. However, both these drugs produce toxic side effects in AIDS patients.

Atovaquone (Mepron), a new drug released in 1993 by Burroughs-Wellcome, is indicated as a possible treatment of mild to moderate PCP in individuals unable to take TMP-SMX. It has been shown to be just as effective in treating PCP as TMP-SMX or pentamidine in those people who respond to the drug. However, a greater number of people failed to respond to Mepron as compared with TMP-SMX. Also, more deaths occurred in the Mepron group than in the TMP-SMX group, probably due to a greater number of fatal bacterial infections in those treated with Mepron.

The side effects of Mepron appear to be temporary and self-limiting. They include skin rash, nausea, vomiting, insomnia, headache, and fever. The physician should be notified if a skin rash occurs. However, only a small number of people have had to discontinue taking the drug due to side effects.

## ▶ Expanded Influenza-Therapy Options

In September 1993, the FDA announced the approval of rimantadine (Flumadine), a new drug that can be used to treat influenza A. This serious form of the flu each year affects millions of people in the United States, causing approximately 20,000 deaths. Although influenza A is not usually fatal, it can be particularly dangerous, especially in the elderly and in people with chronic illnesses and other health problems.

## Search for New Class of Drugs

A variety of drugs are currently in development that have potential to treat many viruses and cancers that elude current therapies. One new class of drugs is the antisense agents, chemicals designed to target and impede messenger RNA from issuing basic directions, in the form of "sense" strands, for the production of specific proteins. The new antisense drugs are being designed to create mirror images of the RNA molecules they target. This allows the antisense strand to bind with the sense strand, halting its production of proteins. The advantage of these drugs is that as long as the genetic sequence of a virus' protein is known, an antisense molecule can be designed to target it.

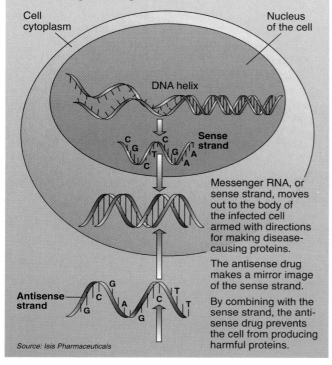

Cell cytoplasm

Nucleus of the cell

DNA helix

Sense strand

Messenger RNA, or sense strand, moves out to the body of the infected cell armed with directions for making disease-causing proteins.

The antisense drug makes a mirror image of the sense strand.

Antisense strand

By combining with the sense strand, the antisense drug prevents the cell from producing harmful proteins.

Source: Isis Pharmaceuticals

Flumadine, if taken within 48 hours after symptoms of the flu begin, can reduce the duration of fever and other flu symptoms. It must be taken twice daily for at least seven days, and is available both in a 100-mg coated tablet and as a syrup. At this time, it is indicated for treatment in adults only.

Vaccination is still the preferred method for preventing the flu, according to the Centers for Disease Control and Prevention (CDC). But for patients who are allergic to vaccine components or those who are taking drugs that suppress the immune system, Flumadine may be a safe, effective alternative.

### ▶ Halting Progression of Multiple Sclerosis

Multiple sclerosis (MS) is a common disease of the central nervous system characterized by periodic attacks followed by periods of no symptoms. The disease usually begins in early adulthood; symptoms of an attack may include impaired vision, decreased perception of the sense of position, lack of coordination of muscle movement, tremors, exaggerated reflexes, bladder problems, and weakness or paralysis of one or more limbs. Eventually attacks get worse and occur more frequently until patients are confined to a wheelchair, with increasing disability finally leading to death. The cause of multiple sclerosis remains uncertain, but it is thought that the disease may be associated with a problem in the immune system; attacks may be triggered by a viral infection.

A new drug, interferon Beta-1B (Betaseron), has just been released by Berlex. Betaseron is approved for the treatment of relapsing-remitting multiple sclerosis, the most common form of the disease.

It is not known how Betaseron works, although interferons have been shown to have effects against viruses and to induce changes in the immune system. A recent study showed that patients who were given injections of 8 million units (mu) every other day for three years had fewer and less serious attacks as well as a longer time between the first and second attacks than those patients given a placebo. It was also found during the study that patients on Betaseron spent fewer days in the hospital over the period. However, the drug does not stop all attacks, and among those in the treatment group and those receiving the placebo, there was no difference in the number of patients who became disabled. More needs to be learned about the long-term effects of Betaseron on the progression of multiple sclerosis. It may be that three years was not a long enough time to see a difference in the disability rates.

However, the positive effects of the drug, such as fewer and less serious attacks and fewer days spent in the hospital, can lead to a better quality of life as well as a reduction in health-care costs for these patients.

### ▶ Migraine Therapy

In the United States alone, 17.6 percent of females and 5.7 percent of males suffer one or more migraine headaches per year. Current therapy for migraine headaches—including ergotamine-containing preparations, narcotic analgesics, simple analgesics such as non-steroidal anti-inflammatory drugs, and drugs used to control nausea—is not always regarded as satisfactory and has many side effects.

Glaxo Pharmaceuticals has recently released sumatripton (Imitrex) for the acute treatment of migraine attacks with or without aura. Imitrex has been shown to effectively relieve the head pain and decrease the incidence of nausea and vomiting commonly associated with migraines. In most cases, relief occurs within 15 to 30 minutes after the drug is administered. This allows the patient to resume a normal lifestyle or return to work.

Imitrex is administered as a 6-mg subcutaneous (just under the skin) injection, either by the patient or by a physician. For people disinclined to give themselves injections, Imitrex is also available with an auto-injector device. The most commonly reported side effects with the drug include pain at the injection site, dizziness, and warm and hot sensations. These symptoms are usually mild and pass quickly.

Imitrex should not be used by people with angina, a history of myocardial infarction, documented silent ischemia, or Prinzmetal's angina. Imitrex may also cause an increase in blood pressure, and should therefore not be used in patients with hypertension.

## ▶ A New Drug for Bronchial Asthma

Asthma is a disease of the respiratory tract that causes difficulty breathing, shortness of breath, and wheezing. As many as 5 percent of adults and 7 percent of children in the United States suffer from asthma. Acute asthma attacks can be brought on by drugs, air pollution, respiratory infections, exercise, or emotional stress.

The best therapy for asthma is prevention. Nedocromil (Tilade), by Fisons Corporation, was recently approved for maintenance therapy in the management of patients with mild to moderate bronchial asthma. Tilade is an inhaled anti-inflammatory agent that is used to *prevent* attacks of asthma. It is important to note that Tilade is not a bronchodilator, and therefore cannot be used to reverse an acute asthma attack. The drug must be used on a regular schedule to prevent attacks.

In clinical studies, Tilade has been shown to be at least as effective as the steroid beclomethasone when added to drug therapy in patients with mild to moderate asthma. Tilade is also as effective as cromolyn sodium (Intal) in preventing cold- and exercise-induced asthma attacks.

## Top 10 Resistant Microbes

| Microbes | Diseases | Drugs |
|---|---|---|
| 1. Enterobacteriaceae (family) | Bacteremia, pneumonia, urinary-tract infections, surgical-wound infections | Aminoglycosides, Beta-lactam antibiotics, chloramphenicol, trimethoprim |
| 2. Enterococcus | Bacteremias, urinary-tract infections, surgical-wound infections | Aminoglycosides, Beta-lactam antibiotics, erythromycin, vancomycin |
| 3. Haemophilus influenzae | Epiglottitis, meningitis, otitis media, pneumonia, sinusitis | Beta-lactam antibiotics, chloramphenicol, tetracycline, trimethoprim |
| 4. Mycobacterium tuberculosis | Tuberculosis | Aminoglycosides, ethambutol, isoniazid, rifampin, pyrazinamide |
| 5. Neisseria gonorrhoeae | Gonorrhea | Beta-lactam antibiotics, spectinomycin, tetracycline |
| 6. Plasmodium falciparum | Malaria | Chloroquine |
| 7. Pseudomonas aeruginosa | Bacteremia, pneumonia, urinary-tract infections | Aminoglycosides, Beta-lactam antibiotics, chloramphenicol, ciprofloxacin, tetracycline, sulfonamides |
| 8. Shigella dysenteriae | Severe diarrhea | Ampicillin, trimethoprim-sulfamethoxazole, chloramphenicol, tetracycline |
| 9. Staphylococcus aureus | Bacteremia, pneumonia, surgical-wound infections | Chloramphenicol, ciprofloxacin, clindamycin, erythromycin, Beta-lactam antibiotics, rifampin, tetracycline, trimethoprim |
| 10. Streptococcus pneumoniae | Meningitis, pneumonia | Aminoglycosides, chloramphenicol, erythromycin, penicillin |

SOURCE: George Jacopy, *Medical World News* November 1992

## ▶ Nighttime Heartburn Therapy

Nighttime heartburn due to stomach-acid reflux, also known as gastroesophageal reflux, causes a burning, irritating sensation in the chest and sometimes an acid taste in the mouth. Cisapride (Propulsid) is the most recent agent to be introduced by Janssen Laboratories for treating this problem. Acid reflux usually occurs when the lower esophageal sphincter at the lower end of the esophagus is not working properly, and the ability of the stomach to empty is compromised. Reflux is most likely to occur when the stomach is full, when a person is lying down, or when stomach pressure is increased (pregnancy, obesity, or tight clothing). In most cases, diet, drug restrictions, weight reduction, and refraining from smoking manage the reflux. In some cases, drug therapy is initiated with antacids if the problem is not too severe. For severer cases, metoclopramide (Reglan) or histamine blockers such as famotidine (Pepcid) may be prescribed. Reglan's usefulness is sometimes limited, however, by such adverse reactions as tremor, agitation, menstrual irregularities, drowsiness, and fatigue.

But Propulsid works in a unique way, and has not been shown to cause these adverse reactions. Propulsid appears to work by increasing the lower-esophageal-sphincter pressure to prevent acid reflux, and by prompting the stomach to empty its contents, therefore reducing the possibility of reflux. Propulsid appears to be safe and well tolerated; complaints of diarrhea and transient abdominal cramping are the most common adverse effects.

## ▶ New Combined Vaccination for Children

Routine immunization of infants and children of school age has contributed to a decline in many childhood illnesses. For example, the use of oral polio vaccine has virtually eradicated polio in the United States. Due to the increasing numbers of vaccines that are now routinely recommended for children, combination vaccines are being developed so that fewer injections are required. Hemophilus B conjugate/DTwP (Tetramune), produced by Lederle-Praxis, is a combination of two vaccines. One component protects against *hemophilus* infections, including meningitis (an infection of the spinal cord), pneumonia, and epiglottitis (a severe swelling in the throat). The second component of the vaccine prevents diphtheria, tetanus, and pertussis. Diphtheria is a serious infection in the respiratory tract. Tetanus, also known as lockjaw, is an infection that causes increased muscle tone and muscle spasm. Tetanus usually occurs after a puncture wound with a nail or other contaminated object. Pertussis, more commonly known as whooping cough, is another respiratory-tract infection that causes sneezing, cough, and fever. Because these are serious but preventable diseases, immunization is extremely important. Tetramune provides protection against all of these infections with one injection instead of two, and is recommended for infants and children two months to five years of age.

## ▶ Drug Therapy for Alzheimer's Disease

Alzheimer's disease develops in as many as 20 percent of people aged 80 years or older. People with Alzheimer's disease frequently suffer from anxiety, depression, or bizarre behavior. But the most debilitating characteristic of the disease is memory loss, particularly for recent occurrences. Tacrine (Cognex), from Warner-Lambert, has recently been approved to improve memory deficits in Alzheimer's patients. Studies have demonstrated that some Alzheimer's patients taking Cognex have shown some improvement in memory and, in some cases, a slower decline in both memory function and ability to perform daily activities. Unfortunately, only a minority of patients with mild to moderate Alzheimer's disease appear to respond to Cognex therapy. Substantial improvements in memory or functional ability should not be expected. It is important to note that Cognex is not a cure for Alzheimer's and will not stop the progression of the disease.

## ▶ Options for Epileptic Seizures

At last there is new hope for patients suffering with epilepsy who have had either poor control of seizures or unacceptable side effects to antiseizure medications. Felbamate (Felbatol), manufactured by Wallace Laboratories, is the first major advance in 15 years for the treatment of epilepsy. It is effective both alone and in combination with other epilepsy drugs in adult patients with either partial or generalized seizures. It can also be used in children more than two years old with seizures associated with Lennox-Gastaut syndrome, a difficult-to-control disorder usually seen in children with mental retardation.

Felbatol has several advantages over traditional antiseizure medications. It has a low level of toxicity, and is not associated with the types of adverse reactions that occur with other anti-epileptics, such as gum problems, weight gain, and problems in concentrating and thinking. The most common side effects are anorexia, vomiting, insomnia, nausea, and headache. These side effects are generally mild and will usually go away even if the drug is continued.

Another advantage over traditional anti-epileptics is that patients taking Felbatol do not have to have their blood taken routinely to monitor for blood levels. The dosage of the drug is changed according to how well seizures are controlled, and not according to blood levels.

*Cheryl A. Stoukides, Pharm.D., and*
*Michelle M. Emery, R.Ph.*

# Mental Health

## ▶ Who Is Troubled

The Epidemiological Catchment Area (ECA) study, the largest and most comprehensive study on mental health ever conducted, was initiated to assess the prevalence of mental and addictive disorders and to learn how individuals make use of mental-health services. Headed by Darrel A. Regier, M.D., M.P.H., director of the Division of Epidemiology and Services Research at the National Institute of Mental Health, the study included interviews with 20,000 men and women in 1980. A follow-up study of 16,000 of these individuals was conducted from 1981 to 1985 to find the number of new cases of mental disorder that occurred in the course of a year.

The study's results, published in the February 1993 issue of the *Archives of General Psychiatry,* shows that, while 52 million adults suffer from a mental disorder at some point during a year, only 28 percent of these people seek help. The study also finds that, over the course of one year, 9 million people develop a new ailment, 8 million have a recurring ailment, and 35 million suffer continuing symptoms.

Trained interviewers questioned participants about symptoms of eight of the most common mental disorders, as defined by the *Diagnostic and Statistical Manual of Mental Disorders (DSM-III).* The study reveals that the most prevalent problems are anxiety disorders, particularly phobias (15 percent); alcohol disorders (15 percent); affective disorders, such as major depression (8 percent); and drug disorders other than alcoholism (6 percent).

The ECA study finds that 7 out of 10 people with a mental disorder do not seek treatment, and those that do seek help are often not recognized as having a psychiatric disorder. Panic disorder, for instance, is often misdiagnosed as hypochondria; alcoholics may not be recognized if they have a high income and good education; and depression is often missed by primary-care physicians. This is particularly noteworthy since more than 50 percent of those with mental disorders choose a general physician for psychiatric care rather than a psychiatrist or other mental-health professional. However, those that do consult mental-health professionals make an average of 14 visits per year. Visits to general physicians for mental disorders averaged just three to four per year. Interestingly, about 18 percent of study participants said that they sought help from nonprofessionals, such as Alcoholics Anonymous or other self-help groups. About 20 percent seek help from clergy or family-health agencies.

Although this is the largest study of the prevalence of mental disorders to date, the ECA results still pose many questions. The total number of cases reported in the study may be on the low side, since only people who met official psychiatric diagnostic criteria were counted. Therefore, those who were a symptom or two away from meeting the full criteria, considered *subthreshold,* were not tallied. But other studies have shown that subthreshold patients were highly likely to eventually develop a full-blown mental disorder and that patients with subthreshold conditions may experience significant distress. Furthermore, the ECA study does not identify those subjects who have a mental disorder but do not seek help, even though they urgently need it.

But the ECA study does provide new insight into the epidemiology of mental disorders, a topic that has taken on new importance as the Clinton administration embarks on a course to overhaul the nation's health-care insurance system. Many mental-health professionals hope that the study will provide the ammunition needed for including mental-health coverage in any guaranteed health plan that is ultimately created.

## ▶ Delayed-Discovery Memories

The number of reported childhood sexual-abuse cases has skyrocketed from 150,000 reports in 1963 to 2.7 million in 1990, according to the National Center on Child Abuse and Neglect. As victims, parents, teachers, therapists, and medical professionals grapple with the inflammatory and complex issues associated with child sexual-abuse cases, a new segment of victims is just now coming to light —adults who recall past sexual-abuse experiences long forgotten from their childhood. The sometimes heated debates over the reliability of these "delayed-discovery" memories have polarized mental-health professionals.

It has been well documented that victims of sexual abuse often *dissociate,* or slip into an altered state of consciousness during the abuse experience. For example, a child exposed to repeated sexual assaults may deaden his or her body to pain or imagine that the abuse is occurring to someone else. Some experts believe that these traumatic experiences may become *repressed,* hidden in the mind until the victims are adults and some event triggers the memory. In the January 1993 issue of the *Journal of Traumatic Stress,* psychologist John Briere, Ph.D., of the University of Southern California School of Medicine in Los Angeles and social worker Jon R. Conte of the University of Washington in Seattle found that, in a survey of 450 female psychotherapy patients who had been sexually abused as children, 59 percent said that they had forgotten about their abuse experiences at some time before age 18. In another study conducted by Linda Meyer

Williams of the University of New Hampshire in Durham, 38 of 100 women did not recall childhood sexual abuse that had been documented in their hospital records 17 years earlier.

"Our minds . . . protect us from what we are unable to bear," says Lynne Finney, a Utah lawyer and therapist who wrote of her own delayed discovery in *Reach for the Rainbow* (Putnam, 1992). "The reason we protect these memories is that when we are abused as children, the emotions are too overwhelming—the sadness, the terror, the betrayal, the shame and guilt and anger and hatred and helplessness and confusion."

Yet critics question if this apparent repression actually exists as a psychological process with the power to act as a trap door for violent memories. Furthermore, in an interview with *Science News*, Elizabeth F. Loftus, Ph.D., a psychologist at the University of Washington in Seattle, stated, "We do not yet have the tools for reliably distinguishing the signal of true repressed memories from the noise of false ones."

Loftus and others worry that memories of child abuse may be fabricated through the suggestions or persuasions of others, from a therapist to self-help books for incest victims. No studies have produced evidence for the reliability of repressed memories. But many studies have indicated that memories of past events are often amended with new events picked up from newspapers, television, or movies. In one study, a group of people ranging from age 8 to 42 were convinced of a memory that they had "forgotten" at the age of 5. The memory was completely fabricated by the experimenter, who then coached the study participants until they "recalled" the event.

In *Hidden Memories* (Prometheus Books, 1992), Robert A. Baker, Ph.D., professor emeritus at the University of Kentucky, suggests that childhood conflicts regarding authority figures may be catapulted into memories of sexual abuse as a result of experiences such as therapy sessions that focus on incest as a cause of adult insecurity or celebrity admissions of past abuse. Baker writes, "Obtaining the truth is never easy, but claims of childhood sexual abuse that emerge only after psychotherapy are particularly suspect."

Many mental-health professionals are concerned that this false memory assertion may have a backlash effect for victims of child abuse seeking justice. They fear that victims who were already traumatized as children will have their feelings of powerlessness and low self-esteem doubly reinforced if they decide to voice their abuse experiences. Still, despite the difficulty of corroborating a victim's accusation, 19 states have passed legislation permitting victims to sue for recovery of damages for injuries suffered from childhood sexual abuse, and other states are considering similar legislation. As a result, at least 300 lawsuits have been filed.

While delayed-discovery memories continue to produce bitter divisiveness in the childhood-abuse research community, it is just this sort of polarity that may eventually spark new, more sophisticated studies on the impact of sexual abuse.

## ▶ Sexual Harassment and Mental-Health Professionals

The reported incidence of sexual harassment has grown in recent years. In a survey of 20,314 federal employees, the largest study ever of workplace sexual harassment, 42 percent of female employees and 15 percent of male employees claim to have been sexually harassed. Other studies have found lifetime prevalence rates of sexual harassment ranging from 52 percent to 100 percent. As cases of sexual harassment become more widespread, the mental-health professional is commonly being called upon to play a role. In an article published in *Psychiatric Annals* in August 1993, Margaret F. Jensvold, M.D., director of the Institute for Research on Women's Health in Washington, D.C., states that these health professionals have very specific roles that constitute appropriate professional behavior. Unfortunately, Jensvold concludes, "the potential for misuse and abuse of psychiatry around sexual harassment is growing."

Jensvold contends that in sexual-harassment cases, mental-health professionals can act as therapists; testify as expert witnesses in lawsuits, providing expertise on issues other than the victim's mental status; and perform psychological evaluations of the victims for court lawsuits claiming emotional damages.

The harassment and retaliation affecting victims of sexual harassment may trigger myriad emotional symptoms. These same symptoms may be used by the harasser as evidence that the victim imagined, caused, or even deserved harassment. Even without emotional symptoms, the victim may become subject to demoralizing accusations. At the Clarence Thomas confirmation hearings, for example, Anita Hill was alternately accused of being mentally unstable, potentially schizophrenic, and of fantasizing. Therapists can play a necessary and vital role by helping victims of harassment cope with the harassment experience and its aftermath.

When a sexual-harassment victim sues for emotional damages, the harasser or the company may institute a variety of coercive tactics to intimidate complaining employees. These tactics may include asking the victim to undergo forced psychiatric evaluation (to establish fitness for duty); and even forced psychotherapy.

These tactics open the door for the misuse of psychiatry in sexual harassment. Whether these tactics are merely threatened or actually realized, the very act of needing to gather information about the victim's psychological state and history of psychopathology reinforces the harasser's contention that the employee imagined, caused, or even deserved the behavior he or she is complaining about.

Furthermore, forcing an employee to take part in a psychiatric evaluation implies that the problem is inherent in the employee—if the employee's flaw is corrected, the problem will be resolved. This approach avoids dealing effectively with the harasser or the problematic interaction between the harasser and the employee, and the harasser's behavior may be permitted to continue. A psychiatric evaluation or psychiatric diagnosis has the added effect of stigmatizing the victim, which may penalize him or her in a later job search or create a "preexisting illness" preventing insurance coverage at a future job.

Mental-health professionals must be careful not to be used as unwitting pawns for the harasser's edification and the victim's detriment. Jensvold recommends that an evaluating mental-health professional dealing with a sexual-harassment case should follow certain guidelines, including: establishing the reasons for and uses of an examination; establishing if the purpose of the session is to provide treatment or to evaluate the patient for the purposes of a third party; and informing the patient about the nature of and limitations to confidentiality.

## ▶ Manic Depression and Genetics

More than 2.5 million Americans suffer from manic depression, a mental-health disease that causes victims to suffer a roller coaster of emotions, alternately rocketing to dangerous highs and plunging to suicidal lows. Some 80 percent of manic depression is thought to have a genetic origin. In 1987 researchers were convinced that they had found a link between this psychiatric illness and a gene on the X chromosome. These preliminary findings had leaders in the field confident that it was only a matter of time before the secret to hereditary mental disorders would be unraveled by straightforward DNA analysis.

Six years later, the confidence of these same researchers has been eroded. In the January 1993 issue of *Nature Genetics*, Miron Baron, M.D., of the New York State Psychiatric Institute at Columbia University headed a study that fails to confirm the earlier link between manic depression and a gene on chromosome X. The 1987 studies had focused on three Israeli families. The researchers used biochemical markers considered very crude by today's standards. In the 1993 study, more-precise genetic probes were used on the same data. As a result, any association between manic depression and the X chromosome vanished.

These results have spurred new, intriguing theories ripe for exploration. In an interview with *The*

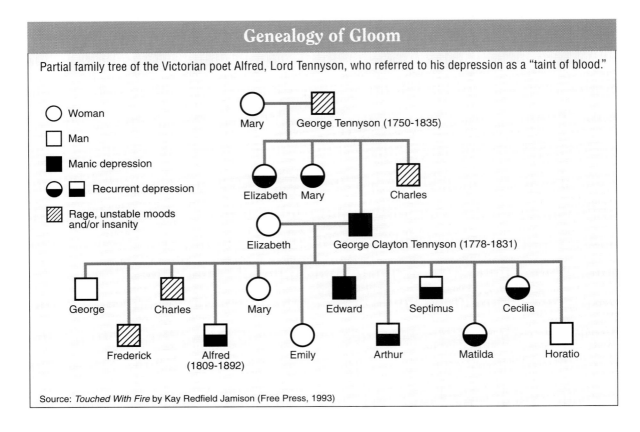

## Genealogy of Gloom

Partial family tree of the Victorian poet Alfred, Lord Tennyson, who referred to his depression as a "taint of blood."

○ Woman
□ Man
■ Manic depression
◐ ◧ Recurrent depression
▨ Rage, unstable moods and/or insanity

Mary — George Tennyson (1750-1835)

Elizabeth  Mary  Charles

Elizabeth — George Clayton Tennyson (1778-1831)

George  Charles  Mary  Edward  Septimus  Cecilia

Frederick  Alfred (1809-1892)  Emily  Arthur  Matilda  Horatio

Source: *Touched With Fire* by Kay Redfield Jamison (Free Press, 1993)

*New York Times,* Dr. Baron said, "We now know that there is no single major gene for psychiatric illnesses. The model of three or four or five interacting genes, operating in tandem to produce an illness, is becoming more and more appealing."

Furthermore, this latest study has opened the door for investigation of other components of psychiatric diseases, particularly environmental factors. Researchers now suspect that a person who has a genetic predisposition to manic depression may not develop the full-blown disease without specific environmental triggers. These triggers may include nutritional factors, exposure to drugs, extreme stresses like the death of a loved one, or even hormonal imbalances.

While the single-gene theory has been discounted, research still continues to identify the genetic origin of the disorder. A team of researchers at The Johns Hopkins Medical Institution is screening families with several members who have manic-depressive illness. Led by J. Raymond DePaulo, Jr., M.D., the Hopkins team is searching for families that have at least three affected siblings. One parent's side of the family must be free of illness so it is clear when creating a family tree which family member is passing along the disease. The search for families that match this criteria is still ongoing, but preliminary research using the family data has spurred some provocative theories. In one family, every woman with manic depression passed the disease to her children, while no man with the disorder passed it on. The researchers propose that manic depression may be linked to mitochondrial DNA, which is only passed along to a child by the mother. More highly detailed family trees will need to be evaluated before these theories can be tested.

## ▶ Hypnosis

Ever since Austrian physician Franz Anton Mesmer first proposed his theory of "mesmerization" 200 years ago, hypnosis has alternately been considered a charlatan's hoax and a useful psychotherapeutic tool. In the last 30 years, hypnosis has gained more credibility, as well-respected researchers from such prestigious institutions as Harvard University and Stanford University pioneered hypnosis research projects, intent on producing clear evidence of the effectiveness of the hypnotic state using proven scientific methods.

In the burgeoning hypnosis field, reports are emerging documenting the effectiveness of hypnosis in a wide variety of medical and psychological applications. For instance, hypnosis has been found to be an effective anesthesia to numb the pain of some surgical procedures; it has been used successfully to alleviate phobias, such as a fear of flying; and numerous studies have shown that hypnosis can treat warts. Since warts are caused by viruses, these studies suggest that hypnosis may mobilize the immune system into action.

But while hypnosis has been credited as a useful medical tool, other hypnosis claims border on downright chicanery. For instance, a Florida doctor has touted hypnosis as a new and safe method for enlarging breasts without the use of breast-augmentation surgery. The doctor, Michael A. B. Stivers, director of the Professional Hypnosis and Research Center in Largo, Florida, hypnotizes patients and makes them regress back to their hormone-raging puberty years. Stivers claims that hypnosis tricks the body into reactivating hormone production so that breasts increase in size.

Other hypnotherapists are not only skeptical about these claims, they are alarmed. No study has shown that hypnosis can stimulate hormonal change, and those in the field are concerned that such claims will sully and even inhibit genuine clinical research in hypnosis. In an interview with *Omni* magazine, William Brink, executive director of the American Association of Professional Hypnotherapists, said, "There are enough eyebrows raised in regard to hypnosis, but when you go using it for these purposes, it raises a lot more—and not usually in a positive manner. While there may be some validity to it, we really don't favor it."

Why does hypnosis flounder as a pseudoscience? Critics contend that most hypnosis studies use flawed methodologies. There is no definition of what constitutes a hypnotic state. Attempts to find any physiological pattern that distinguishes hypnosis from a waking state, such as brain-wave patterns or rapid eye movements, have failed. In the absence of a standard physiological definition, it is impossible to evaluate the hypnotic state using traditional scientific methods. So there is no way to discern whether patients under hypnosis remain pain-free during surgery due to hypnosis or because they are adept at focusing their attention elsewhere.

Furthermore, practitioners of hypnosis do not employ consistent procedures for inducing a hypnotic trance. As a result, hypnotherapy is often the umbrella term used by therapists for a wide variety of techniques, including psychoanalytic age regression, direct suggestion for symptom removal, and systematic desensitization. It is therefore difficult to discern whether a problem is treated by hypnosis or as a result of verbal suggestions.

While exaggerated claims for hypnosis abound, many of the effects attributed to hypnosis really do occur. And even though the hypnotic state may be more of a subjective realm than an objectively measurable altered state of consciousness, many mental-health professionals feel that to toss hypnosis out of a therapist's repertoire would be doing many patients an injustice.

*Lisa Holland*

Two Massachusetts molecular biologists shared the 1993 Nobel Prize in Physiology or Medicine. Richard J. Roberts and Phillip A. Sharp were honored for their 1977 discovery of "split genes." The two scientists, working independently of one another, achieved profound insights into genetic structure and function that opened a new chapter in modern biology. In the words of the Nobel committee, "Roberts' and Sharp's discovery has changed our view on how genes in higher organisms develop during evolution. The discovery of split genes has been of fundamental importance for today's basic research in biology, as well as for more medically oriented research concerning the development of cancer and other diseases."

The awarding of the Nobel Prize to Drs. Roberts and Sharp came as no great surprise to their fellow scientists, who had recognized the importance of their discovery immediately. One prominent scientist even remarked that it would not be an understatement to call their work "the single most surprising and illuminating experiment that has ever been done in biology."

▶ **Split Genes**

Through research on bacteria, scientists have formed a picture of how the genetic information in deoxyribonucleic acid (DNA) is translated into the proteins that regulate all the living functions of an organism. In bacteria, individual genes exist as continuous, unbroken segments of nucleotides within the double-stranded DNA. When a gene is activated, its information is copied into a single-stranded molecule called *ribonucleic acid,* or *RNA.* This *messenger RNA,* as it has come to be known, translates the information into the synthesis of a specific protein.

Scientists observed that there was a direct correspondence between the structure and chemistry of individual genes (the continuous, uninterrupted stretches of DNA) and that of the resulting proteins. It was widely believed that this general scheme applied, not only to bacteria, but also to higher organisms such as humans. In 1977 Drs. Roberts and Sharp announced findings that turned this assumption upside down.

Rather than using the simple bacteria on which previous researchers had worked, Drs. Roberts and Sharp chose to experiment with a more complex organism, a kind of virus called *adenovirus.* In humans, adenovirus is known to cause such ailments as the common cold and conjunctivitis, or pinkeye. Because this virus is relatively simple and yet also has properties that are similar to those found in the cells of higher organisms, the scientists believed that adenovirus would be an ideal model in which to observe how genetic information is processed in the synthesis of proteins in higher organisms, such as humans and other mammals.

The two scientists worked separately with their own teams of researchers—Dr. Roberts at the Cold Spring Harbor Laboratory on New York's Long Island, and Dr. Sharp at the Massachusetts Institute of Technology (MIT) in Cambridge, Massachusetts. The two teams created special mole-

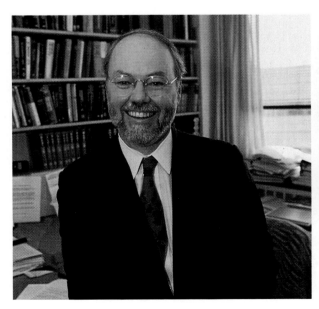
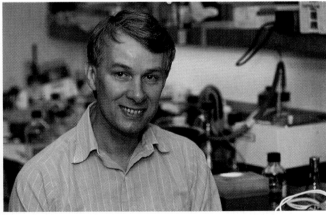

*Two molecular biologists, Phillip A. Sharp, Ph.D. (left) and Richard J. Roberts, Ph.D. (above), were awarded the 1993 Nobel Prize in Physiology or Medicine for their discovery of "split genes." Their research has led to a better understanding of how cancer and other diseases develop.*

cules in order to study the process by which the adenovirus DNA binds a complementary strand of messenger RNA. The expectation, based on the general scheme of gene structure obtained from work in bacteria, was that the genetic information in the messenger-RNA molecule would correspond exactly to continuous segments of genes along the DNA strand.

To their surprise, however, the researchers found that this theoretical correspondence was not the case. Roberts and Sharp and their colleagues used very powerful electron microscopes to examine their experimental molecules. They found that the messenger RNA of the adenovirus actually corresponded to no less than four separate regions of DNA. With the aid of the electron microscope, they could see that there were long stretches of DNA that did not seem to play a part in the making of the messenger RNA. Clearly, these areas of DNA were not involved in the formation of proteins.

From the evidence in their experiments, Drs. Roberts and Sharp concluded that adenovirus genes do not take the form of unbroken strands of DNA. Instead, the genes are organized in discontinuous strands—they are, in effect, "split"—interrupted by stretches of DNA that do not code for any specific protein. When Drs. Roberts and Sharp and their teams announced their findings at a meeting of biologists in June 1977, it became clear to the scientific community that genetic structure and function in higher organisms such as human beings and other mammals was vastly more complicated than scientists had previously thought.

After Drs. Roberts and Sharp announced their findings, other researchers began their own explorations of gene structure in other viruses and cells. These other researchers corroborated Drs. Roberts' and Sharp's findings by determining that the "split-gene" structure was in fact the most common gene structure in higher organisms.

In discussing the process by which genetic information is translated into the synthesis of proteins, scientists now use the term *exons* to refer to those regions of DNA that code for a specific protein (since these regions "express" genetic information). As Drs. Roberts and Sharp first demonstrated, these coding regions are interrupted by other segments of DNA that do not seem to contain genetic information. To convey the idea of "intervening" regions, scientists refer to these noncoding segments as *introns*. As the genetic information from DNA is translated into RNA code, these intron regions appear to be edited out. The remaining exons are combined to form messenger RNA. The process by which exons are joined together in the formation of messenger RNA is known as "splicing." Gene splicing has become one of the most active and important fields in biological re-

search today. Scientists are intensely interested in examining how the coding and noncoding regions of DNA are shuffled and combined in the formation of different proteins.

## ▶ Insights into Evolution and Disease

The concept of split genes that was introduced by the discoveries of Drs. Roberts and Sharp has caused scientists to change their ideas about the process of evolution. Previously scientists believed that organisms evolve primarily through mutation —that is, by a series of small accumulated changes in DNA over many generations. Following the discovery of "split genes," some biologists now theorize that an organism's capacity to shuffle different regions of DNA into many new protein combinations might in itself serve as a very powerful and rapid mechanism in driving evolution.

The work of Drs. Roberts and Sharp has also made it possible for researchers to obtain insights into certain hereditary diseases. A form of anemia known as beta-thalassemia, for example, occurs when genetic material is improperly spliced together in the assembly of a protein called beta-globin, which makes up part of the hemoglobin in red blood cells. The beta-globin formed by the faulty splicing will not function properly. This shortens the life span of red blood cells, giving rise to anemia. Similarly, a form of cancer known as chronic myelogenous leukemia also results from errors that occur during the editing and splicing of introns and exons. In the case of this disease, the faulty joining of two genes results in an RNA molecule that directs the formation of a cancer-causing protein. Understanding more about the splicing errors that cause these and other diseases may one day help scientists to develop better treatments.

*Richard J. Roberts,* Ph.D., was born on September 6, 1943, in Derby, England. After earning his bachelor's and doctoral degrees in chemistry at the University of Sheffield, England, he moved to the United States and undertook a research fellowship at Harvard University in Cambridge, Massachusetts. In 1972 Dr. Roberts joined the staff of the Cold Spring Harbor Laboratory, leaving in 1992 to become director of research at New England Biolabs in Beverly, Massachusetts.

*Phillip A. Sharp,* Ph.D., was born on June 6, 1944, in Falmouth, Kentucky. He earned his undergraduate degree in chemistry and mathematics from Union College in Barbourville, Kentucky, and his doctorate in chemistry from the University of Illinois. In 1974, after completing postdoctoral fellowships at the California Institute of Technology in Pasadena and at Cold Spring Harbor Laboratory, Dr. Sharp joined the faculty of MIT, where he now heads the biology department.

*Christopher King*

# Nutrition and Diet

## ▶ Pesticides in the Diet

A committee of the National Academy of Sciences (NAS) released a report in June 1993 recommending that changes be made in regulating pesticide residues in children's diets. While there is limited knowledge regarding children's vulnerability to pesticide exposure, the committee believes that enough data on other toxic substances exists to show that children may be more sensitive than adults to some pesticides.

Current pesticide regulations are based on tolerances set by examining food surveys and conducting laboratory tests. The Environmental Protection Agency (EPA) defines a *tolerance* as the legal limit of a pesticide residue allowed in or on a raw agricultural product or a processed food. These methods do not take into account certain factors that may make children more susceptible than adults to pesticide exposure. For example, children and infants eat fewer foods than adults, and tend to consume more of certain foods per unit of body weight. In addition, information on children's food intake has been categorized into broad age groups, such as from age 1 to age 6. Yet these broad groupings do not reflect constant changes in diet that occur as children grow. Furthermore, current food-consumption surveys focus on average food intake, which may ignore ethnic and geographic factors that affect pesticide exposure.

The committee recommends that toxicity testing on immature animals should be undertaken to evaluate the pesticide sensitivity of children, particularly any dangers to the developing immune, nervous, and reproductive systems.

Food-consumption surveys should also be altered to reflect the difference between the diets of children and adults. The committee advises the use of food surveys for children at seven age levels: at every one-year interval up to age 5, between ages 5 and 10, and between ages 11 and 18.

The committee also recommends that measurements of pesticide residues be standardized across the country, and that a database be established for gathering data from different laboratories. Pesticide regulations should also consider increased testing of foods eaten by infants and children, the different methods of pesticide application, and how food processing affects pesticide levels.

In order to estimate cancer risk more accurately, the committee recommends designing new techniques that evaluate the changes in pesticide exposure and susceptibility that occur throughout a person's life. Children exposed to a carcinogen early in life have much more time ahead of them than do adults to develop a cancer.

A report by the Environmental Working Group (EWG), a nonprofit consumer group, echoes the concerns of the NAS. The EWG's analysis of 24,629 foods reveals low, but measurable, residues of at least one pesticide in half of the samples. The Department of Agriculture's (USDA's) analysis of pesticides in 1992 found detectable residues in 58 percent of 2,859 produce samples tested. Two or more pesticide residues were evident in 30 percent of the apples sampled, and 19 samples were in violation of federal standards.

The NAS and EWG reports encourage parents to continue to include fruits and vegetables in children's diets. The best advice for now is to wash produce well or, better yet, peel the skin. Consider purchasing organic produce, and, if possible, grow organic vegetables in the summer.

On September 21, 1993, the EPA, the Food and Drug Administration (FDA), and the USDA announced a joint proposal of regulations to implement the recommendations of the NAS. Their goal is a 50 percent reduction in the use of pesticides by the end of the decade. It is likely that this proposal will come up in Congress for a vote during 1994.

## ▶ The Designer Foods Program

Researchers at the National Cancer Institute (NCI) are analyzing the phytochemicals (defined as any chemical produced by a plant) in fruits, vegetables, herbs, and spices to investigate their ability to prevent disease. This project, called the Designer Foods Program, is also exploring how these substances work together and how they can be used to enrich common foods.

### Folic Acid Fortification

In 1993 the Food and Drug Administration (FDA) announced a proposal to fortify flour, breads, and other grain products with folic acid, a B vitamin, to reduce the risk of neural-tube defects, such as spina bifida. This proposal will also allow a health claim stating this beneficial effect on products that are good sources of folic acid.

In 1992 the U.S. Public Health Service recommended that women of childbearing age consume 0.4 milligram of folic acid daily to lower the risk of neural-tube defects in their infants. Since overconsumption of folic acid can mask pernicious anemia, a $B_{12}$ deficiency, the fortification amounts have been planned to stay within safe levels even for women who consume large quantities of grain products. The FDA proposes a health claim on grain products that states the reason for fortification, lists other dietary sources of folic acid (such as oranges and dark-green leafy vegetables), and warns that daily folic acid intake should not exceed 1.0 milligram from all sources.

Currently researchers are studying garlic, citrus fruits, flax, soybeans, licorice, and umbelliferous vegetables, which include carrots, parsnips, celery, and parsley. Garlic, for example, contains several phytochemicals, some of which are released only after cooking. Raw garlic appears to have antibiotic properties. When garlic is sautéed, two sulfides are produced—one will be used in a drug to treat asthma, and the other may prevent hormones from transmitting pain. When garlic is added to boiling water, another sulfide is released that has been shown to inhibit cancer of the colon. In order to have a standardized form of garlic containing as many phytochemicals as possible, the researchers now use aged garlic extract for their studies. The garlic extract, approved by the FDA, also has anti-inflammatory and antioxidant properties, and controls synthesis of cholesterol.

The NCI is working closely with private companies, research institutions, and the FDA to develop and test foods containing various phytochemicals. One designer food already being tested by NCI is a vegetable juice that combines carrot, celery, and tomato juices with garlic, basil, rosemary, pepper, and paprika. According to Herb Pierson, M.D., former director of the Designer Foods Program, the technology exists to develop an orange juice that contains the beneficial phytochemicals of 10 to 20 different oranges. Research has shown that the phytochemicals in oranges may fight cancer, lower cholesterol, and reduce inflammation.

What lies ahead for the Designer Foods Program? Researchers will continue to analyze other foods for phytochemicals. Green tea, rosemary, cruciferous vegetables (such as broccoli), cucurbits (the family of squash, melons, and cucumbers), and solanaceous vegetables (tomatoes, peppers, and eggplant) are some of the targeted foods. Once all the information is collected in a database, computer programs will be used to sort out the most-significant results, including identifying any synergistic qualities between certain phytochemicals.

Any designer foods developed will undergo rigorous safety testing via feeding trials in animals. In humans, scientists will first study the effects of these foods on cancer-related chemical pathways in healthy people. Eventually intervention trials will be conducted in which people at high risk for cancer will consume foods specifically developed to ward off the chemical processes that lead to cancer.

Since some of the designer foods will contain naturally occurring chemicals at levels much higher than normal, the FDA will need to decide whether to classify these products as foods or drugs. It may be several years before any of these designer foods reach the supermarkets. In the meantime, beneficial phytochemicals are, of course, present in foods we eat daily.

## ▶ The *Fresh Start* Program

The National School Lunch Program operates in 95 percent of the country's schools, and feeds approximately 25 million children lunch daily, and more than 5 million children breakfast at school. School lunches currently derive about 40 percent of their calories from fat, 10 percent higher than the level recommended by the U.S. Dietary Guidelines published by the USDA. Saturated fat contributes 15 percent of the total fat, which is 50 percent higher than recommended. The sodium content of school lunches is approximately 1,200 milligrams (mg), twice the amount recommended by the National Research Council.

According to one report, more than half of the children in the School Lunch Program eat less than one serving of fruit per day, and one-fifth eat less than one serving of vegetables per day. Moreover, one-third of the lunches the children choose themselves do not include any fruits or vegetables.

Children's lack of interest in these foods is likely due to the unpalatability of canned or frozen products, and perhaps to their poor nutritional knowledge. In some schools the menus do not even offer a vegetable, or else such condiments as ketchup are classified as vegetables. Since the school lunch is the only decent meal some children eat daily, the need to improve the nutritional quality of these meals is essential.

In September 1993, the *Fresh Start* Program was established to improve school meals across the nation. Led by Ellen Haas, the assistant secretary of Agriculture for Food and Consumer Services, this program has already implemented some changes in the School Lunch Program. The amount of fresh fruits and vegetables offered to schools will be doubled from 8.8 billion pounds to 16 billion pounds. The variety of fresh produce will also increase to include more than just the fresh apples, pears, grapefruits, oranges, tomatoes, and baking potatoes now available. Schools will offer beef patties with only 10 percent fat, and ground turkey averaging 11 percent fat. In addition the USDA is developing a low-fat turkey sausage. The sausage, along with low-fat Cheddar and mozzarella cheese, was made available on a trial basis in some schools during the 1993–94 school year.

Nutrition education in schools has been sorely lacking. During the late 1970s, approximately 50 cents per child per year—a total of $26 million—was appropriated for nutrition education. Although only $5 million was earmarked for this purpose by 1990, funding had already increased to $10 million in 1993. According to Ellen Haas, funding for nutrition education must be increased as a component of the *Fresh Start* program. It seems necessary that children have a better understanding of the connection between good nutrition and disease prevention.

## ▶ Fat and Breast Cancer

Researchers continue to look for the link between dietary fat and breast cancer. Epidemiological studies have shown that women living in countries such as Japan and China, where dietary fat is less than 20 percent of total calories, have a much lower incidence of breast cancer than women in the United States, where fat consumption averages 37 percent of total calories. However, recent U.S. studies examining the fat and breast-cancer link have had conflicting results.

In October 1992, results of the Nurses' Health Study headed by Walter Willet, M.D., from Harvard Medical School were published in the *Journal of the American Medical Association.* Almost 90,000 female registered nurses were followed for eight years via a detailed questionnaire that included a dietary assessment. Newly diagnosed cases of breast cancer were identified by the questionnaire as well as by follow-up telephone calls. The women were grouped into categories based on the percentage of total fat in their diets. The researchers found no difference in the incidence of breast cancer between the group consuming nearly 50 percent of their calories from fat compared to the group consuming less than 30 percent of their calories from fat. Some researchers hypothesize that only diets that are very low in fat (20 percent of total calories or less) can lower the risk for breast cancer. The Harvard study did not have a subgroup of women following a diet with only 20 percent of the calories from fat.

An NCI study examined the effects of dietary fat on the length of the follicular phase of the menstrual cycle. The follicular phase is the time from the first day of menses until the luteinizing hormone peaks. A group of 31 premenopausal women, ages 20 to 40, was followed for nine menstrual cycles. The women had no dietary restrictions for one menstrual cycle. Each woman was then placed on a high-fat diet (40 percent of the calories from fat) for four more cycles.

The results revealed that when fat consumption was reduced from 40 percent of total calories to 20 percent (during the last four cycles), two-thirds of the women increased their follicular phase by almost two days. The researchers suggest that lengthening the follicular phase permits a woman to have fewer menstrual cycles throughout her life, thus limiting her total exposure to estrogens. Certainly further research on this dietary fat and menstrual cycle link needs to be done to establish a conclusive association between fat intake and breast-cancer incidence.

As part of The Women's Health Initiative, a large, 14-year study launched by the National Institutes of Health (NIH), researchers will examine whether a diet with fat constituting 20 percent of total calories will lower the risk for breast cancer. Since a low-fat, high-fiber diet has definitely been proven to reduce one's risk for heart disease, colorectal cancer, and obesity, it only makes sense to follow these habits now. In the meantime, we await more news on the diet and breast-cancer link.

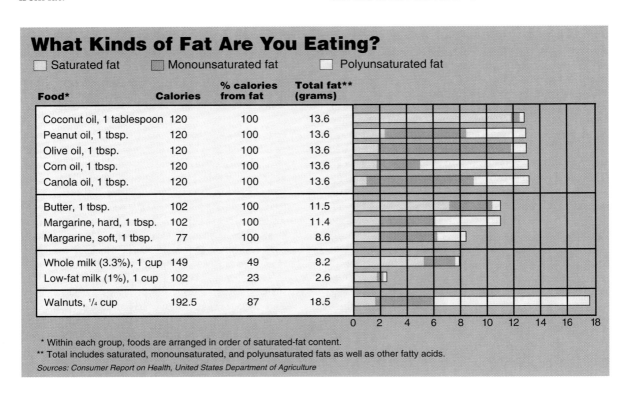

## What Kinds of Fat Are You Eating?

☐ Saturated fat   ■ Monounsaturated fat   ☐ Polyunsaturated fat

| Food* | Calories | % calories from fat | Total fat** (grams) |
|---|---|---|---|
| Coconut oil, 1 tablespoon | 120 | 100 | 13.6 |
| Peanut oil, 1 tbsp. | 120 | 100 | 13.6 |
| Olive oil, 1 tbsp. | 120 | 100 | 13.6 |
| Corn oil, 1 tbsp. | 120 | 100 | 13.6 |
| Canola oil, 1 tbsp. | 120 | 100 | 13.6 |
| Butter, 1 tbsp. | 102 | 100 | 11.5 |
| Margarine, hard, 1 tbsp. | 102 | 100 | 11.4 |
| Margarine, soft, 1 tbsp. | 77 | 100 | 8.6 |
| Whole milk (3.3%), 1 cup | 149 | 49 | 8.2 |
| Low-fat milk (1%), 1 cup | 102 | 23 | 2.6 |
| Walnuts, ¼ cup | 192.5 | 87 | 18.5 |

0  2  4  6  8  10  12  14  16  18

\* Within each group, foods are arranged in order of saturated-fat content.

\*\* Total includes saturated, monounsaturated, and polyunsaturated fats as well as other fatty acids.

*Sources: Consumer Report on Health, United States Department of Agriculture*

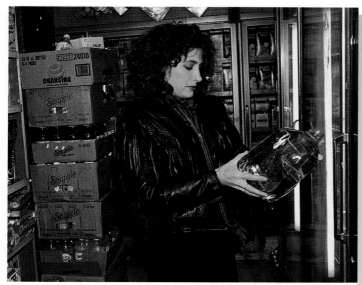

## ▶ Bottled Waters

Gone are the days when thirst for water was synonymous with just pouring a cold glass from the tap. Beginning in the early 1980s, Americans began turning to bottled water to quench their thirst. According to figures from the International Bottled Water Association (IBWA), per capita consumption of bottled water increased from 1.5 gallons in 1976 to 8 gallons in 1991. Today there are more than 700 different brands of bottled water available in the United States, with 75 brands made from imported waters.

Consumer-attitude surveys conducted by the IBWA have shown that taste is the main reason why many people prefer bottled water. Ozone, a form of oxygen, is used by most of the bottling manufacturers as a final disinfectant. While chlorine often leaves an aftertaste or odor in tap water, ozone does not. Another reason people prefer bottled water is that they believe (sometimes erroneously) that it is safer than tap water. Increased interest in health, weight control, and alcohol moderation has also turned people away from higher-calorie beverages to bottled waters, most of which are calorie-free.

Without a doubt the bottled-water industry, in its labeling and advertising, has capitalized on Americans' interest in health and fitness. Undefined terms such as "natural springwater" or "glacier water" are often misleading. Advertisements showing lean men and women downing a bottle after an invigorating workout imply that bottled water has special restorative properties.

Over the past few years, the bottled-water industry's wholesome image has taken its share of licks. In 1990 traces of benzene were found in samples of Perrier mineral water, forcing the manufacturer to recall 160 million bottles. The company has not yet completely recovered, with sales only half of what they were prior to the recall. A second, more pervasive blow came in 1991, when the U.S. House Energy and Commerce Committee began a comprehensive investigation of the bottled-water industry. The committee's findings include: 25 percent of expensive bottled waters come from the same source as plain tap water; another 25 percent of the companies could not document their water source at all; and 31 percent of the waters contained microbiological contamination at levels higher than allowed.

**FDA cracks down.** Although 23 states have passed legislation that regulates quality and labeling standards for the bottled-water industry, widespread variations persist in how different types of waters are defined. In January 1993, the FDA proposed regulations that would set standard definitions for various terms used on the labels of these waters. The terms that have been defined include: *spring, mineral, artesian, well, distilled,* and *purified.* For example, *springwater* would be defined as bottled water taken from an underground formation from which water flows naturally to the surface, or would if it were not collected underground. (See the sidebar for additional definitions.) The FDA's proposal would also require that water bottled from a municipal water supply must be clearly labeled as such. "Seltzer" and "soda" waters were excluded from the proposed regulation since they are classified as soft drinks.

At the same time, the FDA established new limits for about 50 contaminants, and, in August 1993, proposed new or revised maximum limits for 24 environmental contaminants that may be present in bottled water. The second set of proposed limits matches limits set for public drinking water in July 1992 by the EPA. The proposal will require each bottled-water manufacturer to analyze its product at least once per year to ensure compliance.

**Nutrition.** With the exception of sweetened seltzer waters, bottled waters are certainly a refreshing and healthy substitute for soft drinks. However, they are not nutritionally superior to tap water. Bottled waters do contain varying amounts of minerals, such as calcium, magnesium, iron, fluoride, chloride, sodium, and potassium, which may result from the water passing over rocks in its natural environment. In addition, during processing, the manufacturer may add or eliminate some minerals. Although touted as a good source of calcium and magnesium, even mineral water does not qualify as a major dietary source for these minerals. For example, one quart of an expensive mineral water contains 141 mg of calcium, only 12 percent of the Recommended Daily Allowance for teenagers.

The sodium content may vary considerably depending on the type of water. According to testing performed by *Consumer Reports,* the sodium content of nonsparkling waters was negligible, but the sodium content of mineral waters varied from 4 mg to over 100 mg per 8-ounce glass. Seltzer water has been filtered and infused with carbon dioxide, but no minerals or salts are added, so the sodium content is usually negligible. Club soda is made the same way as seltzer water, but has added minerals and salts. Consequently, the sodium content in club soda is significant, ranging from about 25 to 65 mg per 8-ounce glass.

Although many sparkling waters with natural flavors are calorie-free, a popular group of these so-called "clear" waters contain sweeteners, usually in the form of fructose or high-fructose corn syrup. Since these "clear" waters are in the same aisle as the calorie-free bottled waters, it is easy to be misled unless you carefully read the ingredient list. These products can contain from 54 to 70 calories in just 6 ounces. People with diabetes should definitely avoid these "clear" waters. Moreover, since there is some evidence from recent studies that high-fructose corn syrup may raise low-density lipoprotein (LDL) cholesterol levels, it is wise for most people to limit their consumption of them.

To obtain detailed information on a specific brand of bottled water, call or write to the manufacturer.
*Maria Guglielmino, M.S., R.D.*

# Obstetrics and Gynecology

As health-care reform takes shape, many types of tests and treatments will be reevaluated with cost-effectiveness in mind. Routine use of ultrasound and fetal monitoring during labor have been called into question for both effectiveness and cost-effectiveness. High-tech interventions for infertile couples will be critically evaluated. New health risks such as HIV infection will make the future even more complicated. But major advances in technology occurring in the contraceptive field and new areas of study initiated to evaluate women's health issues will ensure that future generations will benefit from the groundwork laid in 1993.

## ▶ Women's Health Initiative Launched
The Women's Health Initiative, a long-term study funded by the National Institutes of Health (NIH) evaluating the health habits and medical treatment of women aged 50 through 80, was launched in 1993. Historically, women have been virtually excluded as subjects from many major clinical trials—particularly women over 50 years old. The Women's Health Initiative should lessen some of the knowledge gap in this age group. In addition, part of the study will randomly choose women to receive estrogen-replacement therapy (ERT), combined estrogen-progesterone-replacement therapy (E/PRT), or placebo. While it is generally accepted in the medical community that estrogen replacement is beneficial in protecting women against atherosclerotic heart disease and osteoporosis (thinning of the bones), the overall health impact of long-term ERT is unknown. This study should ultimately answer important questions about how mature women can maintain their health.

## ▶ AIDS and Women
In the United States, acquired immune deficiency syndrome (AIDS), a disease caused by the human immunodeficiency virus (HIV), is the sixth-leading cause of death overall, and the fastest-growing cause of death in women aged 25 to 44. The death rate represents only a fraction of the infection rate, since women can be infected for many years before death occurs. Seventy-five percent of women with AIDS are black or Hispanic; such women often lack access to diagnostic and treatment programs. The Centers for Disease Control and Prevention (CDC) has launched programs in several cities to study various forms of counseling and intervention to avoid continued spread of the disease. Historically,

HIV spread has been attributed to homosexual contact, sharing of contaminated needles during intravenous drug use, and transfusions of contaminated blood; however, for women, unprotected heterosexual intercourse is a common route of infection. The use of latex condoms (including the new female condom) could help in preventing new infections. Nonetheless, the world is facing an enormous global epidemic. (For more information on women and AIDS, turn to page 50.)

### ▶ Menstruation Controversy

A controversial new theory contends that a primary function of menstruation is to protect the womb from infection. Margie Profet, an evolutionary biologist from the University of California at Berkeley, writing in the *Quarterly Review of Biology,* believes that the menstrual flow helps fight off bacteria that may have attached to sperm as a means to travel through the uterus and up the Fallopian tubes. Menstruation accomplishes this feat in one of two ways: by carrying off the bacteria with the sloughed-off uterine lining, and through the action of immune cells contained within the menstrual blood itself.

If Profet's theory is proved correct, it would force physicians to rethink their recommendations for women who suffer from irregular periods. Currently such women are routinely diagnosed as having an endocrine-system problem, and are often put on a regimen of hormones. Profet asserts that such treatments could actually be counterproductive to the patient's health.

Profet's theory has generated much debate within the medical and scientific community. For example, gynecologists point out that the occurrence of pelvic infections increases after a woman's period, and that, in fact, women seem to be more susceptible to infection while menstruating—trends that run counter to Profet's findings. Her scientific method has also caused some scientists to look askance at her theory. Instead of offering a body of statistical evidence and data derived from extensive double-blind studies, Profet backs her theory largely with electron micrographs that show bacteria attached to sperm. Finally, her claim that menstruation among mammals is widespread has raised a number of scientific eyebrows.

Whatever the outcome of the controversy, Profet's theory has caused researchers to take another look at the process of menstruation and the as-yet-unknown roles it may play in a woman's health.

### ▶ New Contraceptives Available

Several new contraceptives and improvements in some older contraceptives have widened the birth-control options available to American women. Oral contraceptive pills (OCPs) have undergone multiple reformulations. In 1993 pills using desogestrel, a progestin with a better impact on the blood-cholesterol profile, were introduced. In addition, the Food and Drug Administration (FDA) has approved low-dose OCPs for women over 40 years old, reflecting the improved safety of currently used pills.

Depo-Provera, a highly effective injectable form of progestin, has also become available in the United States. While potential side effects—weight gain, possible bone loss with long-term use, and adverse effects on cholesterol levels—do not make Depo-Provera ideal for all women, its effectiveness and ease of administration (one injection lasts for three

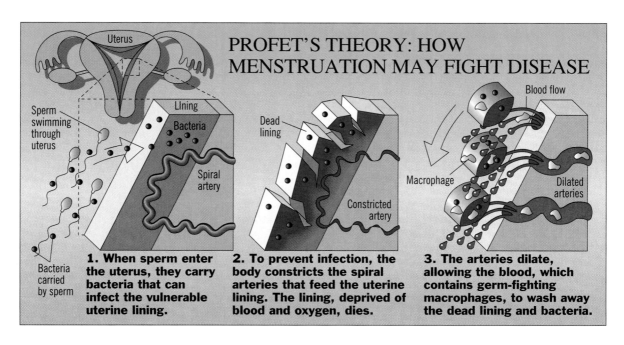

PROFET'S THEORY: HOW MENSTRUATION MAY FIGHT DISEASE

**1. When sperm enter the uterus, they carry bacteria that can infect the vulnerable uterine lining.**

**2. To prevent infection, the body constricts the spiral arteries that feed the uterine lining. The lining, deprived of blood and oxygen, dies.**

**3. The arteries dilate, allowing the blood, which contains germ-fighting macrophages, to wash away the dead lining and bacteria.**

months) make it very useful for some women who cannot tolerate the estrogens in OCPs or who frequently forget to take OCPs. Another progestin-based method, the Norplant capsules, offers an option for women desiring reliable long-term, but reversible, contraception. These capsules, placed under the skin on the upper arm, are more than 99 percent effective and can be used for up to five years. However, the initial cost of Norplant makes this form of birth control too expensive for many women.

The medical abortifacient RU-486 has been used by more than 60,000 women in Europe. When taken within 72 hours of unprotected intercourse, a dose of RU-486 blocks the normal action of the hormone progesterone in the uterus and prevents implantation of a fertilized egg. Two days later a prostaglandin drug, such as misoprostol, is administered to the woman to increase uterine contractions and induce an abortion.

The drug has long been blocked from the U.S. market by the controversy surrounding the abortion issue. In early 1993, however, the Clinton administration cleared RU-486 for investigational use in the United States, based on preliminary research that found the drug could be useful in treating breast cancer, brain tumors, and some female reproductive disorders. The French manufacturer of the drug, Roussel-Uclaf, had agreed in principle to allow a group called The Population Council to arrange for U.S. manufacture of the drug. And in November 1993, the FDA approved clinical tests of RU-486 to treat women with advanced breast cancer. The tests will be conducted by the Breast Center and Cancer Institute at Long Beach Memorial Medical Center.

Preliminary research performed by Mitchell Creinin, M.D., and Philip Darney, M.D., at the University of California at San Francisco may have found an alternative for RU-486. Methotrexate, a drug widely used in the United States for treatment of cancer and arthritis, may also be effective in inducing medical abortions. In their study, methotrexate was combined with misoprostol. While the combination was not as effective as RU-486 combined with misoprostol, methotrexate has the advantage of being currently available in the United States, and could be used if RU-486 does not become available.

### ▶ Ultrasound During Pregnancy

Bernard G. Ewigman, M.D., of the University of Missouri at Columbia led a multicenter study of the use of routine ultrasound on pregnant women that failed to demonstrate any significant benefits of this imaging technique. The 55,744 women selected for the study were screened for high-risk factors; 32,000 of those women demonstrated medical indi-

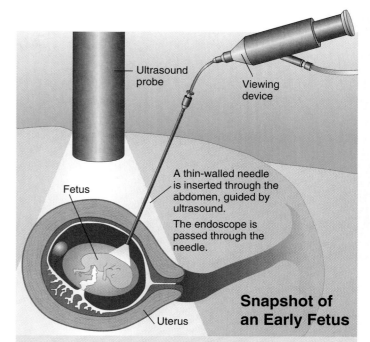

Ultrasound probe

Viewing device

Fetus

A thin-walled needle is inserted through the abdomen, guided by ultrasound.

The endoscope is passed through the needle.

Uterus

**Snapshot of an Early Fetus**

An experimental technique called embryoscopy permits doctors to view a fetus in an earlier stage than has been possible before. The tiny scope is adapted from an endoscope used by cardiologists to see inside blood vessels. Carried in an ultra-thin needle that is inserted into the abdomen, the scope can diagnose fetal abnormalities during the first trimester of pregnancy, when ultrasound is generally uninformative or inconclusive. This technique may be helpful for women who have already had pregnancies complicated by genetic disorders that cannot be detected by the usual methods of prenatal diagnosis – chronic villus sampling or amniocentesis. In the future, embryoscopy may be used to deliver treatment, such as certain types of surgery or even gene therapy.

cations for ultrasound, and were thus excluded from the study. Ultimately 15,500 women were randomly selected to receive either no ultrasounds or two ultrasounds. The "ultrasound" group of women had an average of 2.2 ultrasounds per pregnancy; the "nonultrasound" group an average of 0.6 ultrasounds per pregnancy. The study failed to find significant improvement in pregnancy outcomes in the ultrasound group.

While these findings may be useful in defending physicians who do not perform routine ultrasounds on pregnant patients, many obstetricians still feel that ultrasound as a screening tool makes sense. A Scandinavian study did show benefits of a universal ultrasound-screening program, mainly because the procedure can identify birth defects prenatally. In Ewigman's study, however, only 9 out of 187 major fetal abnormalities were detected prenatally, well below the expected detection rates. It should be noted, however, that more than two-thirds of the original group was excluded from the study, often because the women were at high risk for pregnancy

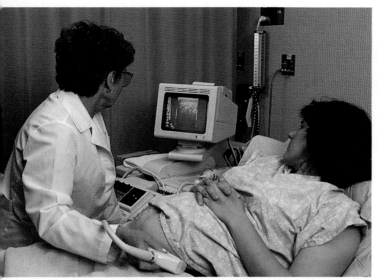

*Some researchers suggest that the use of routine ultrasound on pregnant women has no real benefit. Many obstetricians disagree, and praise ultrasound's ability to identify prenatal problems.*

problems, and hence physicians felt ultrasound was medically indicated and presumably beneficial. For the time being, the effectiveness of ultrasound during pregnancy in establishing pregnancy dating, detecting twins, guiding procedures such as amniocentesis, and in identifying birth defects and growth problems prenatally will continue to make the procedure a key component of prenatal care.

## ▶ Ovarian Cancer

The lifetime risk of developing ovarian cancer is approximately 1.7 percent, making it a rare but lethal cancer; some 12,000 women die of ovarian cancer annually. There are no screening tests for early detection. Several groups of researchers are looking at combinations of ultrasound and blood "markers" to see if these can be combined to detect early ovarian cancer, but, to date, no method can be recommended for routine screening.

A report linking fertility-drug use with a slightly increased risk of ovarian cancer generated a great deal of public concern. However, there was only a small increase in risk in the study, and there could be multiple explanations as to why women with fertility problems might stand at heightened risk. The National Cancer Institute (NCI) has called for more study on the issue, but no changes in current patient care have been recommended based upon this very small number of patients. In the meantime, women with family histories of ovarian cancer or women who have taken fertility drugs need to be monitored regularly with gynecologic exams. Women at high risk may also want to consider using birth-control pills since they provide protective effect against ovarian cancer.

*Linda Hughey Holt, M.D.*

## Occupational Health

### ▶ Toxic Substances

Shoe-manufacturing workers, potentially exposed to solvents and solvent-based adhesives, show statistically higher rates of mortality due to cancer of the trachea, bronchus, and lung, according to a study in the April 1993 *Scandinavian Journal of Work and Environmental Health*. However, the workers did not show elevated rates of death due to leukemia and aleukemia, the researchers found.

The 7,814 white workers, followed from 1940 through 1982, were probably exposed to solvents like toluene and benzene. Chronic nonmalignant respiratory disease was significantly elevated among males, but was less than expected among female employees. Given the greater incidence of smokers among men than women, this finding suggests that smoking is a possible contributing factor to the mortality from respiratory cancer. But, the researchers note, even an adjustment for the potential effects of smoking does not completely eliminate the increased risk for lung cancer.

Despite a comprehensive Occupational Health and Safety Administration (OSHA) standard for lead exposure, this hazard still exists in many industries. In New York City, a blood-screening and education program for automobile-radiator-repair workers and their families revealed that 67 percent of the workers in 89 percent of the shops tested had blood-lead levels in excess of 25 micrograms per deciliter —lower than the OSHA standard for this group of workers, but still very significant.

The results of the program, reported in the *American Journal of Industrial Medicine*, also reveal that the vast majority of workers had neither been tested previously nor had received health and safety training regarding occupational lead exposure. The study concludes that lead exposure in the automotive radiator repair industry continues to be widespread.

### ▶ Stress and Firefighters

Few studies have investigated the stress factors affecting firefighters and the potential psychological and emotional consequences. Recently, 145 firefighters were studied to determine possible stress factors and to assess psychological distress and problems with alcohol use. As reported in the April 1993 *Scandinavian Journal of Work and Environmental Health,* learning that children are in a burning building was the highest-ranked stress factor.

Between 33 and 41 percent of the firefighters experienced significant psychological stress on the job, and some 29 percent had possible or probable problems with alcohol use. These figures are significantly higher than would be expected in a typical community or working population, the researchers say. However, no relationship was found between the 10 most highly ranked emotional-stress factors and measures of emotional stress or alcohol use.

## ▶ Hazards at Sea

Fishing has long been identified as a hazardous industry. Annual work-related death rates ranging between 26 and 260 per 100,000 fisherman have been reported in studies from Great Britain, Canada, and New Zealand. In the *American Journal of Public Health,* researchers using death certificates, presumptive death certificates, and U.S. Coast Guard records presented their findings on occupational-injury deaths in the Alaska fishing industry from 1980 through 1988.

About 45,000 people are employed annually in the Alaska commercial-fishing industry. The investigation found that for the years 1980 though 1985, fishing was a major contributor to occupational mortality in the state, accounting for 19 percent of the deaths. For the period 1980 through 1988, 278 fishing-related deaths were identified, with an average of 31 deaths per year.

The average annual fishing-related fatality rate was 414.6 per 100,000 fisherman, five to eight times higher than the rates found in Alaska's other high-risk industries like transportation, communication, and public utilities (73.1 per 100,000); mining (53.1 per 100,000); and construction (49.1 per 100,000), the study says.

In other findings the *British Medical Journal* reports a mortality study involving 27,884 Icelandic merchant sailors and fisherman over a nearly 30-year period, focusing on fatal accidents that occurred other than at sea. Mortality ratios were significantly greater than the standardized norm. This was particularly true for accidents other than those at sea, such as traffic accidents, poisonings, homicides, and other violence. The researchers conclude that seamen seem to be a special group with a high risk of fatal accidents, and that length of employment seems to be a contributing factor. As a group, they appear to be modified by their occupation toward hazardous behavior or risky lifestyle.

## ▶ Construction Work

In spite of new building techniques designed to make working conditions safer, construction work around the world remains a very dangerous occupation, according to the International Labor Organization (ILO). As reported in the July/August 1993 issue of *The Futurist,* ILO figures show that in Great Britain an average of one construction worker is killed on the job every three days, and 59 are injured each day. Within the European Community (EC), construction accounts for 15 percent of the work-related accidents and 30 percent of the fatalities. During 1990 the number of accidents for construction workers in France rose 23 percent from the previous year, and the number of fatalities was up 12.5 percent, the ILO says.

In the United States, deaths and disabling injuries are more common in construction than in any other major industrial sector. The trend reached a high in 1985 with 2,400 deaths.

According to the ILO, high levels of noise and vibration, operational errors with lifting machines, safety problems in demolition and electrical-installation jobs, and exposure to dusts and dangerous chemicals are among the factors that contribute to accidents and deaths.

A study in the September 1993 *Journal of Occupational Medicine* on fatal occupational injuries in the

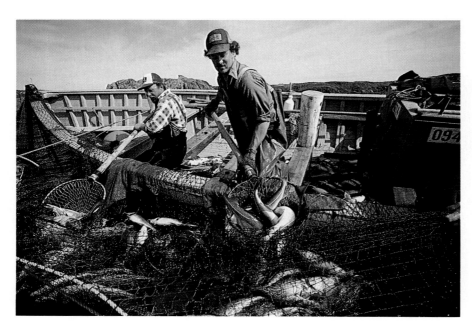

*Studies have documented that the accident and mortality rates for fishermen are significantly greater than for other occupations. In Alaska alone, the fishing-related fatality rate is five to eight times higher than that in other industries.*

New Jersey construction industry confirms the ILO data. Researchers found that work in the construction industry involves an approximately threefold increase in risk of fatal injury compared with all New Jersey industries combined.

Of 200 construction-related fatalities identified in New Jersey from 1983 to 1989, all were men. The death rate was 14.5 per 100,000 employed person-years during the study period. Death rates diminished with increasing age after 34, but picked up again at age 65, when death rates were the highest, at 27.7 per 100,000. Fatality rates were higher for Hispanics and blacks than for whites.

Ironworkers and roofers had the highest rates of death, general construction workers the lowest. The leading cause of death was falls (47 percent), followed by auto-related fatalities (15 percent), electrocutions (14 percent), and cave-ins (7 percent).

## ▶ Women Veterinarians

Veterinarians are exposed to an imposing group of hazards in the workplace. Many of these hazards are exclusively, or more significantly, detrimental to women, particularly in regard to their reproductive systems, says a study in the March 1993 *American Industrial Hygiene Association Journal*. The researchers note that a more focused awareness of these potential health risks is in order because an increasing number of women practitioners and para-professionals have entered the field during the past few decades.

*Female veterinarians are exposed to a number of work-related hazards that are potentially detrimental to their reproductive systems. For instance, a pregnant vet who contracts toxoplasmosis from an infected cat may transmit the disease to her fetus.*

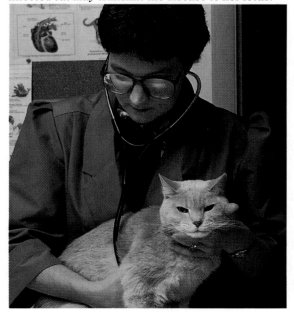

For pregnant workers, maternal stress, the fatigue associated with pregnancy, and even physical imbalance in advanced pregnancy increase the likelihood of job-related injury, the researchers say.

Occupational hazards affecting veterinarians comprise four main categories: physical hazards like radiation and physical trauma; animal-borne infections; chemicals; and drugs. The study focused on select hazards of importance to all veterinarians, with special attention to female practitioners.

Ionizing radiation—which is used in the diagnosis of gastrointestinal ailments, tumors, and pneumonia, as well as in the treatment of some tumors—represents a safety hazard. Earlier researchers, using data on veterinarians who died between 1947 and 1977, reported an excess of leukemia for those whose practices spanned the periods when radiological procedures were commonly used.

Veterinarians and their staff members are susceptible to many sources of physical trauma. Lifting heavy animals can cause lower-back injury, for example. Large and small animals can cause injury through kicking, biting, or crushing. In a previous study conducted by the American Veterinary Medical Association, 35 percent of the veterinarians said they required laceration sutures during their careers; 10 percent required fracture or dislocation treatment; and 5 percent required dental work.

## ▶ Environmental Tobacco Smoke

The adverse health effects of exposure to second-hand tobacco smoke are well recognized. The Environmental Protection Agency (EPA) has estimated that such exposure causes around 300 lung-cancer deaths each year in nonsmokers. Many state and local governments have prohibited smoking in public places (including restaurants) and in private workplaces. A July 1993 study in the *Journal of the American Medical Association* assessed the relative exposure to environmental tobacco smoke (ETS) for bar and restaurant employees, compared with office workers and with nonsmokers exposed in the home. They found that ETS is a significant occupational health hazard to food-service workers, and does contribute to elevated lung-cancer risk.

Using previously collected data on more than 1,000 offices, more than 400 restaurants, and more than 600 homes, the researchers determined that ETS exposure for restaurant workers was estimated to be 1.6 to 2.0 times higher than for office workers, and at least 1.5 times higher than for persons who live with a smoker. For bar employees, ETS exposure was estimated to be 3.9 to 6.1 times higher than for office workers, and at least 4.4 times higher than for persons exposed in the home.

The study tried to correct for active smoking by restaurant and bar employees; for vital statistics like age, sex, and race; and for the exposure to other carcinogens like cooking fumes. Even after these corrections, the study finds it plausible that an elevation in lung-cancer risk is attributable to ETS in the restaurant workplace. An excess lung-cancer risk of more than 30 percent could be expected for restaurant workers compared with unexposed nonsmokers in domestic settings. In six previous studies that controlled for active smoking, an excess lung-cancer risk of around 50 percent was found for food-service workers compared with the general population.

### ▶ Hotel and Motel Workers

Some 1 million to 1.5 million Americans are employed at hotels and motels, most of them either serving or preparing food, cleaning rooms, or otherwise maintaining grounds and premises. They work round-the-clock shifts, and face a variety of safety and health risks, including falls on slippery floors, burns from preparing food and from caustic cleaning compounds, and sprains from handling heavy objects, reports the Bureau of Labor Statistics (BLS) in its July 1993 *Monthly Labor Review.*

According to a 1991 BLS survey, the hotel industry—which includes ski lodges, tourist cabins, and inns—was one of nine industries reporting at least 100,000 cases of injury and illness that year. The latest survey shows that a trend toward safer hotels and motels is not evident, given the data collected from 1980 to 1991. At the start of the study period, the injury and illness rate for hotels and for private industry as a whole each stood at around 9 cases per 100 full-time workers. By 1991 the rate for hotels increased to 10.4, while that for private industry decreased to 8.4.

In addition to becoming disabled more often, hotel workers are sustaining injuries that take longer periods of recuperation. For each injury or illness in 1991, hotel workers spent an average of 20 workdays away from the job or on light duties, compared with only 14 days in 1980.

Sprains and strains were the most frequently reported injury, accounting for almost 50 percent of the 21,700 reported cases in one 1987-to-1988 database. Other disabling conditions included contusions, crushing, and bruises; cuts, lacerations, and punctures; fractures; and burns—each accounting for between 5 percent and 10 percent of the total.

Women sustained slightly more than half of the 21,700 injuries or illnesses. Most of the injured women were maids; most of the men were employed in various food-service positions. The study said that women appear to be at comparatively higher risk in hotels than in private industry as a whole. Women make up about half of the workforce in each group, but their share of injuries in private industry was only around 25 percent.

*Neil Springer*

# Pediatrics

### ▶ Immunizations

Immunizations against polio, diphtheria, whooping cough (pertussis), tetanus, measles, and mumps have been widely available in the United States for years. New vaccines to protect children from *Hemophilus influenzae* meningitis and from hepatitis B have also been introduced. Yet increasing numbers of children are not receiving them. Low vaccination rates among preschool children are causing a resurgence of these formerly common and debilitating diseases.

Nationwide, one-third to one-half of two-year-olds are not fully immunized, according to the Centers for Disease Control and Prevention (CDC). This problem has been attributed to difficulties in reaching urban poor and racial and ethnic minorities, failure by medical

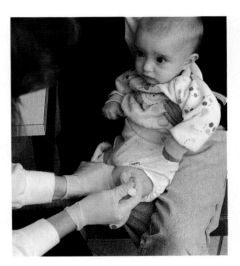

*By some estimates, one-third to one-half of all two-year-olds in the U.S. are not fully immunized, causing a dangerous and costly resurgence of some debilitating but preventable diseases.*

providers to administer the vaccines appropriately, and the lack of insurance coverage for vaccines.

In 1993 the federal government approved an immunization-entitlement program (effective October 1, 1994) that guarantees free vaccines for children who are Medicaid-eligible, uninsured, or Native American. Although this falls short of President Clinton's original proposal for free immunizations for all children in the United States, the American Academy of Pediatrics sees the program as an important first step in improving childhood immunization rates. The next steps are to create a nationwide computerized tracking system and public-information campaign to ensure that all eligible children participate.

### ▶ Lorenzo's Oil

Adreno-leuko-dystrophy, a rare and fatal hereditary disease of the nervous system, was highlighted in the 1992 movie *Lorenzo's Oil*. In the film, based on a true story, Augusto and Michaila Odone develop a concoction of vegetable oils that they believe improves the condition of their 14-year-old son, Lorenzo, who is afflicted with adreno-leuko-dystrophy. The Odones fight the doctors they believe are slow to accept the possibility that their remedy really does work in slowing the boy's steady deterioration.

Writing recently in the *New England Journal of Medicine*, Patrick Aubourg, M.D., and his colleagues from the St. Vincent de Paul Hospital in Paris conclude that the "remedy" is worthless, at least for the milder, adult form of the ailment. They could find no improvement in 24 patients who had taken Lorenzo's oil for up to 48 months.

Even though it may cut down on the level of toxic compounds in the blood that are believed to cause the disease, Lorenzo's oil apparently cannot reverse already-sustained nerve damage, which often results in blindness and paralysis.

Nonetheless, there are believers. Hugo Moser, M.D., an expert in metabolic diseases at the Kennedy Krieger Institute in Baltimore, Maryland, believes that Lorenzo's oil may delay the onset of symptoms. "We know that it's not 100 percent preventive," says Moser, who is conducting a five-year study of 80 boys who have inherited the gene for the disease but started taking Lorenzo's oil while still healthy. "The question that still needs to be answered is whether it's partially preventive."

## ▶ Fetal Alcohol Syndrome

Fetal alcohol syndrome (FAS) is a leading cause of congenital mental retardation, but little is known about the long-term development and adolescent outcome of children with FAS. In a 10-year follow-up study of 60 patients diagnosed as having FAS in infancy and childhood, Hans-Ludwig Spohr, M.D., and his colleagues in Germany and Switzerland found that the characteristic head and facial appearance of FAS, such as narrow eye openings, small upper jaw, and thin upper lip, diminish with time, but small head size and, to a lesser degree, short height and low weight (in boys) persist; in female adolescents, body weight normalizes. Persistent mental retardation is the major outcome of intrauterine alcohol exposure in many cases, and environmental and educational factors do not have strong compensatory effects on the intellectual development of affected children.

## ▶ Attention-Deficit Hyperactivity Disorder

Attention-deficit hyperactivity disorder (ADHD) is a well-recognized behavioral condition. The major symptoms are motor restlessness, impulsiveness, inattention, and distractibility.

**Thyroid-hormone resistance.** The cause of ADHD is unknown, but there is evidence of a familial predisposition. Symptoms suggestive of this disorder have been reported in individuals resistant to thyroid hormone, which their own body produces. In a study of 49 affected and 55 unaffected family members with resistance to thyroid hormone, all were evaluated with structured psychiatric questionnaires by interviewers who were unaware of the medical diagnosis. The likelihood of having ADHD was 10 to 15 times higher for those with the thyroid-hormone disorder. While the reasons for this discovery are not clear, researchers suggest that studies of thyroid function should be done as part of the evaluation for ADHD. Furthermore, they speculate that there may be a role for thyroid hormone in the treatment of ADHD, even in those who do not have resistance to thyroid hormone.

**ADHD among adolescents.** Much of the research on ADHD has focused on children, but recently there has been recognition that the disorder persists into adolescence and adulthood at least 60 percent of the time. In the United States, motor vehicle crashes account for nearly half of all deaths of adolescents between the ages of 16 and 19 years, and two-thirds of deaths among individuals between 15 and 24 years old. Many interrelated factors have been proposed to contribute to automotive crashes and related fatalities among adolescents, including their excessive risk taking, lack of driving skills and experience, greater attention to objects rather than activities in their field of vision, infrequent use of seat belts, alcohol and/or drug intoxication, familial stress, and the presence of persistent behavioral or emotional difficulties. Russell Barkley, M.D., at the University of Massachusetts Medical Center in Worcester, found that ADHD, and especially its association with oppositional/defiant and conduct disorders, was associated with the substantially increased risks found among teenager and young-adult drivers. Subjects with ADHD used less-sound driving habits and had four times the rate of traffic citations compared to those in control groups. They were also far more likely to have auto crashes resulting in bodily injuries. Part of the long-term treatment for ADHD should include counseling for adolescents and their parents about these risks.

## ▶ Traumatic Brain Injury

Some 30,000 children become mentally and physically disabled from accidental brain injury each year. Over 7,000 die from trauma to the head. While the most desirable goal of head-injury management is prevention, recent advances in the understanding of what happens to the brain immediately after injury provide new directions for treatment in the intensive-care setting.

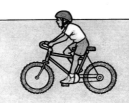

## Fitting a Helmet for Safety and Comfort

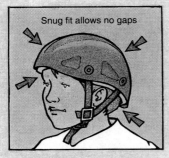

Snug fit allows no gaps

A properly fitting helmet should touch the head at the crown, sides, front, and back. Buy the smallest comfortable size and use sizing pads (usually included) to fine-tune the fit. An assortment of pads that attach to each point is the most flexible arrangement. If the helmet moves enough to create a gap when pushed sideways, get thicker pads or a smaller helmet.

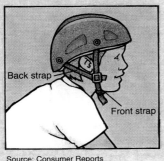

Back strap

Front strap

With the helmet level across the fore-head, just above the eyebrows, adjust the straps so the front strap is nearly vertical. The back strap should lie straight, just below the ear, with no slack. The straps should meet just below the hinge of the jaw, in front of the ear, and be equally tight. The helmet should not roll backward or forward on the head when you push up.

Source: Consumer Reports

**Prevention through helmet use.** Each year 600,000 persons visit emergency rooms for bicycle injuries. Most of the 1,300 deaths to bicyclists (half in children and adolescents) are due to head injury. Many survivors are left with lifelong mental and physical impairments.

Recent efforts to prevent traumatic brain injury in children have been impressive. Thanks to a bicycle-helmet campaign in Seattle, Washington, the incidence of such brain injuries fell by 88 percent. The campaign included television, radio, and billboard advertising; the distribution of coupons that enabled parents to buy helmets at half-price; and attempts to dispel the "nerd" factor (wearing helmets appears "uncool"). Manufacturers were approached to put NFL insignia or Ninja Turtle figures on the helmets to make them more acceptable. The Seattle project estimated that health-care insurers could save impressive sums by providing modest subsidies for helmet purchases, thereby reducing head injuries and the immense costs of rehabilitation.

**New approaches to acute care.** The immediate results of head injury, say following an automobile accident in which the head strikes the windshield forcefully, include skull fracture, brain contusion, and hemorrhage around or within the brain. However, in the next few days, the brain reacts to these injuries in ways that can cause further, and even more serious, injury. Deep within the brain, neuronal axons, the tracks along which electrical impulses travel, are partially injured by shearing forces from the impact. If conditions are unfavorable within the hours to days following initial injury, these axons die. Conversely, if the conditions can be improved, the axons may survive and recover. Three events that determine axonal viability are now known to be of particular importance.

All tissues of the body respond to injury with swelling. However, since the skull is a closed space in older children and adults, there is very little area to accommodate expansion. When the brain swells, pressure within the skull increases, reducing the blood flow into the brain. Standard medical practice in severe head injury is to insert an intracranial pressure monitor. If the monitor indicates that pressure is rising from swelling, medications and other techniques can be used to lower it.

On a biochemical level, it is now known that certain normally present substances in the brain can increase to toxic levels following brain injury. One such substance, an excitatory neurotransmitter called glutamate, is responsible for increasing the electrical activity of the brain and helping electrical impulses travel from one neuron to another. When too much glutamate is released, the equilibrium of the brain's metabolic activity is disturbed, leading to further damage.

Another response to injury is an increase in prostaglandin release, which leads to excessive peroxidation of fats and release of oxygen-free radicals, substances that are very toxic to tissues if they are not neutralized and carried away. Injured brain tissue has limited capacity to carry out this important function. A vicious cycle is initiated in which injury and the brain's attempts to fix it lead to further injury.

Much current research has focused on finding treatments to prevent or at least dampen these secondary events. One interesting group of compounds now under study called "lazeroids" (after the biblical character Lazarus, who was raised from the dead) have demonstrated some protection against tissue damage. Other compounds scavenge and neutralize the toxic oxygen-free radicals. When administered intravenously following head injury, the hope is that these compounds may prevent further damage and improve chances for full recovery.

## ▶ The Boy in the Bubble

David, a Texas boy who spent 12 years living in a sterile environment, suffered from a rare immune disease called X-linked severe combined immuno-deficiency (SCID). From early life, victims of this disorder are afflicted with severe and persistent infections because they lack the immune function that would normally offer resistance to disease.

David died a decade ago. But thanks to body cells researchers removed from the boy and saved for future research, doctors have discovered the gene defect that causes X-linked SCID using technologies that were not available 10 years ago. According to Warren Leonard, M.D., of the National Institutes of Health (NIH), this finding opens the door to the development of better tests for prenatal and postnatal diagnosis, identification of female carriers of the disorder, and even gene therapy (insertion of a normal gene into a SCID patient's blood cells).

## ▶ Breast Is Still Best

Accumulating evidence shows indisputably that, for most infants, breast milk is better than artificial formulas. Breast-fed babies have less diarrhea and fewer upper-respiratory infections due to protective immunoglobulins and other substances in the mother's breast milk that ward off infection. These advantages are particularly significant in developing areas of the world where sanitation is poor and death rates among infants from diarrhea and dehydration are high. Children's-advocacy groups have led boycotts against companies that market artificial formulas in underdeveloped countries, and the groups are fighting the practice of advertising formulas directly to consumers, which the advocacy groups feel may discourage breast-feeding.

A new study from the University of Arizona in Tucson shows that breast-fed infants have half the number of ear infections compared to artificial-formula-fed infants. There are several reasons for these findings. Secretory IgA, an immunoglobulin contained in breast milk, blocks the attachment of bacteria to the respiratory-tract lining, thus preventing infection.

Also, when a mother nurses her baby, the infant is likely to be in a head-up position so that the milk and other mouth secretions drain into the esophagus toward the stomach. When formula is given, some mothers prop the bottle into the mouth while the infant lies flat. In this case the milk has a tendency to pool in the mouth and nasal passages. These fluids can carry bacteria up the Eustachian tube into the middle-ear chamber, where ear infections evolve. For these and many other reasons, pediatricians strongly recommend breast-feeding through the first year of life, and especially during the first six months.

*James A. Blackman, M.D., M.P.H.*

# Plastic Surgery

## ▶ Microsurgery

The ability to utilize "spare parts" of one's own body has become a reality for victims of trauma or patients with deformities from birth. Surgeons are now able to use one part of the body to reconstruct another. The many possible options include the process of transforming the great toe to reconstruct a previously amputated thumb; re-creating, from abdominal skin and fat, a breast lost from cancer surgery; or recontouring a missing jawbone after its removal for cancer in the mouth.

All of these state-of-the-art procedures can be performed routinely in most plastic- and reconstructive-surgery centers. All that is required is the disconnection of muscle, skin, or bone from one area, and the reconnection of their blood vessels and nerves at the new site. Using sutures as thin as a human hair, and powerful magnifying microscopes, it is possible to replant missing fingers, arms, legs, or even the entire scalp. The surgeons choose a site that can be donated from the same individual where he or she will not sacrifice important function.

These concepts are not actually new: doctors have been utilizing the microscope to reconnect blood vessels and nerves since the early years of this century. However, the expansion of training in these disciplines, the advent of better needles and suturing materials, and the improved optical properties of the modern microscopes have advanced the surgeon's ability to perform these delicate procedures.

## ▶ Endoscopic Plastic Surgery

In 1993 techniques borrowed from general surgeons were advanced to revolutionize the manner in which aesthetic or cosmetic plastic surgery is performed. In the past, most cosmetic surgical procedures were performed by making incisions, which tended to be long but well hidden. Now, by employing lighted tubes and video technology, surgeons are able to make very small incisions, raise the desired flaps of skin tissue, and allow it to re-drape to a new, more youthful position. These procedures are routinely being utilized for face-lifts and forehead brow lifts. The surgeons watch a video monitor while manipulating the endoscopic (lighted-camera) instruments. Advanced training is now being offered to doctors who will learn this different type of surgery and continue to adapt the technology to new cosmetic applications.

By eliminating long incisions and their resultant scars, this new technology has revolutionized the world of cosmetic surgery, as it had already in the realm of abdominal surgery. It will also enable more people to have access to surgical opportunities for rejuvenative surgery.

### ▶ Suction-assisted Lipectomy

Body fat provides insulation, serves as a source of nutrition, and furnishes a place for energy storage. It also contributes to the contour of the external appearance of the body. As our culture and society dictate the norms of beauty, the current trend toward thin and athletic body features compels individuals to seek better ways to achieve their desired shape.

It has been shown scientifically that the total number of body-fat cells remains relatively constant throughout one's lifetime, and that only the size and shape of these cells change with weight gain or loss. There are also hormonal variations in the specialization of these fat cells; for example, the fat cells in the buttocks of pubescent girls enlarge during this dynamic period involving major changes in body morphology.

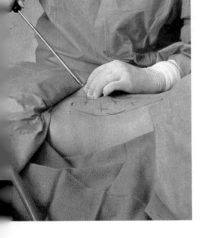

The most commonly performed cosmetic procedure in the United States has now become the removal of unwanted fat cells by vacuuming. This technique, called liposuction (photo at left), allows plastic and reconstructive surgeons to reduce localized areas of fatty deposits that have been unresponsive to reduction by conventional weight-control and exercise programs.

After this technique was introduced, it quickly gained popularity as a cosmetic procedure, particularly on the abdomen and thighs. Beyond the purely cosmetic, however, liposuction is also finding important applications in reconstructive surgery, such as for the face or breast, and it may be used as a therapeutic technique. After anesthesia, a cannula, or slotted tube, is placed into an area of desired fat reduction; suction is then applied to the end of the cannula. This can be accomplished by syringe or machine vacuum. The cells of fat, along with some blood, are removed. By utilizing blunt-ended tubes, the vital structures—nerves and arteries—are pushed aside by the advancing probe.

*C. Andrew Salzberg, M.D.*

## Podiatry

### ▶ Referred Pain

That undiagnosed pain in your jaw, knee, or lower back that your doctor told you was all in your head may actually be all in your feet. Pain that originates at one site in the body but is felt elsewhere is called referred pain. This medical conundrum can drive patients and their physicians to wit's end as they try to diagnose the source of the pain. Symptoms often mimic other illnesses or disorders and the actual cause of pain may only be identified by trial and error.

Some podiatrists have become expert sleuths at discovering the source of referred pain. In one case, Howard J. Dananberg, D.P.M., a podiatrist in Bedford, New Hampshire, linked a patient's excruciating jaw pain with a foot condition called functional hallux limitus (FHL), in which the big toe stays locked during walking. FHL causes some people to develop an abnormal walking gait that produces structural imbalances throughout the body. This imbalance, in turn, creates tension or pain elsewhere in the body, such as in the jaw. The patient diagnosed with FHL was examined in Dananberg's gait analysis lab and prescribed with orthotics, devices worn in the shoe to alleviate pressure or change the placement of the foot and its motion. Within one week, the patient's jaw pain was gone.

While FHL may be a culprit in some undiagnosed pains, other structural abnormalities may also trigger walking patterns that cause stress and ultimately pain in the ankle, knee, lower back, or even jaw or head. One abnormality is an uneven leg length in which the shorter leg causes postural imbalances. A fused joint in the foot limits motion at that site and causes other parts of the body to work beyond their range to compensate.

In a preliminary study, Dananberg and colleagues examined patients with chronic postural symptoms like lower-back pain, but who had no foot problems. Seventy-seven percent of those patients who were treated with foot orthotics reported that their pain improved 50 to 100 percent.

While orthotics may not be the answer for all undiagnosed pain, patients who have tried conventional treatments with no success may want to be examined by a podiatrist.

### ▶ Liposuction

Liposuction, the surgical removal of fat deposits, and lipoinjection, using fat deposits as graft material, have been used by plastic surgeons since 1977 to artfully reduce body volume and sculpture body parts. Typically considered a mere cosmetic procedure to reduce an overly large girth or wide hips and thighs, liposuction and lipoinjection are also used for more serious medical purposes, such as breast reconstruction after mastectomy. And more recently, podiatric physicians have employed these two techniques to improve and restore the plantar fat pads of the foot.

The internal bones, muscles, and joints of a healthy foot are naturally protected by fibrous fat tissue that runs along the bottom of the foot. These fat pads brace the arch and absorb stress, particularly those points where the foot receives the most stress from standing, walking, and running—the sole area just below the toes, and the heel area. Occasionally these fat pads become atrophied, due to injury, disease, or age. When this occurs, walking and standing for any length of time becomes very painful. Orthopedic shoes or orthotics may or may not help the symptoms.

Liposuction and lipoinjection can repair these fat pads, in many cases with long-term excellent results. Using instruments especially adapted for liposuction, fat is removed from the abdomen, thighs, or calf and transferred to the affected area of the foot. Because some of the transferred fat is typically lost via absorption into the body, the podiatrist generally transfers more fat to the site than is needed, causing the area to become slightly overinflated.

After surgery, sterile gauze strips help prevent the newly injected fat from moving from the initial site. For fat-pad replacement below the toe area, a platform shoe is worn by the patient, and weight-bearing can begin the same day. But for fat-pad replacement of the heel, no weight-bearing is allowed for six weeks, and crutches are necessary.

## ▶ AIDS and Podiatry

Human immunodeficiency virus (HIV) infection is typically accompanied by a variety of neurological disorders affecting virtually every level of the central and peripheral nervous system. Early neurological symptoms frequently develop in the legs and feet, causing such problems as leg weakness, reduced ankle and knee reflexes, extreme muscle stiffness, unsteady gait, uncoordinated muscles movements, and spasticity. As a result of these motor problems, the podiatric physician may be an AIDS patient's first medical contact.

Prompt diagnosis using computerized tomography (CT) scans and magnetic resonance imaging (MRI) to identify brain lesions and other problems characteristic of neurological diseases typically associated with AIDS, such as AIDS dementia complex, myelopathy, and painful sensory neuropathy, can help the alert podiatrist to rule out other disease causes and identify HIV infection. This diagnosis can then be followed by appropriate therapy.

*Lisa Holland*

## Public Health

## ▶ Cholera

Periodically the severe dysentery disease known as cholera begins a new march around the world, mostly in the tropical climates. The most recent global outbreak, or pandemic, first hit sub-Saharan Africa in 1970, and has continued to trouble the continent ever since. In 1992 and 1993, Burundi and Zimbabwe were heavily afflicted by the disease. Where possible, governments closed off known sources of polluted water to citizen access, a step that quickly controlled outbreaks.

The anticholera campaign in at least one African country, Angola, has been hampered by the theft of anticholera drugs, supplies, and equipment. In Luanda, the nation's capital, up to 1,200 people per week were being admitted to hospitals; about 200 people were dying per week, largely due to the lack of medicines and equipment.

*A new strain of cholera.* In 1993 a new strain of cholera appeared and began spreading across the Indian subcontinent. In the city of Calcutta alone, more than 13,000 cases have been reported. In the neighboring country of Bangladesh, more than 10,000 cases of cholera have been reported, with a mortality rate of 5 percent. The disease now has spread throughout most of the coastal region around the Bay of Bengal.

The new organism is different from the 138 previously known strains of the *Vibrio cholerae* bacterium, and it has been labeled group 0139.

Because there apparently is little or no cross-reactivity with either the other 138 strains or with the antigens in the cholera vaccine, public-health authorities cannot use vaccines to control the outbreak, nor can they depend on previous immunity to help. The only prevention is good sanitation, especially of water and seafood. Primary treatment of cholera is simply to replace the water and salts lost through diarrhea until the body's defenses reject the organism. Although the new strain of cholera may be sensitive to tetracycline, it is resistant to the other antibiotics traditionally used to treat cholera. The new strain of cholera was brought back to the United States by a U.S. traveler to India. The person recovered, and the disease is not expected to spread in the United States, thanks to the country's good sanitation.

## ▶ *Vibrio vulnificus*

The cholera organism is not the only vibrio bacterium that can cause disease. From March through December 1993, *Vibrio vulnificus* regularly caused serious illness in Florida. In the past dozen years,

125 Floridians have been reported ill with the disease; 35 percent of these people died, a higher case-fatality ratio than for cholera. The organism is especially dangerous to persons with liver disease or immune deficiency.

The infections were acquired through eating raw shellfish. Consuming raw shellfish is always a risky endeavor unless the diner has personal knowledge that the shellfish beds are safe. Shellfish can easily cause dysentery because they concentrate and eat any sewage in the water they filter, making them potentially very dangerous to eat raw.

## ▶ Milwaukee Water Problem
Most Americans live with the assumption that the water coming into their home is safe to drink. In the spring of 1993, residents of Milwaukee, Wisconsin, discovered that this is not necessarily true. Thousands of people in Milwaukee contracted dysentery due to *cryptosporidium,* an intestinal parasite. The spores of this parasite are very small, and any breakdown in the water-filtration system can let them through. Although the source of the parasites in the water is unclear, the spread of the disease could be traced to temporary changes in one of the city's water-treatment plants—changes that made the filtering system less effective. The disease, common in developing countries, has occasionally occurred in the United States, but not quite so spectacularly as it did in Milwaukee.

*Many people in the Milwaukee, Wisconsin, area were forced to obtain their water from wells when the public water supply became contaminated.*

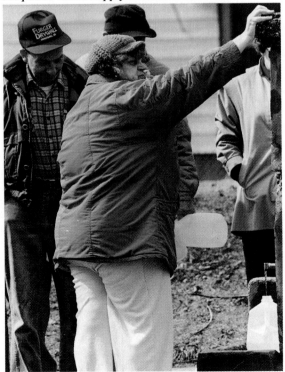

## ▶ *Escherichia coli*
*E. coli* bacteria used to be considered mostly harmless occupants of the intestinal tracts of animals and humans. They were used in most tests for sewage pollution of water and food, not because it was thought that they were causing disease, but because their presence indicated fecal contamination, which might very well contain other dangerous bacteria, viruses, or parasites. However, *E. coli* are considered harmless no longer.

About a decade ago, one particular strain of the organism (called 0157:H7) was found to cause a severe infection called *hemolytic uremic syndrome,* marked by low levels of blood platelets (which help to control bleeding), a hemolytic anemia that damages small blood vessels, and acute kidney failure.

Early in 1993 a major outbreak of disease due to the *E. coli* 0157:H7 strain occurred on the West Coast. It was caused by contaminated meat in hamburgers served by a chain of fast-food restaurants. Another outbreak, in southeastern New England, arose from contaminated fresh-pressed apple cider. Some of the apples used in making the cider may have been contaminated by falling on ground that contained animal feces. The apples were apparently not washed before the cider was made.

## ▶ Rabies
Epidemic raccoon rabies has been spreading north and east from Virginia since 1976, and has reached into New York, Connecticut, and western Massachusetts. In 1992 New York State had 1,761 rabies cases, the highest reported. When an 11-year-old girl in upper New York State died of rabies, it was assumed she must have acquired the infection from a raccoon. However, there was no evidence of her having been exposed to raccoon, and a culture of the virus that killed her showed it to be from the strain carried by bats, not the strain carried by raccoon. Bat rabies in human beings is very rare, but does occur occasionally, usually among cave explorers. Sometimes the rabid bats infect other animals (such as cats who try to catch them) which, in turn, infect human beings. It is not known how the young girl was exposed.

## ▶ Tuberculosis
Tuberculosis (TB) was thought to be on its way to extinction in the United States in the early 1980s. Its decline stopped in 1984, and since then the number of TB cases has increased by 18 percent. Even more critical, a growing number of reported cases are of the multiple-drug-resistant tuberculosis (MDRTB), against which antibiotics sometimes are ineffective. A significant part of the resurgence is due to human immunodeficiency virus (HIV); HIV-infected persons are much more susceptible to TB than are others. Perhaps 15 million Americans are

infected with TB bacteria, but their immune systems are keeping them dormant. If such a person acquires HIV, the existing TB in his or her body is very likely to become active and cause an overwhelming infection.

The World Health Organization (WHO) has called the TB situation a global emergency. About 9,000 persons die each day from TB throughout the world. The TB situation is much worse in areas with high HIV infection rates. In New York City, which has more people infected with TB than does any other U.S. city, about 40 percent of those infected with TB are co-infected with HIV.

### ▶ Immunization

*Poliomyelitis.* Not all of the news about infectious diseases has been discouraging. For example, progress continues toward the eradication of the polio viruses around the world. In 1988 WHO established the goal of achieving worldwide polio eradication by the year 2000.

China, with the largest population in the world, has been among the leaders in providing supplemental immunization to children. Accordingly, the paralytic poliomyelitis rates there have been falling rapidly in the 1990s. The wild poliomyelitis virus appears to have been eradicated from North America; the few paralytic cases reported in recent years have been vaccine-associated, and the disease has usually been mild.

*Measles.* In 1993 the United States reported the lowest number of measles cases since reporting began in 1944. The cases that did occur were concentrated in population groups who either had only one dose of the vaccine or had had no vaccine (sometimes because of medical or religious objections to the vaccine).

*New U.S. immunization law.* After long debate, Congress passed, and President Clinton signed, a new immunization program that will go into effect on October 1, 1994. It will guarantee free vaccines to children who are Medicaid-eligible, Native American, or uninsured. Underinsured children will be eligible for free vaccines at public clinics. States will also have the option of buying extra vaccine for noneligible children at the price the federal government pays for the vaccines (half of what private physicians have to pay).

### ▶ Valley Fever

Disease due to an infectious fungus called *Coccidioides immitis* has been increasing rapidly in the southwestern United States since 1991, and it achieved epidemic proportions in 1993. It has long been known that one form of the type of fungus called arthroconidia resides in the soil of the San Joaquin Valley in California, where, when the soil is dry and the wind blows, it becomes airborne. When inhaled, arthroconidia produces occasional cases of serious disease (called "valley fever" because of its origin.) Cases of the disease have also occurred sporadically in Arizona, New Mexico, Nevada, Utah, and Texas. Although the San Joaquin Valley has been hardest hit, the rates have been rising rapidly in the Phoenix and Tucson, Arizona, areas.

Although not all the reasons for the latest outbreak are known, the recent droughts in the Southwest have produced the dusty conditions ideal for the organism to spread. It should be added that many people previously unexposed to the infection and who, therefore, have not developed resistance to it, have been moving into the San Joaquin Valley and other areas of the Southwest.

### ▶ Four Corners Disease

Beginning in July 1991, cases of an unexplained, often fatal respiratory disease began to appear near the "Four Corners" area of the United States, where Arizona, New Mexico, Utah, and Colorado meet. Affected persons developed fever, muscle aches, headaches, and cough, followed by rapidly developing respiratory failure; more than 60 percent of the cases so far have proved fatal. The youngest victim was 12 years old, and the oldest age 69, but the majority have been teenagers or young adults. Slightly over half of the cases were of Native American background, and most of the other victims were Caucasian.

The symptoms initially caused physicians to worry that the new disease might be pneumonic plague, but tests were negative for the bacterium that causes that condition, and negative as well for all of the other bacteria and viruses that commonly cause lung problems. However, by comparing blood-antibody levels from when the patient first became ill to those from approximately two weeks later, it was discovered that the only consistent rise in antibody levels occurred for a specific antibody that fights a type of virus called *hantavirus*. This group of viruses was first identified in Korea in 1978, but has rarely caused illness in the United

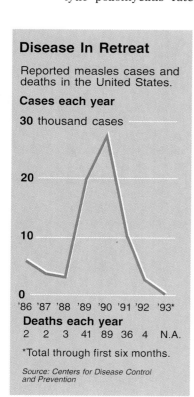

**Disease In Retreat**

Reported measles cases and deaths in the United States.

**Cases each year**

30 thousand cases

20

10

0

'86 '87 '88 '89 '90 '91 '92 '93*

**Deaths each year**

2    2    3    41   89   36   4    N.A.

*Total through first six months.

*Source: Centers for Disease Control and Prevention*

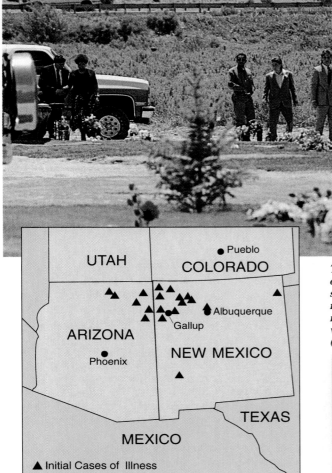

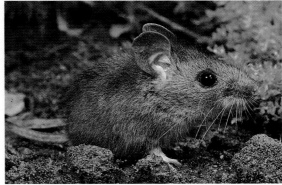

The so-called Four Corners disease has taken dozens of lives, the majority of them in the area where the states of Utah, Colorado, Arizona, and New Mexico meet (see map). The disease, officially known as pulmonary syndrome hantavirus, is transmitted by a virus found in the droppings of the deer mouse (below), and perhaps in those of other rodents.

States. At first nobody suspected hantaviruses, because, prior to the current outbreak, they had been known to cause only hemorrhagic disease and/or kidney failure, but not respiratory failure. Even though the antibodies of patients with the disease react with the antigens of several Korean varieties of the virus, it seems probable that the new disease is caused by a strain of hantavirus that is different from all those previously recognized.

Rodents are the hosts for all known hantaviruses. When hantaviruses were recognized as having caused the so-called Four Corners disease (officially called pulmonary syndrome hantavirus), public-health personnel soon found the primary rodent carrier: the deer mouse *Peromyscus maniculatus,* a creature found in most parts of continental North America except the Southeast U.S. and Canada. The deer mouse as the chief carrier has public-health experts dismayed. The reason: this animal's habitat is very wide and the virus may well infect the animals throughout their range. People at particular risk of exposure include rural dwellers, agricultural workers, and others likely to disturb rodent burrows or rodent droppings.

In one study of mice in the Four Corners states, about 30 percent in each state were infected, a very high rate. Some Centers for Disease Control and Prevention (CDC) experts speculate that the virus infected the deer-mouse population years ago and has achieved a steady state in the Southwest, and perhaps elsewhere.

Now that physicians have been alerted to hantavirus and an antibody test for it has become available, many more hantavirus infections are being identified. As of early 1994, there have been 20 cases in New Mexico, 12 in Arizona, and five in Colorado; three each in California, Kansas, Idaho, Nevada, and South Dakota; two in both Montana and North Dakota; and one each in Indiana, Louisiana, Minnesota, Oregon, Texas, and Rhode Island.

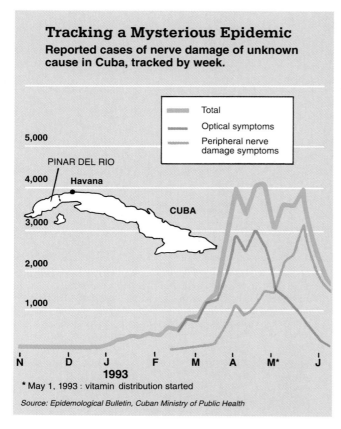

## Tracking a Mysterious Epidemic
Reported cases of nerve damage of unknown cause in Cuba, tracked by week.

Total
Optical symptoms
Peripheral nerve damage symptoms

PINAR DEL RIO
Havana
CUBA

5,000
4,000
3,000
2,000
1,000

N    D    J    F    M    A    M*    J
**1993**
* May 1, 1993 : vitamin distribution started

*Source: Epidemiological Bulletin, Cuban Ministry of Public Health*

## ▶ Outbreak of Blindness in Cuba

The year 1993 saw the peak, and probably the solution, of an outbreak of a mysterious neurological disease in Cuba that has affected more than 50,000 persons. One form of the disease involved the optic nerves, predominantly in men in the western part of Cuba, and frequently resulted in blindness. The other form of the disease involved the peripheral nerves, predominantly in women in central and eastern Cuba, leading to pain and weakness in the legs. The outbreak began slowly in 1991, baffling medical authorities, who could not find a cause or suitable treatment. The disease reached a peak in 1993, at which time more than 4,000 new cases were occurring each week.

Eventually Cuban authorities, with the assistance of international experts, were able to conclude that the underlying cause of the outbreak was a nutritional deficiency, particularly of B vitamins, resulting from the severe economic conditions in Cuba. Although there was little frank malnutrition, there was a significant drop in the intake of proteins and vitamins. In addition, many patients in western Cuba admitted to drinking homemade rum, which was found to contain small amounts of cyanide and varying amounts of methanol, both of which are toxic to the nerves of the eye. Others have questioned if pesticides were a causative factor. Although there is no final answer, the most likely scenario now seems to be that the optic neuropathy was a toxic-nutritional disease due to ingestion of methanol or cyanide in the presence of a deficiency of B vitamins, particularly of folic acid.

The peripheral (arm and leg) neuropathy was mostly in middle-aged women who consumed large amounts of cassava, beans, cabbage, and manioc, which contain some cyanide. The amount of cyanide in these foods is small enough that they probably do not cause nerve damage if the diets also include adequate amounts of B vitamins.

In May 1993, Cuban authorities began a program of vitamin supplementation among the entire Cuban population, and thereafter the rates of these nerve diseases fell rapidly.

## ▶ Diphtheria in Russia

Diphtheria was brought under control in the first half of this century by immunizing children against the toxin produced by the diphtheria organism. This toxin is what causes the very sore throats and the heart and nerve damage that characterize the disease and produce death in approximately 10 percent of its victims. During the initial decades of diphtheria control, the organism was still common enough to give adults frequent "booster" infections (without symptoms), so that most adults retained high antibody levels and were protected against symptomatic disease.

By the second half of this century, the majority of diphtheria cases in the United States were occurring in adults. Apparently, with the diphtheria organism now fairly rare, adults do not get the booster effect of being reexposed to the organism. Thus, in the absence of booster shots against diphtheria, their immunity levels gradually wane.

This is what appears to be happening in Russia. Despite having excellent immunization programs for school-aged children, Russia is in the midst of a several-year outbreak of diphtheria. The diphtheria rates are now about 25 per million per year, the highest reported rate of diphtheria in the world since the 1960s, perhaps 25 times as high as in the U.S.S.R. in 1970, and about comparable to the United States in the 1950s. However, most of the cases have occurred in persons over age 14, suggesting that declining immunity in older persons may be the biggest cause of the outbreak. The Russian government has begun a campaign to immunize people of all ages against diphtheria. Unfortunately, the country is also suffering from severe economic and social upheaval, a situation that may decrease the individual resistance of many people, and certainly makes immunization programs more difficult to find.

*James F. Jekel, M.D., M.P.H.*

# Rehabilitation Medicine

### ▶ Traumatic Brain Injury in Children

One-fourth of the hospitalizations for children under 15 years of age are for traumatic brain injuries. Annually, about 30,000 children are admitted to hospitals and rehabilitation centers in the United States for closed brain injuries. Motor vehicle accidents are still the leading cause of brain injury, but a high percentage of such cases result from bicycle riders hitting or being hit by motor vehicles. Trailing closely behind as causes of brain injury are falls from bicycles, skateboards, and roller skates. The chances of a brain injury for a child under the age of 15 are 4 percent for boys and 2.5 percent for girls.

Fortunately, the young brain has vast rehabilitative potential and is able to overcome even rather severe injuries with structured rehabilitation efforts. Traumatic-brain-injury units established by health agencies are improving the odds for children with brain injury. Furthermore, wearing a bicycle helmet can significantly decrease the risk of brain injury (by about 80 percent) and decreases the severity of brain damage by about 60 percent.

### ▶ Growing Pains

Growing pains, often a major concern for parents, usually occur bilaterally (on both sides of the body) and tend to occur at the end of the day and during the night. Often, children awake during the night and complain about the pain. The incidence of growing pains is highest between ages 4 and 12, after which the growth rate declines somewhat as compared to the growth rate between ages 1 and 4.

Usually the pains are located between the knees and the thighs, and often affect the groin. Sixty-five percent of a child's growth takes place in the lower body, mainly in the growth centers at the lower end of the thighbone and the upper end of the shinbone. But only a very small percentage of children actually have pain in the knee region. Children with growing pains have the same rate of growth in their limbs as do children without them.

Studies have shown that passive leg-stretching exercises performed on the child by the parents in the evening decrease the incidence of growing pains to such a degree that these children have an episode only once every three or four months. These exercises may increase the blood flow into the muscles, although at times the beneficial results of the stretching exercises are so dramatic that some experts feel that the time the parent spends with the child also may fulfill an emotional need for the child.

Whatever the cause for the success of the method, the rehabilitation of this at times disconcerting problem should be done by the parents themselves at home after some instructions by a therapist or physician. The parents must be assured that the growth of the child is not impaired.

### ▶ Treatment of Spasticity

Spasticity often limits the functioning of people with cerebral palsy and other conditions and often causes a spastic gait. It is traditionally treated with oral antispasmodic medication, which can produce side effects. Now, the exotoxin produced by the food-poisoning bacteria *Clostridium botulinum* is being used successfully to inactivate the nerve fibers that cause spasticity in the striated or skeletal muscles. This botulinum toxin, called Botox, blocks the release of the neurotransmitter acetylcholine, providing a more selective treatment of this condition with no side effects.

### ▶ Living on Easy Street

An innovative rehabilitation program is being instituted in hospitals across the nation to help patients with disabilities, mobility restrictions, or other problems prepare for everyday situations. The program, called "Easy Street," creates mock kitchens, supermarkets, or even automatic teller machines within the hospital environment. Patients can then use these practice arenas before they are released into the real world.

In a typical Easy Street scenario, a person recovering from hip-replacement surgery may learn how to juggle a walker or four-pronged cane while shopping in a recreated supermarket (below). Therapists teach the patient such techniques as picking up fallen objects without bending. Living on Easy Street also bolsters a sense of independence in patients that the pain and fear produced by their disabilities may have erased.

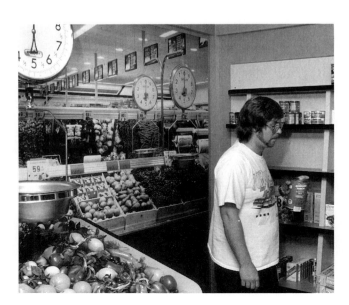

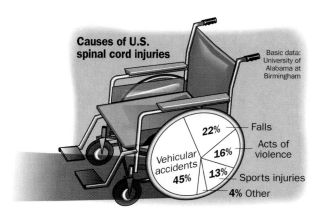

Causes of U.S. spinal cord injuries

Basic data: University of Alabama at Birmingham

Vehicular accidents 45%

Falls 22%

Acts of violence 16%

Sports injuries 13%

4% Other

## ▶ Spinal-Cord Repair

Spinal-cord injuries afflict close to 10,000 Americans each year, often resulting in partial or complete paralysis and irreversible nerve damage. But researchers are slowly unlocking the secrets of nerve growth and regeneration. In a January 1994 issue of the British journal *Nature,* two teams of scientists report that they may have found evidence that nerves in the spine can be coaxed back to life. In one study, a European research group found that a combination of natural chemicals enhanced spinal-nerve growth in young rats. A Japanese scientist found that newborn rats with severed spinal cords transplanted with embryonic nerve tissue were eventually able to walk and climb. While these studies are too preliminary to offer hope for humans in this decade, they do suggest new methodologies that may make the words "You'll never walk again" obsolete.

## ▶ Treatment of Burn Scars

A long-term study of 151 burn patients suggests that the need for repeated plastic and reconstructive surgery can be reduced by about 50 percent with modern scar-softening treatment, which may include compression devices, daily stretching, and scar treatment. This is especially good news for children, since reconstructive surgery always means hospitalization and time away from school. The application of silastic gel sheets for softening of the scar contributes in large measure to the success rate.

One major concern is still the compliance rate in wearing a compression device, which must be worn 23 hours a day to prevent the formation of a scar due to deprivation of oxygen. Otherwise, ischemia develops; also, the scar must not be given enough room to form blood vessels for oxygen transfer and to expand. Intense patient follow-up and a full explanation of the consequences that may result if the devices are not properly used, including illustrations about the possible poor cosmetic and functional outcome, may improve compliance.

*Willibald Nagler, M.D.*

# Respiratory System

## ▶ Treating ARDS

Acute respiratory distress syndrome (ARDS) usually represents the final, fatal stage of many lung diseases. It often occurs with sepsis (blood infection), but may also be associated with such conditions as aspiration, near drowning, smoke inhalation, head injury, and pancreatitis, among others. The treatment of this disease is supportive. Patients with ARDS require high concentrations of oxygen and are placed on ventilators. Basic vital signs and organ functions are closely monitored, and medications and antibiotics are administered as indicated. Nonetheless, the mortality rate remains high (70 to 90 percent), and physicians are eager for new approaches to treat ARDS. Early enthusiasm for corticosteroid drugs has been tempered by studies that failed to reveal a benefit, and suggested that mortality may even be increased. The use of monoclonal antibodies has met with mixed results. Other anti-inflammatory agents (such as ibuprofen and indomethacin), prostaglandins, antioxidants (vitamin E, vitamin C), pentoxyfilline, and, most recently, inhalation of nitric oxide (a potent pulmonary-artery dilator) have also been tried. While nitric oxide has shown partial success in ameliorating the condition, it appears that no single agent is capable of arresting ARDS once it begins.

## ▶ Cystic Fibrosis Update

Lung disease manifested by obstruction of the airways by thick mucus, leading to infections and airway-wall dilation and destruction (bronchiectasis), is the most debilitating and life-threatening aspect of cystic fibrosis (CF). Treatment for CF has traditionally involved the maintenance of pulmonary hygiene, aggressive antibiotic therapy, and the use of bronchodilators. Newer approaches are directed at improving the water content of the mucus through medications or by breaking down certain proteins in the secretions and making the mucus thinner and thus more easily expectorated. DNAse, an enzyme administered by inhalation, is capable of this latter type of action. For those whose disease has advanced to respiratory insufficiency, lung transplantation is now an option with promising results.

Unfortunately, none of these forms of therapy addresses the basic cause of CF in most patients: a defective gene that does not produce a specific cell protein, which scientists have successfully identified. Gene therapy for CF in which a healthy gene is transferred to the upper-respiratory-tract cells of a patient to produce the necessary protein is a reality within reach. A few human trials are under way.

## ▶ Asthma and COPD

Our understanding of the cause of asthma has been furthered by the finding of substances called cytokines in fluid from the lungs of patients with acute asthma. Cytokines cause inflammation, and their presence in patients underscores the role of inflammation in the generation and propagation of asthma. For those with moderate to severe asthma, the National Asthma Education Program recommends the use of inhaled steroids or cromolyn for maintenance therapy, supplemented by inhaled beta agonists as needed. There is concern, however, that regular use of beta agonists may ultimately make asthma more difficult to control, although this is not yet proven. Nedocromil (Tilade), an anti-inflammatory agent whose mechanism of action differs from that of steroids, has been released for use in patients with moderate to severe asthma.

Other drugs recently used for asthma include methotrexate, gold, and cyclosporine. These agents have anti-inflammatory and immunosuppressant properties. Unfortunately, serious side effects limit their usefulness on a daily basis. Patient education and self-monitoring play an essential role in the management of asthmatic conditions.

Chronic Obstructive Pulmonary Disease (COPD) is a term used to denote diseases characterized by chronic airflow obstruction. These include chronic bronchitis, chronic asthmatic bronchitis, and emphysema. Various risk factors have been associated with such illnesses, including smoking, family history, air pollution, and nonspecific bronchial reactivity. Of these, smoking is by far the greatest single cause of COPD. Smokers show a dramatically accelerated yearly decrease in flow rates (a measure of progressive airway obstruction) when compared to nonsmokers. To a large extent, this rate is reversible with cessation of smoking.

Education of COPD patients as to the nature of the disease, the course, prognosis, and the steps necessary to help in preventing it is extremely important. The use of inhalers, anticholinergic and beta agonists, as well as inhaled or oral steroids in certain patients, is also important. Oxygen supplementation in patients whose oxygen has fallen below a certain level is essential to forestall complications. During air travel patients may require an increase in their oxygen concentration. Vaccination against influenza (once a year) and against pneumococcus pneumonia (at least once in a lifetime and perhaps every five years) is highly recommended. Physical reconditioning and breathing exercises should form part of any regimen for treatment of COPD.

Mucoactive agents (drugs that alter the thickness of mucus) have been evaluated in large clinical studies. The value of these drugs in reducing such symptoms as cough, chest discomfort, dyspnea (sensation of breathlessness), and difficult expectoration has been well demonstrated. Mucoactives appear to work best in patients whose condition is more consistent with chronic bronchitis and in those who have an element of reversibility to their obstruction. Nutrition also plays a central role in patients with COPD. A recent study shows a significant depletion of magnesium in the red blood cells of patients with COPD. Magnesium acts as a bronchodilator and as a vasodilator, and is important in muscle function as well. Therefore, a deficiency of this element could play a role in the manifestations of COPD. Ideal body weight should be maintained with the use of diet supplements (especially fat-fortified ones) and the addition of adequate antioxidant vitamins (such as beta carotene, vitamin C, and vitamin E). Calcium and magnesium replacement is desirable.

In a small percentage of patients, emphysema is caused by alpha-1-antitrypsin deficiency. Alpha-1-antitrypsin is a protein produced in the liver to prevent the breakdown of lung tissues by enzymes released from white blood cells. Lack of this protein (a genetic defect for which the responsible gene has been identified and cloned) leads to an early onset of emphysema and limited respiratory reserve. The treatment for this disease includes replacement of alpha-1-antitrypsin. We still do not know whether augmenting the level of this enzyme will prevent or alter the progression of emphysema. Gene therapy has been demonstrated experimentally and awaits

**How Chronic Obstructive Pulmonary Disease Affects the Lungs**

In healthy lungs, millions of alveoli exchange oxygen for carbon dioxide. A fine web of blood vessels picks up oxygen to be used by tissues and organs throughout the body.

**Normal**

Air exchange

Bronchioles

Alveolar sacs

Air exchange

Mucus

**COPD**

Narrowed bronchioles

Aveolar sacs (shown in section)

In patients with emphysema, air sacs rupture, blood vessels are lost, and stale air is trapped. When chronic bronchitis is also present, the bronchioles narrow and are clogged by mucus.

Trapped air

human trials. The young patient with emphysema should be tested for deficiency of this enzyme.

## ▶ Interstitial Lung Disease

Idiopathic pulmonary fibrosis (IPF) is a chronic and often fatal interstitial lung disease. It occurs in susceptible individuals after exposure to an inciting agent, which precipitates a cascade of events involving inflammation, immunologic responses, and other reactions that lead to fibrosis (scarring) of lung tissue and respiratory insufficiency. Viral infection may be involved, but this theory is as yet unproven. Certain drugs (bleomycin, nitrofurantoin, and methotrexate) are known to induce pulmonary fibrosis as a dose-related side effect. In some instances the pulmonary manifestations are due to a hypersensitivity or allergic condition produced by the inciting agent. A syndrome of pulmonary disease associated with the ingestion of the amino acid supplement tryptophan has been recognized and recently studied by the Centers for Disease Control and Prevention (CDC). Fluid from the lungs of patients with IPF is rich in various cells and inflammatory agents, assorted enzymes, and cytokines. Patients exhibit progressive shortness of breath, cough, and an abnormal chest X ray. A high-resolution CAT scan of the chest is often helpful in determining the extent of the disease. IPF is treated with corticosteroids and immunosuppressive drugs and in certain patients, unresponsive to medical therapy, by using transplantation.

## ▶ Lung Transplantation

Advances in immunosuppression, surgical techniques, organ preservation, and therapy for complications have increased the success rate and survival of patients undergoing lung transplantation. Single-lung, double-lung, and heart-lung transplantation are the three procedures that have been performed. The choice of procedure is dictated by the underlying disease and the secondary effects on the heart. The most common underlying lung diseases have been pulmonary fibrosis, emphysema, cystic fibrosis, bronchiectasis, and pulmonary hypertension.

Complications after lung transplantation include perioperative pulmonary edema, graft failure, and —later on—infection and rejection. Repeated bronchoscopies are performed to diagnose and treat early rejection and/or infection. In some patients, a late complication after lung or heart-lung transplantation is obliterative bronchiolitis, a form of chronic rejection affecting the small airways; it leads to symptoms of cough, phlegm expectoration, and shortness of breath. One-and two-year survival rates of 75 percent or better are being reported; it is likely that as experience accumulates, the long-term survival will improve even more dramatically.

*Maria L. Padilla, M.D.*

# Sexually Transmitted Diseases

## ▶ Drug-resistant Gonorrhea Strains

Although the overall reported incidence of gonorrhea in the United States has been decreasing since the mid-1970s, antibiotic resistance in gonorrhea strains has increased during the same period. The most prevalent antibiotic-resistant gonorrhea *(Neisseria gonorrhoeae)* produces a penicillin-cleaving enzyme, making the bacteria resistant to all penicillins and first-generation cephalosporins. (Fortunately, it remains susceptible to second- and third-generation cephalosporins.) A less common gonorrhea variant is tetracycline-resistant *and* cephalosporin-resistant. According to the Gonococcal Isolate Surveillance Project (GISP), established by the CDC in 1986 to monitor drug-resistant gonorrhea trends, the problem has been growing progressively worse.

GISP is a surveillance system involving 26 publicly funded sexually transmitted disease (STD) clinics and five regional laboratories. At each clinic, urethral cultures are obtained from the first 20 men diagnosed with gonorrhea each month; these isolates are shipped to one of the regional laboratories, where the properties of the gonorrhea organisms (including resistance to antibiotics) are determined. In 1988, 14.6 percent of the cultures were resistant to antibiotics, primarily penicillin and tetracycline. That figure rose to 32.4 percent of the GISP sample in 1991; 34.7 percent in 1992; and 39.8 percent of the sample as of October 1993—with resistance to cephalosporins and other drugs also showing significant increases. On the positive side, no documented clinical-treatment failures have yet occurred with the antibiotics ceftriaxone or ciprofloxacin—so these antibiotics have become the drugs of choice for treating gonorrhea.

## ▶ STDs and Youth Gangs

Sexual behaviors occurring among adolescent gang members pose increasing danger of sexually transmitted disease outbreaks among the nation's most vulnerable population, ages 10 to 19. Practices of initiating adolescent girls into youth gangs increasingly involve "sexual roulette"—girls being asked to perform sexual acts with groups of males, including those infected with STDs. For boys, gang initiation/acceptance rituals, some including heterosexual and homosexual activity, are also becoming prevalent.

The spread of drug-resistant gonorrhea and other STDs among the adolescent population of Colorado Springs, Colorado, is representative of the current national trends. In April 1990, the county health department serving that city, the state's second largest, reported an outbreak of drug-resistant gonorrhea and other sexually transmitted diseases. A high percentage of the reported cases occurred among black and Hispanic youths involved in street gangs. The outbreak revealed a previously unidentified core group of persons with STDs in Colorado Springs. The youth gangs, originating in Los Angeles and associated with the crack-cocaine trade in the United States, had not been observed in Colorado Springs before May 1988. In 1990, of a total of 578 adolescents found to be engaging in sex with multiple partners, 410 were involved in street gangs; over 300 of them tested positive for antibiotic-resistant gonorrhea, so-called "normal" gonorrhea, chlamydia, and syphilis. More recently the outbreak has increased to epidemic levels in Colorado Springs, with the local health department reporting over 1,000 new STD cases since January 1992. A relatively high proportion of those infected with gonorrhea strains (37 percent of total cases reported) were coinfected with chlamydia.

In Colorado the number of reported cases of gonorrhea increased 19.9 percent from 1991 to 1992, after declining steadily during the 1980s. Persons in the 10- to 19-year-old age group accounted for the highest number of reported cases of gonorrhea during 1992, and the highest age-group-specific rate (639 per 100,000). Gang and drug involvement occurring in Colorado Springs and the Denver metropolitan area was believed to be putting an increasing number of adolescents (especially young blacks) at risk for contracting STDs. In all regions of the United States in 1991, some of the highest rates of STDs occurred among black and Hispanic adolescents involved in gangs.

### ▶ Preventing Chlamydia
In August 1993, the Centers for Disease Control and Prevention (CDC) in Atlanta, Georgia, announced an updated national strategy for preventing chlamydia *(Chlamydia trachomatis)* infections. More than 4 million chlamydial infections occur annually in the United States, mostly among sexually active adolescents and young adults. Infection by this organism is insidious—initial symptoms are absent or minor among most infected women and many men, many of whom become carriers and spread the disease. Most carriers (as well as other infected persons) are at risk for acute infection and serious long-term consequences including penile and vaginal discharges and, eventually, infertility and sterility. Up to 25 percent of infants exposed to chlamydia develop neonatal conjunctivitis and pneumonia; infants with chlamydia pneumonia are at risk for serious lung disorders later in childhood. Among other prevention strategies, the CDC recommends

education-based chlamydia-public-awareness programs in schools (and programs targeted to out-of-school adolescents) and early screening by health-care providers—especially of sexually active women less than 20 years of age.

### ▶ The "Magic" Johnson Announcement
A 1993 CDC report documented the effect on sexual-risk behaviors of Earvin "Magic" Johnson's announcement that he had tested positive for the human immunodeficiency virus (HIV). The report summarizes findings concerning patients with STDs at a Maryland clinic in a Washington, D.C., suburb. Comparisons were made of the patients' responses during the 14 weeks before and the 14 weeks after the basketball star's press conference on November 7, 1991. In recent years, media and public interest had been sparked by periodic accounts of persons infected with HIV—but the effect of these stories on sexual behaviors has been largely unknown. In the Maryland study, participants were predominately male (60 percent) and black (73 percent); their average age was 25.1 years. While the random-survey report shows no substantial differences in sexual behaviors measured over long periods before and after Johnson's announcement, trends toward fewer sex partners and fewer "one-night stands" in the postannouncement period are observed, although self-reported condom use (or the lack of it) appears unchanged.

### ▶ Condom Effectiveness and STDs
How effective is condom use as a protection against sexually transmitted diseases? An August 1993 CDC report summarized the effectiveness of penis-

*Members of youth gangs have a higher incidence of sexually transmitted diseases than do adolescents who do not belong to gangs.*

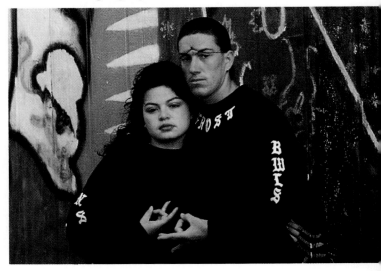

**Number of sexually active young men and measures of condom use, by race or ethnic group**

| Measure and race/ethnicity | All | | Ages 17.5–19 | |
|---|---|---|---|---|
| | 1988 | 1991 | 1988 | 1991 |
| **NUMBER** | | | | |
| All | 1,198 | 1,355 | 655 | 616 |
| Black | 533 | 544 | 267 | 250 |
| White | 422 | 526 | 255 | 230 |
| Hispanic | 214 | 244 | 114 | 116 |
| **CONDOM USE** | | | | |
| **% who used at last intercourse** | | | | |
| All | 56.2 | 44.2*** | 53.0 | 56.1 |
| Black | 66.6 | 49.2*** | 63.4 | 60.5 |
| White | 53.5 | 42.7*** | 50.8 | 55.9 |
| Hispanic | 50.6 | 48.1 | 43.2 | 57.3* |
| **Consistency of use** | | | | |
| **with last partner†** | | | | |
| All | 53.9 | 46.0*** | 50.4 | 55.5* |
| Black | 62.0 | 50.6*** | 58.5 | 60.9 |
| White | 51.7 | 45.6* | 48.6 | 56.1 |
| Hispanic | 51.3 | 40.5** | 43.9 | 45.7 |
| **Consistency of use** | | | | |
| **in last year†** | | | | |
| All | 55.6 | 45.6*** | 51.0 | 54.7 |
| Black | 61.4 | 50.3*** | 57.2 | 58.1 |
| White | 54.4 | 44.7** | 49.9 | 54.8 |
| Hispanic | 51.1 | 42.6** | 42.6 | 48.3 |

*Difference between columns is statistically significant at p<.05. **Difference between columns is statistically significant at p<.01. ***Difference between columns is statistically significant at p<.001. †The percentage of acts of intercourse in which a condom was used.

sheathing latex condoms and polyurethane "female condoms" in preventing STDs. The report found that latex and polyurethane condoms substantially reduce the risk of STDs among heterosexual couples, though the importance of consistent use (i.e., use of a condom with each act of intercourse) and correct condom use were emphasized. Condom use was found to reduce the risk of gonorrhea, herpes simplex virus (HSV) infection, genital ulcers, and pelvic inflammatory disease (PID). In addition a recent CDC laboratory study indicates that intact latex condoms provide a continuous mechanical barrier to HSV, hepatitis B virus, chlamydia, and drug-resistant gonorrhea strains. Three other recent international studies conducted indicate that latex condoms are unlikely to break or slip during proper use. Reported breakage rates in the studies were 2 percent or less for vaginal and anal intercourse. One study reports complete slippage off the penis during intercourse, for one of 237 (0.4 percent) latex condoms, and reported the same rate (0.4 percent) of slippage during withdrawal.

Laboratory studies indicate that the female condom—a lubricated polyurethane sheath with a ring on each end that is inserted into the vagina—is an effective barrier to sexually transmitted viruses, including HSV.

*Gode Davis*

# Skin

## ▶ Allergy to Topical Steroids

The medications most commonly used by dermatologists are the topical steroids. Their potency in relieving inflammation of the skin, their relative safety, and their convenience of use make them the dermatologist's first choice in treating inflammatory diseases of the skin. Unfortunately, there has been an increased incidence of allergic reactions to corticosteroids. This type of allergy is a deceptive, difficult-to-diagnose problem. When the topical-steroid cream is applied to inflamed skin but fails to resolve the inflammation, the dermatologist may be inclined to conclude that the steroid was ineffective. The actual underlying steroid allergy can thus remain totally undetected.

Allergy to topical steroids was first described in 1950. The mechanism of this reaction is the same as that by which poison ivy causes a skin rash. Thus, giving topical steroids to a steroid-allergic individual is like having a poison-ivy-sensitive patient rub poison ivy on his or her skin.

Because topical-steroid allergy frequently goes unrecognized, these patients are sometimes inadvertently treated with oral steroids or injections of steroids. The resulting reaction can vary from an annoying flare-up of the localized skin inflammation to a sudden, full-body, potentially lethal allergic reaction. Even more alarming is the possibility that once patients are sensitized to topical-steroid medications, they may end up reacting to their own naturally produced steroids.

Efforts are now being made to improve the methods for diagnosing these patients. Allergic contact-patch testing is the standard diagnostic technique. Small amounts of the suspected allergen are placed on the skin to test for a reaction. Unfortunately, there are hundreds of different types of topical steroids in widespread use; allergic patients frequently react to only a few of these steroid molecules. Patch testing of all of these molecules is impractical. Fortunately, a study by A.D. Burden and M.H. Beck from the department of dermatology, West Infirmary, Glasgow, Scotland, reports that patch testing with a single agent—tixocortol privalate—can identify 90.8 percent of allergic patients. The hope is that dermatologists can identify a few patch-test chemicals that can be easily used to identify the steroid-allergic patients. This work may eventually lead to an understanding of steroid allergy that makes possible the formulation of hypoallergenic topical steroids. Such steroids could be used without fear of the patient developing this deceptive form of contact allergy.

## ▶ Gene Therapy for Metastatic Melanoma

A creative form of gene therapy shows promise in the treatment of metastatic melanoma. Because of its accessibility in the skin, melanoma has been used frequently as a model for new cancer therapeutic trials. Thus, it is not surprising that trials of the new, dynamic medical technique called gene therapy would be used against metastatic melanoma. Unfortunately, the application of gene therapy to melanoma and to all types of cancer has proven far more challenging than its use in the treatment of metabolic diseases. In many metabolic diseases, a single gene defect can be identified and the normal gene can be substituted. Melanoma, like most forms of cancer, probably results not from a single genetic defect, but as a result of multiple gene defects. Furthermore, even if all of these genetic defects could be identified, it would be necessary to replace the genes in all of the tumor cells. This probably makes standard gene therapy for melanoma and most types of cancer impossible.

Thus, attacks on cancer via gene therapy require a more innovative approach. Gary Nabel, M.D., from the University of Michigan Medical School has demonstrated such an approach to treating metastatic melanoma. He uses gene therapy to boost the ability of the melanoma patient's immune system to recognize the tumor cells as foreign. Dr. Nabel inserts a new, foreign gene into metastatic melanoma cells. This causes the melanoma cells to express a new foreign marker on their surface. Because of this new surface marker, the patient's immune system is able to recognize the tumor cells as foreign. The host immune system rapidly mounts a white-blood-cell response to fight these changed tumor cells. Importantly, this immune response attacks not only the changed tumor cells with the new gene, but also the unchanged melanoma cells. In other words, by increasing the antigenicity or foreignness of some of the tumor cells, a host defense is triggered against all of the tumor cells. Preliminary human experimentation with this creative variation of gene therapy for melanoma was begun in 1993. It is hoped it will become an effective form of therapy not only for metastatic melanoma, but also for other forms of cancer.

## ▶ Alpha₁-Proteinase Inhibitor to Treat Eczema

Eczema is a common skin disease characterized by inflammation of the skin and severe itching. The disease takes many different forms, from a localized hand inflammation to generalized, full-body skin inflammation. For many years, topical corticosteroid preparations have been the mainstay of eczema therapy. Unfortunately, because eczema is a chronic disease, patients are forced to use large quantities of increasingly potent topical steroids in order to maintain control of the skin inflammation. This results in a virtual addiction to topical steroids; on each attempt to discontinue steroid therapy, flare-ups of eczema occur. Furthermore, the chronic use of potent topical steroids is associated with such adverse effects as progressive thinning or atrophy of the skin and dangerous suppression of the body's own natural production of steroids. Thus, the development of an effective nonsteroid therapy would be an important discovery for dermatological patients.

*Alpha₁-proteinase inhibitor* is a naturally occurring chemical produced by liver cells and by specialized forms of white blood cells. This chemical has the ability to inhibit *serine proteinases,* an important class of enzymes that contribute to inflammation. It is believed that an inability to properly neutralize these enzymes is an important factor in many different inflammatory diseases of the skin, including eczema. Dan K. Chalker, M.D., and Beverly B.

## New Skin for Burn Patients

Burn patients typically undergo a skin autograft, in which skin is taken from elsewhere on the patient's body. The graft is perforated (below) to allow it to stretch. But for a person with extensive burns, healthy skin may be in short supply. Fortunately, clinical trials now underway are testing an artificial dermis, which could be stored in hospitals to be used as needed to close wounds and to speed skin regeneration.

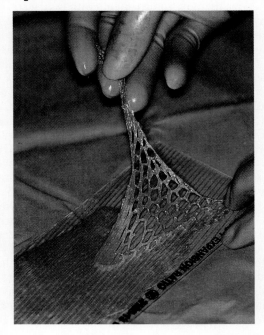

Sanders, M.D., of the Medical College of Georgia presented preliminary data at the American Academy of Dermatology's 1993 summer meetings in Toronto, Ontario, that show a dramatic benefit from the topical application of alpha$_1$-proteinase inhibitor. Improvement of eczema was noted within weeks of initiating therapy, and at the end of the six weeks, the alpha$_1$-proteinase inhibitor had produced significant improvement in all treated patients.

It was suggested by Dr. Chalker that the proper formulation of alpha$_1$-proteinase inhibitor in a moisturizing-cream base rather than in the primitive liquid spray used in the studies would increase its efficacy. It is hoped that this new therapy may also prove effective for many other inflammatory diseases of the skin.

## ▶ Hepatitis C and Porphyria

The porphyrias are a group of diseases that result from abnormalities in the metabolism of hemoglobin. Of the group, porphyria cutanea tarda (PCT) is the most common, occurring in both a hereditary form and in a sporadic form. PCT patients frequently seek help from dermatologists because they develop a distinctive skin rash (including sun-induced blistering on the back of the hands) and increased hair growth on the face. The disease and its various symptoms result from an enzymatic defect that causes a buildup of an ultraviolet-light-absorbing chemical, uroporphyrin, in the body. In the sporadic form of PCT, the enzymatic defect is localized in the liver.

Standard therapy for PCT focuses on lowering the uroporphyrin level. However, in spite of this effective therapy, some patients with PCT go on to develop chronic progressive liver disease, and even liver cancer. Separate studies by J. Ph. Lacour in the *British Journal of Dermatology* and C. Herrero in *Lancet* published in 1993 suggest a strong association between PCT and the hepatitis C virus (HCV). In both studies, approximately three-quarters of all patients with sporadic PCT had evidence of HCV infection. More importantly, all of the patients with PCT and the associated progressive liver disease were infected with HCV. It is very likely that HCV is the cause of the progressive liver disease and occasional liver cancer in PCT patients, and in some cases it may be the causative agent for PCT itself.

Certainly all previously diagnosed patients with PCT should now be screened for this virus. This is particularly important because a type of interferon is recognized as an effective treatment for HCV-infected patients with chronic liver disease. In the future, many patients with PCT will be treated not only to lower their level of uroporphyrin, but also with interferon to help battle the hepatitis C virus infection.

*Edward E. Bondi, M.D.*

# Substance Abuse

## ▶ Health-Care Costs and Substance Abuse

A study conducted by N. G. Hoffmann and colleagues at the University of Minnesota in Minneapolis indicates that the costs of medical care for substance-abuse patients who are abstinent are substantially lower than are the costs for patients who continue to use drugs and alcohol. The researchers examined the medical-care utilization of 3,572 patients who received substance-abuse treatment from 1983 to 1986, and compared it to their utilization of medical care in the year prior to entering treatment. Those who remained totally abstinent had significant reductions in hospitalizations and health-care costs as compared to those in the year prior to treatment, and compared to those substance abusers who continued to use drugs or alcohol. The findings suggest that prevention of substance use and substance-abuse treatment can greatly reduce health-care costs.

A close examination of the relationship between type of substance-abuse treatment and its success was conducted by researchers from the University of Pennsylvania School of Medicine in Philadelphia. The data show that different treatment settings may vary considerably in their effectiveness and quality. The researchers, led by A. T. McLellan, followed 198 adults referred for drug treatment through their workplaces. The subjects entered into one of four different, privately funded treatment programs that varied in intensity of treatment and treatment philosophy, but which were similar in treatment duration and accreditation. Dropout rates ranged from a low of 4 percent in one inpatient program to a high of 26 percent in one outpatient program. At six-month follow-up, abstinence rates ranged from a low of 71 percent in the least intensive outpatient program to a high of 98 percent in the most intensive inpatient program. The findings suggest that the quality and range of services delivered during substance-abuse treatment vary considerably from program to program, and this factor may well account for differences in treatment success. More research needs to be conducted on the factors that determine successful treatment.

## ▶ Female Alcoholics

Only in the past few years has much attention focused on identifying and understanding alcoholism in women. While several studies have shown that alcoholism in men is strongly influenced by genetic factors, there are few comparable studies on the genetic factors for alcoholism in women. Kenneth

Kendler and his colleagues from the Medical College of Virginia studied over 1,000 pairs of female identical and fraternal twins. The researchers found that the probability of both twins having alcoholism was greater for the identical twins than for the fraternal twins, indicating a genetic influence. By factoring in environmental factors, the researchers estimate that at least half the risk for alcoholism in women is a result of genetic factors.

It is well known that women are less likely to seek alcoholism treatment than are men, although the reasons for these differences are unclear. Two recent studies examined the influence of gender in alcoholism treatment. Constance Weisner and Laura Schmidt of the University of California at Berkeley investigated alcoholism treatment in female heavy drinkers over a period of several years. They found that, compared to men, women are less likely to receive treatment early in the course of their problem drinking, and they are more likely to delay treatment until their problems become severe. In addition, alcoholic women avoided specialized alcoholism-treatment programs and were more likely to seek help in primary-care and general mental-health programs. The women were found to be economically less well off than comparable men. The authors express concern that alcoholic women may not be receiving as effective treatment as their male counterparts, perhaps due in part to their relative lack of financial resources.

In another study comparing male and female alcoholics in treatment, Tracy Jarvis of the University of New South Wales in Australia reviewed 20 published alcoholism-treatment-outcome studies. The review found that treatment success in men usually occurred in inpatient treatment programs that included group psychotherapy in conjunction with Alcoholics Anonymous (AA). In contrast, women treated successfully were involved in more individually based, behaviorally oriented programs. The author found that women did better in all-female groups, and often felt isolated and stigmatized in treatment settings in which males predominate.

## ▶ Substance Use and Abuse in the Elderly

Another population group not well studied as to use of alcohol and other drugs is the elderly. Alcohol use is common in the elderly, particularly in those seeking medical treatment. A study by W. Adams and colleagues from the Medical College of Wisconsin in Milwaukee found that 14 percent of patients aged 65 or more who sought treatment in a university-hospital emergency room were alcoholics. However, the emergency-room staff was able to detect alcoholism only in about one of five of these patients. In a related study, the researchers analyzed Medicare records of elderly patients hospitalized during 1989. The data showed that over 87,000 (1.1 percent) of the hospitalizations were for alcohol-related problems, with a median cost of over $4,500 per hospitalization. Thus, the costs of these potentially preventable problems are considerable.

A study from the University of Hawaii in Honolulu further underscores the seriousness of substance abuse among the elderly. A retrospective review of records from 383 patients who underwent comprehensive geriatric assessments found that 29 percent of the sample reported alcohol use; 69 percent of these patients showed cognitive impairment. For those whose drinking represented a problem, 100 percent showed cognitive impairment. Again, alcohol problems were not usually detected by the regular staff. During the initial assessment fewer than half of these patients were diagnosed as having alcohol problems.

The use of prescription psychoactive medications in elderly nursing-home patients is another significant problem. A study from the Schools of Medicine and Public Health at the University of California at Los Angeles (UCLA) shows that over 40 percent of nursing-home patients received at least one inappropriate medication, and 10 percent received two or more inappropriate medications. The most frequently misused medications were long-acting benzodiazepines, antidepressants, and antipsychotics that were prescribed at excessive doses.

Other research suggests that the overmedication of nursing-home patients is a correctable problem. Researchers from Harvard Medical School in Cambridge, Massachusetts, examined medication use in nursing homes after starting an educational program for staff on appropriate drug use. Medication use in the six homes was then compared with six matched homes that did not receive the educational program. The administration of drugs in the nursing homes that received the educational program significantly decreased, and the patients showed improved cognition. There were no changes in the frequencies of dangerous or disrupted behavior on the part of the patients.

## ▶ AIDS and Intravenous Drug Use

It is estimated that there are 1 million intravenous (IV) drug users in the United States, most of whom use heroin on a regular basis. In the IV drug abuser, human immunodeficiency virus (HIV) infection resulting in acquired immune deficiency syndrome (AIDS) has become a major public-health problem. In these people, HIV appears to be transmitted primarily by blood retained in shared needles, syringes, or other drug paraphernalia. Unfortunately, needle sharing occurs commonly among IV drug users. HIV may also be spread via sexual contact between addicts and between addicts and their sexual partners who do not use drugs. The potential for rapid increases of HIV in the blood of IV drug users, and the ability of these people to be a conduit of infection into the general population, underscores the need to develop strategies to remedy this situation.

Fortunately, evidence suggests that concern about HIV and AIDS is reducing the rates of IV drug use in opiate users. In a study comparing IV drug use in 1986 and 1988, Richard Schottenfeld, M.D., and other researchers at the Yale University School of Medicine in New Haven, Connecticut, found a reduction in the rates of current IV drug use from 86 percent to 61 percent. The rates of addicts who never used IV drugs rose from 7 percent in 1986 to 22 percent in 1988. Over this time period, addicts reported increasing awareness of AIDS, and changed their drug-use habits because of this. Of concern, however, was the observation that some users reverted back to IV drug use because of the lack of availability of immediate treatment. The authors point out that additional research is needed to determine the factors that result in behavioral change in opiate addicts, and to improve the effectiveness of interventions to reduce the risk of acquiring AIDS.

▶ **Smoking, Depression, and Genetics**

A recent study from the Federal Office of Disease Prevention and Health Promotion finds that the use of tobacco is the number one health problem in the United States. The authors estimate that in 1990, 400,000 deaths occurred due to the use of tobacco products—more deaths than occur from firearms, alcohol, motor-vehicle accidents, and illegal drugs combined. The health consequences resulting from the use of tobacco products include cardiovascular and respiratory disease and cancers, especially lung cancer. Many of the harmful effects of tobacco are not due to nicotine, but are due to other toxic and carcinogenic compounds present in tobacco extract or smoke.

The nicotine patch has been widely used to assist patients who wish to quit smoking. The patch releases a controlled amount of nicotine through the skin and into the bloodstream, which helps to reduce withdrawal symptoms (craving, tension, etc.), and thus assists in the process of stopping smoking. A review of studies on the

nicotine patch's utility by M. Fiore, M.D., and colleagues from the University of Wisconsin in Milwaukee reports that the nicotine patch was found to be effective in reducing smoking in almost all studies. However, effectiveness of the patch is significantly improved by incorporating such behavioral-modification programs as counseling, social support, and follow-up into the treatment process.

Over the past several years, clinicians and researchers have observed that some individuals who stop smoking develop clinical depression. Naomi Breslau and researchers at the University of Michigan School of Medicine in Ann Arbor followed 995 young adults, 389 of whom were smokers, for a period of 14 months. The subjects with nicotine dependence were more than twice as likely to develop depression during the period of the study. The heavier smokers were more likely to have experienced depression in the past compared to lighter smokers. The findings suggest that individuals with a history of depression are more likely to develop nicotine dependence.

A possible link between depression and smoking is further supported in a study of the relationship between depression and smoking in twins conducted by K. S. Kendler and colleagues from the Medical College of Virginia. The authors found that rates of depression increased with the number of cigarettes smoked. Identical twins were more likely than fraternal twins to have similar smoking pat-

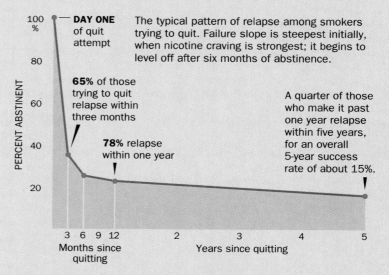

**The Relapse Curve:**
**If you can make it past the first 90 days . . .**

DAY ONE of quit attempt — The typical pattern of relapse among smokers trying to quit. Failure slope is steepest initially, when nicotine craving is strongest; it begins to level off after six months of abstinence.

**65%** of those trying to quit relapse within three months

**78%** relapse within one year

A quarter of those who make it past one year relapse within five years, for an overall 5-year success rate of about 15%.

PERCENT ABSTINENT

3 6 9 12
Months since quitting

2    3    4    5
Years since quitting

*Sources: Centers for Disease Control; American Cancer Society; Marion Merrell Dow Inc.; Richard Clayton, Ph.D., University of Kentucky; David Sachs, M.D., Palo Alto Center for Pulmonary Disease Prevention*

terns and similar histories of depression, suggesting that genetic factors play a role in the development of smoking and depression.

## ▶ Drug Use During Pregnancy

A health-care problem of considerable magnitude and concern is the use of illicit drugs by pregnant women. In 1989 it was estimated that as many as 375,000 infants per year born in the United States were exposed to illicit drugs in utero. In a study by Lawrence Slutsker from the Centers for Disease Control and Prevention (CDC), the researchers examined records of all women who gave birth in the state of Oregon in November 1989. The CDC study found that 5.2 percent of the women used an illicit drug. The most frequently used drug was marijuana (41 percent), followed by cocaine (23 percent). Drug use was found to be associated with lower socioeconomic status; when this factor was taken into consideration, there were no differences in usage due to race or residence.

Over the past several years, a number of research studies had reported that pregnant addicts and their infants are at risk for medical and behavioral complications, with implications for mothers and infants and for society at large. In the case of cocaine, several studies on women using this drug during pregnancy showed associations between cocaine use and severe obstetric complications, such as neurological damage, early placental separation, and extreme prematurity. However, other researchers have questioned whether the poor outcomes are due to the effect of the cocaine itself, or are due to other factors such as poverty, poor nutrition, and poor prenatal care, which are also common problems in this population. A study of 2,810 inner-city newborns by D. A. Bateman and colleagues from Columbia University in New York City confirmed that crack-cocaine use by a pregnant woman was associated with small birth weight and size, and prematurity. However, the researchers did not observe evidence of placental separation, severe prematurity, or neurological abnormalities, obstetric complications which had been previously reported in cocaine babies.

In an encouraging study on drug and alcohol use by pregnant adolescents, M. J. Lohr and colleagues at the University of Washington School of Social Work in Seattle found that substance abuse dropped significantly during pregnancy. Important determinants of drug use were use by friends, boyfriends, and other family members. The researchers also found that the girls' belief in the harmful effects of drugs on the unborn child was an important determinant in cutting down on substance abuse. The study suggests possible educational interventions that may be helpful in treatment.

*Robert M. Swift, M.D., Ph.D.*

# Teeth and Gums

## ▶ Periodontal Regeneration

Periodontitis is a common disease of the gums and bones surrounding the teeth. Left unchecked, periodontitis will destroy the bone that anchors the teeth into the mouth; ultimately teeth are lost. Surgical procedures to treat periodontitis have one of two objectives: to remove the region of bacteria and associated products, and therefore halt the progression of the destruction; or to stimulate the remaining bone to regenerate its lost structure. Regeneration surgery has traditionally involved the implantation of one or more types of bone-grafting material. These grafting procedures have demonstrated varying levels of success.

In the 1980s a new approach to periodontal regeneration emerged, based on studies that demonstrated that specific cells associated with the ligament attached to the tooth root were responsible for regenerative growth. It was found that the placement of a semipermeable membrane (which allows the passage of tissue nutrients, but not cells), over the gums could guide the growth of the appropriate cells to facilitate regeneration of periodontal tissues. This concept was given the name *guided tissue regeneration* (GTR). Unfortunately, the membranes had to be sutured in position, and—worse—following healing, a second surgical procedure was needed to remove the membrane. The necessity of this second procedure represented a significant obstacle for patient acceptance, and added expense to the entire process.

Recently research has focused on developing *resorbable* membranes that can be secured to the surgical area and remain intact for several weeks—long enough to ensure appropriate guiding of the healing response. The membrane would then be degraded by natural enzymes of the body. Collagen, dura mater, polylactate acid, oxidized cellulose, and synthetic materials are among the materials being investigated for this purpose. Some of the materials demonstrate the appropriate characteristics, but long-term clinical efficacy must still be documented.

## ▶ CAD/CAM Technology

The traditional method for restoring tooth structure destroyed by trauma or decay is by the creation and placement of a cast-gold-alloy restoration. This casting methodology has been used for decades and is capable of producing quality dental restorations. However, the procedure is very labor-intensive, and thus costly. There are also multiple steps at which errors can occur, potentially leading to an unsatisfactory product.

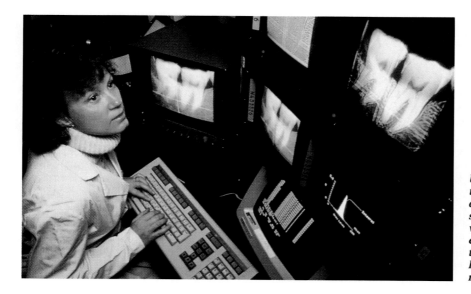

*Using advanced computer technology, restorations of decayed or missing tooth structure can be created with a precision and fit equal to or better than those of the traditional, labor-intensive casting method.*

The computer-assisted design/computer-assisted manufacturing (CAD/CAM) technology offers new approaches to the fabrication of dental restorations. Using this technology the region of missing tooth structure is prepared by the dentist in a conventional manner. A thin layer of opaque powder is then applied to the surface of the preparation, and a digital three-dimensional image of the prepared tooth is acquired by optical scanning with an intraoral camera. The obtained image is stored in a computer. The digitized dimensions are transferred to an electronic milling machine, which creates a restoration from a block of appropriate material (currently ceramic, porcelain, composite resin, or metal). The completed restoration is secured to the tooth with a traditional dental luting material or a hybrid composite material.

Dimensional precision and fit of CAD/CAM restorations have been shown to be equal to those of traditionally created cast restorations. As further refinements and modifications increase usage, the CAD/CAM approach will likely emerge as an efficient, cost-effective method of restoring decayed or missing tooth structure.

### ▶ Bonded Restorations

Early dental restorations, primarily made of metal, are not as aesthetically pleasing when used in the front of the mouth. In the 1950s and 1960s, tooth-colored restorative materials became popular, especially for use in the front teeth. While in their initial soft state, these materials were packed into "undercuts" created by the dentist during removal of decay; they were retained by mechanical interlock until they hardened.

During the 1970s the concept of chemical and mechanical adhesion of resin-based filling materials to the adjacent enamel structure of the tooth became very popular. It was shown that conditioning the enamel with an acid solution created thousands of microscopic pores (microporosities) on the tooth's surface to which the resin material can cling and ultimately seal.

This technique is very successful in regions where the removal of decay leaves intact enamel surrounding the cavity margins. Unfortunately, many areas of dental decay are not surrounded by intact enamel, but instead are bordered by tooth dentin. Dentin, unlike enamel, consists of tubules filled with organic material. The composition of dentin varies from person to person.

Initial attempts to condition dentin by acid treatment and to adhere restorations to the tooth's surface had mixed results for several reasons. The rotary instruments used by the dentist produce a "smear layer" of debris on the dentin surface. Acid conditioning with the smear layer in place results in formation of porosities in the smear layer, and bonding of the restorative material into those porosities. Unfortunately, the smear layer is only weakly attached to the underlying healthy dentin. Moderate stresses may dislodge the smear layer and the attached restoration.

Another early problem of dentin bonding was that dentists assumed that all dentin was equally mineralized, and thus responded in a similar manner when acid-conditioned. A third problem in early dentin bonding was the fact that the early resins in dentistry penetrated effectively only if the region of adherence was totally dry. Drying a region of enamel was no problem, but dentin, because of its organic component, may not be totally dried.

Recent attempts to place dentin-bonded restorations have proven to be much more successful because: 1) new techniques carefully remove or penetrate the dentin smear layer, giving uniform exposure of the healthy dentin matrix; 2) conditioning methods are modified dependent upon the factors that may influence the mineralization of the dentin; and 3) new dentin adhesive resins contain hydrophilic monomers that easily penetrate the moisture inherent in the tooth dentin.

These advances in dentin bonding over the past few years now allow the dentist to predictably place an aesthetically pleasing, tooth-colored dental restoration in a variety of locations not before possible.

## ▶ Lasers in Dentistry

Two decades ago, researchers began to explore a wide range of oral laser applications. During the past 20 years, refinement of technology and techniques has resulted in the development of specific intraoral laser instruments and a greater understanding of laser/oral tissue interactions.

At the present time, dental lasers are approved by the Food and Drug Administration (FDA) for use only in intraoral soft-tissue surgery. When the waveform of the laser is appropriately matched with the characteristics of the tissue and precisely adjusted, it is possible to perform a soft tissue incision with little heat production, thus minimizing tissue damage. While these soft-tissue surgical procedures may be performed effectively with a laser, the high cost of the instruments and the general availability of effective alternative methods of soft-tissue surgery do not warrant routine use of a laser at this time.

*Although their applications in dentistry are now quite limited, lasers will likely be used someday soon to remove tooth decay, vaporize tartar, and seal grooves on the tooth surface.*

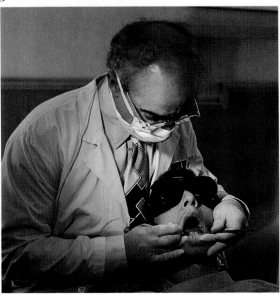

Active research continues to explore the applicability of the laser for oral hard-tissue procedures. Refinement and control of the techniques may eventually allow the dentist to safely and easily seal small grooves on the tooth surface before decay begins. It may also facilitate removal of dental decay and etching of the remaining tooth structure for retention of an appropriate filling material. Eventually dentists may use a laser to vaporize calculus (tartar) deposits from the tooth's root surface with minimal impact upon the adjacent root surface, or remove the pulp from a tooth during root-canal therapy while leaving a maximum amount of tooth structure intact for follow-up restoration.

## ▶ Rigid Fixation for Orthognathic Surgery

Orthognathic surgery, used to correct facial and jaw irregularities, has been used by oral and maxillofacial surgeons for decades. These surgical procedures involve the sectioning and repositioning of the major bones of the jaw. Traditionally the bones were stabilized during the healing period using stainless-steel sutures between adjacent bone segments. Immobilization of the jaws during the initial eight weeks of healing was achieved by wiring the jaws together. Obviously, this approach compromised nutrition, oral hygiene, speaking, and breathing during aerobic activity. The patient also faced an extremely difficult situation should nausea or extreme apprehension arise. In addition, immobilization of the temporomandibular joint for a long period of time was a concern.

Recently surgeons have begun to use rigid internal fixation of the bone segments as an alternative approach for stabilization. Rigid fixation involves exact positioning of each bone segment during the surgical procedure, and stabilization of these segments with metal bone plates secured in place by screws. Following the completion of surgery, the jaws are further steadied by fastening them together with elastic loops for a few days. Following this initial period, the elastics are removed to allow careful jaw movement. Within three to four weeks, the patients may begin opening exercises and other physiotherapy.

While speech, nutrition, and oral hygiene are greatly enhanced with the rigid-fixation approach, the procedure is technique-sensitive. Trauma may occur to the nerves of the jaw and adjacent teeth during screw placement. In addition, postoperative infections, malocclusion, or temporomandibular-joint trauma may occur if the bones are positioned inappropriately. Despite these potential drawbacks, the rigid-fixation approach to orthognathic surgery has led to benefits and enhanced outcomes for individuals undergoing the procedure.

*Kenneth L. Kalkwarf, D.D.S., M.S.*

# Tropical Medicine

## ►Malaria

Malaria's resurgence has continued as researchers have gone back to basics, seeking new strategies to attack the disease. More than 1 million—perhaps nearly 2 million—people now die of malaria each year. Most victims are children in poor equatorial countries. More than 100 million people suffer from malaria in a given year. The resurgence is a result of many factors: failure to control or eradicate mosquito hosts; resistance of malarial parasites to drugs; political unrest in malaria-plagued countries; and decline in funding of malarial research.

Much of the biochemistry of the malarial life cycle remains unknown. The disease is transmitted when an infected *Anopheles* mosquito bites a human and injects *Plasmodium,* a protozoal parasite, into the blood. Researchers are attacking various stages of the plasmodium's life cycle (see artwork below), which includes developmental periods within mosquito and human hosts.

At the National Institutes of Health (NIH), researchers have been developing an "altruistic vaccine." Such a vaccine, if present in a person, would not protect from malaria; instead, it would transfer to a biting mosquito a protein that prevents development of new malarial offspring. That mosquito would then be incapable of infecting other people. Hence, the vaccine is "altruistic," or "transmission-blocking." The protein, known as Pfs25, has been effective when transmitted by mice. If successful with humans, it may serve to halt the spread of mutant forms of malaria—that is, new forms that can defeat old vaccines.

British researchers discovered how malaria can, in part, evade the human immune system. The plasmodium parasite mutates into forms that can stick to the walls of human blood vessels, thereby avoiding travel to the spleen and subsequent destruction by immune cells. This discovery can conceivably lead to methods for blocking the parasite's ability to stick to blood vessels. Researchers at Washington University School of Medicine in St. Louis, Missouri, devised a strategy whereby a drug administered to humans can attract malaria in the bloodstream by imitating hemoglobin molecules, which plasmodium parasites ordinarily seek out and consume. Without the hemoglobin the parasites become starved for energy.

Researchers at Harvard University in Cambridge, Massachusetts, and at the Centers for Disease Control and Prevention (CDC) in Atlanta, Georgia, have pursued the genetic front. They have completed a linkage map of the X chromosome of

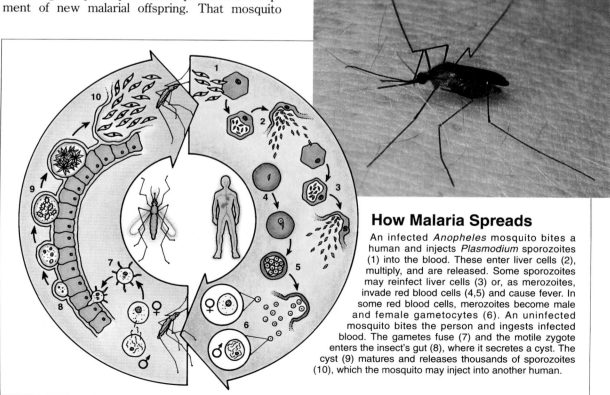

## How Malaria Spreads

An infected *Anopheles* mosquito bites a human and injects *Plasmodium* sporozoites (1) into the blood. These enter liver cells (2), multiply, and are released. Some sporozoites may reinfect liver cells (3) or, as merozoites, invade red blood cells (4,5) and cause fever. In some red blood cells, merozoites become male and female gametocytes (6). An uninfected mosquito bites the person and ingests infected blood. The gametes fuse (7) and the motile zygote enters the insect's gut (8), where it secretes a cyst. The cyst (9) matures and releases thousands of sporozoites (10), which the mosquito may inject into another human.

*Anopheles gambiae,* the mosquito most responsible for transmitting malaria in Africa. Maps of the other two chromosomes of this species should soon follow. Armed with these maps, researchers will search for genes that influence biochemical aspects of the mosquito that affect the visiting parasite. Altering such genes can conceivably lead to mosquitoes that are resistant to malaria.

## ▶ Trypanosomiasis

Trypanosome parasites infect fewer people than do malarial parasites, yet trypanosomes present researchers with greater technical obstacles. Each species of *Trypanosoma* comprises a vexing diversity of strains. The two most prevalent species of the parasite are *Trypanosoma cruzi,* which causes the heart ailment known as Chagas' disease, and *Trypanosoma brucei,* which causes African sleeping sickness.

Epidemiologists believe that, in the United States, infection with *T. cruzi* continues to be restricted to residents who have emigrated from Central and South American countries. The number of infected residents is now estimated to be more than 100,000. The number of infected people worldwide is between 16 million and 18 million.

Scientists have documented more than 100 strains of *Trypanosoma cruzi,* which is transmitted by bloodsucking insects known as "kissing bugs." French and U.S. researchers recently discovered one reason for the great variety of strains of *T. cruzi.* The parasites can reproduce by cloning, a process that leads to the separate lines, or strains— which then respond differently to antiparasitic drugs and vaccines.

The findings by these researchers should prompt drug and vaccine developers to address the problem in terms of multiple strains of the parasite, rather than just a single strain. This approach might lead to more-effective medicines for patients, who usually are infected with more than one strain. At this point, four strains of *T. cruzi* are known to be particularly common. Researchers also noted that other tropical parasites, including *Trypanosoma brucei,* appear to reproduce by cloning.

Researchers at Johns Hopkins Medical School in Baltimore, Maryland, recently made gains in studies of *Trypanosoma brucei,* spread by the tsetse fly, which inhabits large parts of Africa. Molecules on the surface of *T. brucei* can mutate, thereby slowing recognition of the parasite by the human immune system. In one case, the researchers at Johns Hopkins developed a drug that interfered with the parasite's surface chemistry, thus disarming it. In another case the researchers altered the genetic makeup of *T. brucei* by replacing a gene with a harmful designer gene.

*Donald Cunningham*

# Urology

## ▶ Minimally Invasive Surgery

With improved instrumentation and visualization, laparoscopic and minimally invasive techniques have been applied to and suggested for many different procedures. These include nephrectomy, adrenalectomy, bladder suspension, tissue welding, ureteral reimplantation, prostatectomy, and construction of a urinary conduit using intestinal segments. Furthermore, using fine telescopes, repair of congenital abnormalities of the kidney and removal of small tumors are possible without incisions. The patient benefits by a shorter hospital stay, a much faster recovery, and a more rapid return to normal activities.

## ▶ Prostate

Interest in alternative therapies for benign enlargement of the prostate continues. Some medications can be helpful. There seems to be a role for laser energy in prostate surgery. Expandable urethral tubes in specific situations may improve urine flow. Screening for prostate cancer using the digital rectal examination and a simple blood test, called the prostate specific antigen (PSA), has been helpful in detecting prostate cancer early in its course. Surgery and radiation therapy continue to be the treatments of choice when the disease is localized. In certain situations, "watchful waiting" seems to be best.

## ▶ Penis Reattachment

Recently a well-publicized incident involving traumatic amputation of the penis served to remind the public of the significant progress made over the past decade in the area of microvascular surgical techniques. Applying principles developed in the replantation or reattachment of severed extremities, the penis was rejoined to the body in a lengthy operation using meticulous microsurgery. Today the penis is viable and is serving well as a conduit for urine. It will require some time before it is known if satisfactory sexual function will be regained.

## ▶ Urinary Incontinence

Incontinence is a very common problem, particularly in the elderly. Medications and surgery have been effective treatments in some cases. The Food and Drug Administration (FDA) recently approved the use of treated bovine collagen for correction of some forms of postsurgical and stress incontinence, and to treat reflux of urine from the bladder to the kidney. The collagen material, injected with a needle, has been shown to be effective.

*Brendan M. Fox, M.D.*

# Index

Main article headings appear in this index as bold-faced capital letters; subjects within articles appear as lower-case entries. Both the general references and the subentries should be consulted for maximum usefulness of this index. Cross references are to entries in this index. A Cumulative Index of feature articles from the 1992, 1993, and 1994 editions of this volume appears on pages 348 and 349.

# Cumulative Index

This listing indexes feature articles that have appeared in the 1992, 1993, and 1994 editions of *Health and Medicine.*

# Acknowledgments

**ALLERGIES: NOTHING TO SNEEZE AT,** page 18
*American Health* © 1993 by Larry Katzenstein.

**A CHILD'S THEORY OF MIND,** page 171
Reprinted with permission from SCIENCE NEWS, the weekly newsmagazine of science. Copyright 1993 by Science Service, Inc.

**DO YOU NEED A NUTRITIONIST?,** page 76
*American Health* © 1993 by Leslie Vreeland.

**EXERCISE MYTHS,** page 128
Reprinted with permission from the *Good Health Report,* October 1993.

**GETTING THROUGH GRIEF,** page 152
Reprinted from *Health* magazine. Copyright © 1991.

**UNKIND MILK,** page 80
Excerpted from the October 1993 issue of the *HARVARD HEALTH LETTER,* © 1993, President and Fellows of Harvard College.

**WOMEN AND AIDS,** page 50
Reprinted from *FDA Consumer,* October 1993.

## Manufacturing Acknowledgments

We wish to thank the following for their services: Typesetting, Dix Type Inc.; Color Separations, Colotone, Inc.; Text Stock, printed on Champion's 60# Courtland Matte; Cover Materials provided by Holliston Mills, Inc., Decorative Specialties International, Inc., and Ecological Fibers, Inc.; Printing and Binding, R.R. Donnelley & Sons Co.

# Illustration Credits

The following list acknowledges, according to page, the sources of illustrations used in this volume. The credits are listed illustration by illustration—top to bottom, left to right. Where necessary, the name of the photographer or artist has been listed with the source, the two separated by a slash. If two or more illustrations appear on the same page, their credits are separated by semicolons.

3 © Tom Stewart/The Stock Market
10 © Ira Wyman/Sygma; © Peter Johansky/FPG International
11 © David Scharf/Peter Arnold; © Tom Hevezi/Allsport
12 © Sygma
15 © David M. Grossman
17 © Jeffrey Sylvester/FPG International
18 © David Scharf/Peter Arnold
19 © David Scharf/Peter Arnold
20 © Dr. Jeremy Burgess/Science Photo Library/Photo Researchers; art: Copyright 1992 Time Inc. Reprinted by permission.
21 © David Scharf/Peter Arnold
22 Copyright 1992 Time Inc. Reprinted by permission.
23 © David Scharf/Peter Arnold
24 © Renee Stockdale/Animals Animals
25 © Jeffrey Markowitz/Sygma
26 © Christoph Blumrich
28 Art based on illustration from *The American Medical Association Encyclopedia of Medicine,* Random House, and redrawn by Leslie Dunlap; photo: © SIU/Peter Arnold
29 Art copyright © 1993 by The New York Times Company. Reprinted by permission. Art redrawn by Leslie Dunlap; photo: © SIU/Photo Researchers
32 © Stephen P. Parker/Photo Researchers
33 © Dan McCoy/Rainbow
34 The Bettmann Archive
35 © Yoav Levy/Phototake; © Dr. Jeremy Burgess/Science Photo Library/Photo Researchers
36 North Wind Picture Archives; © Barts Medical Library/Phototake
37 © Stan Sholik/FPG International
38 © L. West/Photo Researchers; © Ray Coleman/Photo Researchers; © John Serrao/Photo Researchers
39 Krames Communications
40 Both illustrations: Krames Communications
41 Illustrations: Krames Communications; photo: © Fabricius-Taylor/Gamma-Liaison
42 Krames Communications
43 © envision; © Frank Herholdt/Tony Stone Images
44 Top: The Bettmann Archive; illustrations: Krames Communications
45 The Bettmann Archive; UPI/Bettmann; © Diana Walker/Gamma-Liaison
46 © Astromujoff/The Image Bank
50 © Bill Binzen/The Stock Market
51 Photo: © Tom Landecker/Tony Stone Images
52 © Chris Harvey/Tony Stone Images
53 © Michael Grecco/Sygma
54 © Joe Traver/Gamma-Liaison
56 © Daniel Bosler/Tony Stone Images
58- All artwork: Krames Communications
59
60 © Custom Medical Stock Photography
61 Krames Communications
63 © Susan Lapides/Woodfin Camp & Associates; © Roy Morsch/The Stock Market; © Dan McCoy/Rainbow
64 © UPI/Bettmann
67 © John Heseltine/Science Photo Library/Photo Researchers
68- © David Stoecklein/The Stock Market
69
70 © S.J. Krasemann/Peter Arnold; © Daniel J. Cox/Natural Selection; © Alan G. Nelson/Animals Animals
71 © Amy Reichman/envision
72 © Craig C. Lorenz/Photo Researchers
73 © Gary Griffen/Animals Animals
74 Both photos: © Melabee M. Miller/envision
76 © Scott Pollack
78 © Scott Pollack
80 © Susanne Buckler/Gamma-Liaison; © Spencer Jones/FPG
81 © Peter Johansky/FPG
82 © Steven Mark Needham/envision; © Peter Johansky/FPG; © Ed McCormick/The Stock Market
83 © Steven Mark Needham/envision
84 © Rick Osentoski/envision
85 Quote background photo: © John Kaprielian/Photo Researchers
86 © Kirk Moldoff
87 © Rick Friedman/Black Star
90 Quote background photo: © John Kaprielian/Photo Researchers

91 © Eric Jacobson/FPG International
92 © Jean Higgins/envision; © Luc Novovitch/Gamma-Liaison
93 © Steven Mark Needham/envision
94 © Craig Hammell/The Stock Market
95 © Jeff Greenberg/Photo Researchers; © Jerry Mesmer/Tony Stone Images
96 Courtesy of Commercial Aluminum Cookware
97 © Arthur Beck/Photo Researchers
98 Both photos: Courtesy of Farberware, Inc.
99 © David Barnes/The Stock Market
100 © James A. Hays/Unicorn Stock Photos
101 © FPG International
103 © Welzenbart/The Stock Market
104 © Markus Boesch/Allsport; © Tim Davis/Photo Researchers
105 © Robert Maass/Sipa Press
106- Photo sequence: © John Kane
107
108 © Richard Balzer/Stock Boston; © Richard B. Levine
109 © Yvonne Hemsey/Gamma-Liaison
111 © Marvy!/The Stock Market
112 © David Barnes/The Stock Market
113 © Tom Hevezi/Allsport; © Will Ryan/The Stock Market
114 © Philip Wallick/FPG International
115 © David Madison
116- Left: © Scott Markewitz/FPG International; center: © Nicholas
117 DeVore/Tony Stone Images; inset: © David Weintraub/Photo Researchers
118 © Henry Horenstein
120 © Henry Horenstein
121 Courtesy National Triathlon Training Camp; Courtesy *Golf Digest*
122 Courtesy Van der Meer Tennis
123 Courtesy Magic Johnson Enterprises
124 © Henry Horenstein
125 © Michael A. Keller/The Stock Market
126 The Bettmann Archive
128- UPI/Bettmann
129
130 © Mark Tuschman
131 © David Wells/The Image Works
133 © David Wells/The Image Works
134 © Vandystadt/Allsport
135 © Mike Powell/Allsport; © Gary Newkirk/Allsport
136 © David Madison/Duomo; © Richard Graham
138 © Scott Weersing/Allsport
139 © Mike Powell/Allsport
140 © Allen Russell/Profiles West
141 © Dawn & Dave Mackay/The Stock Market
143 © Lunagrafix/Photo Researchers
144- © D. Goldberg/Sygma
145
146 © Greg Smith/Saba; © Acikalin/Sipa
147 © Lawrence Manning/Black Star
148 Both photos: AP/Wide World Photos
149 © Akhtar Hussein/Sipa
150 © J.P. Laffont/Sygma
152 © John David Fleck/Gamma-Liaison
153 © Roy Gumpel/Gamma-Liaison
155 © Bob Krist/TSW
156 © Bill Swersey/Gamma-Liaison
159 © Mark Downey
161 © Dan Bosler/TSW
162 Copyright © 1992 Time Inc. Reprinted by permission.
165 © Bob Daemmrich/Stock Boston
167 UPI/Bettmann; illustrations: © George Stewart
168 © Nina Berman/Sipa; © Les Stone/Sygma
169 Both photos: © Nina Berman/Sipa
170 © W. Snyder/Gamma-Liaison
171 © Anthony Edgeworth/The Stock Market
172 Both photos: © Laura Dwight/Peter Arnold
173 © Lawrence Migdale
174 © Andrew Cox/Tony Stone Images
175 © Dale Durfee/Tony Stone Images
177 © Andy Sachs/Tony Stone Images
178 © D&I MacDonald/Unicorn Stock Photos
179 © Ron Chapple/FPG International